CAMBRIDGE LIBRARY COLLECTION

Books of enduring scholarly value

History of Medicine

It is sobering to realise that as recently as the year in which On the Origin of Species was published, learned opinion was that diseases such as typhus and cholera were spread by a ‚Äòmiasma‚Äô, and suggestions that doctors should wash their hands before examining patients were greeted with mockery by the profession. The Cambridge Library Collection reissues milestone publications in the history of Western medicine as well as studies of other medical traditions. Its coverage ranges from Galen on anatomical procedures to Florence Nightingale‚Äôs common-sense advice to nurses, and includes early research into genetics and mental health, colonial reports on tropical diseases, documents on public health and military medicine, and publications on spa culture and medicinal plants.

A Treatise on Plague

The bubonic plague, in various forms, has been devastating human populations and affecting the very course of history for over 3000 years. This 1905 study by a renowned expert in the field represents the extent of early twentieth-century knowledge of a disease which was still killing millions at the time of first publication. Charting the history of the plague and its spread across the world, Simpson examines the causes of the disease, including the role of living conditions and poverty, as well as strategies for quarantine, prevention and treatment. Featuring autopsy reports, statistical data, photographs illustrating the symptoms and accounts of medical investigation of all aspects of the plague, this is a comprehensive and arresting overview of the disease. The book also features the full text of the 1903 International Sanitary Convention of Paris which was a response to the 1896 outbreak in India and China.

Cambridge University Press has long been a pioneer in the reissuing of out-of-print titles from its own backlist, producing digital reprints of books that are still sought after by scholars and students but could not be reprinted economically using traditional technology. The Cambridge Library Collection extends this activity to a wider range of books which are still of importance to researchers and professionals, either for the source material they contain, or as landmarks in the history of their academic discipline.

Drawing from the world-renowned collections in the Cambridge University Library, and guided by the advice of experts in each subject area, Cambridge University Press is using state-of-the-art scanning machines in its own Printing House to capture the content of each book selected for inclusion. The files are processed to give a consistently clear, crisp image, and the books finished to the high quality standard for which the Press is recognised around the world. The latest print-on-demand technology ensures that the books will remain available indefinitely, and that orders for single or multiple copies can quickly be supplied.

The Cambridge Library Collection will bring back to life books of enduring scholarly value (including out-of-copyright works originally issued by other publishers) across a wide range of disciplines in the humanities and social sciences and in science and technology.

A Treatise on Plague

*Dealing with the Historical,
Epidemiological, Clinical, Therapeutic and
Preventive Aspects of the Disease*

W.J. Simpson

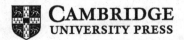
CAMBRIDGE
UNIVERSITY PRESS

CAMBRIDGE UNIVERSITY PRESS

Cambridge, New York, Melbourne, Madrid, Cape Town, Singapore,
São Paolo, Delhi, Dubai, Tokyo, Mexico City

Published in the United States of America by Cambridge University Press, New York

www.cambridge.org
Information on this title: www.cambridge.org/9781108015899

© in this compilation Cambridge University Press 2010

This edition first published 1905
This digitally printed version 2010

ISBN 978-1-108-01589-9 Paperback

A TREATISE ON PLAGUE

CAMBRIDGE UNIVERSITY PRESS WAREHOUSE
C. F. CLAY, Manager.
London: AVE MARIA LANE, E.C.
AND
H. K. LEWIS,
136, GOWER STREET, W.C.

Glasgow: 50, WELLINGTON STREET.
Leipzig: F. A. BROCKHAUS.
New York: THE MACMILLAN COMPANY.
Bombay and Calcutta: MACMILLAN AND CO., Ltd.

A
TREATISE ON PLAGUE

dealing with the Historical,
Epidemiological, Clinical, Therapeutic
and Preventive aspects of the
Disease

by

W. J. SIMPSON,

M.D. Aberd., F.R.C.P. Lond., D.P.H. Camb.

Professor of Hygiene, King's College, London ; Lecturer on Tropical Hygiene,
London School of Tropical Medicine; formerly Health Officer, Calcutta ;
Medical Adviser to the Government of Cape Colony, during the
Outbreak of Plague in 1901 ; Commissioner for the Colonial
Office to Inquire into the Causes of the Continuance of
Plague in Hongkong

Cambridge:
at the University Press
1905

Cambridge:

PRINTED BY JOHN CLAY, M.A.

AT THE UNIVERSITY PRESS.

TO ALL THOSE
WHO ARE ACTIVELY INTERESTED IN PLAGUE
AND ITS PREVENTION THE AUTHOR DEDICATES
THIS WORK

PREFACE.

THIS volume has been written at the request of the Syndics of the Cambridge University Press with the object of bringing within a moderate compass the principal facts concerning plague, from its historical, epidemiological, clinical, therapeutic and preventive aspects. Eleven years ago, plague as an epidemic disease was merely of historical interest. Confined to some remote places in China, in India, in Persia, in Arabia, and in Africa, its power was generally believed to be extinct. To-day plague is a matter of concern to many countries and has been the subject of two International Conferences. These Conferences have met, discussed and agreed to the carrying out of measures which, while inflicting the least injury on commerce, might reasonably be expected to protect Europe from an invasion of the disease, and during the past eight years Europe has, notwithstanding one or two alarms, had little reason to doubt that the adoption of these measures has been most serviceable in preventing the permanent lodgement of plague. Europe is however but a small part of the world and other continents have not been so fortunate, and although no great outburst has occurred on the American, African, or Australian Continent, yet there remains the fact that the disease has acquired a lodgement in these and necessitates the greatest vigilance. Plague takes its own time and opportunities for its development, and it is unwise to be lulled into a sense of security by its apparent impotency to spread in a particular country. That it is capable of spreading is seen too plainly in India. Few thought it possible, when plague broke out in Bombay in 1896 after an absence of 200 years, that the disease would not be controlled, checked and stamped out in a short time. It was a rude awakening when the deaths began to mount up to a few thousands to find the old scenes associated with plague epidemics reappear. The closed houses, the deserted streets, and nearly half of the population of Bombay fleeing panic-stricken from the city, testified to the fact that plague had lost none of its old terrors, and recalled the condition of affairs described in the old epidemics of plague. Later, when, owing to the decline of the epidemic, confidence was restored and the people had in consequence returned, there were congratulations as to the lightness of the attack compared with the mortality in the great epidemics of the past, yet, the next year and every year since 1896, the disease has recrudesced in the city of Bombay, and the number of deaths is fast mounting up beyond the mortality of any epidemic of plague in any single city in the past with the exception of those of Constantinople and Grand Cairo. And still the disease continues. Plague has moreover spread from Bombay to the Bombay Presidency, and from the Bombay Presidency to a large portion of India. Slow in its progress it has steadily advanced; and now the 30,000 deaths from plague which occurred in India in the first year, and which created so much alarm, has reached during the past two years over three-quarters of a million per annum. In 1903 the number of deaths from plague in India was 853,000, and in 1904 it was over a million, being 1,040,429. Of the million deaths in 1904, over 350,000 occurred in one Province. The Punjaub is not a large Province; it has a population of under 27 millions[1], or less than that of England, and yet it lost in the course of 12 weeks in 1904 over a quarter of a million of its inhabitants. If in the Province of Manchuria either the Russian or Japanese army now opposed to one another were by some misfortune completely destroyed, the catastrophe would not be greater than what happened to the inhabitants of the Punjaub from plague, and if both armies were destroyed it would not compare with the destruction of human life from this disease in India in 1904. These are the official figures, and are admitted to be below the mark on account of concealment on the part of the inhabitants. The total number of deaths in India officially recorded from plague since 1896 was, up to the end of December 1904, three millions one hundred and fifty thousand.

Figures give a very inadequate representation of the amount of misery which plague has brought and is continuing to bring to India. Medical men and other workers engaged in plague epidemics may have some conception of its intensity when they see whole families swept away by the disease, but for most, and for those outside its sphere, it is difficult to realise the full extent of suffering and desolation that has

---

[1] Census of India 1901 gives 26,880,217.

befallen hundreds of thousands of families in India and threatens the homes of hundreds of thousands more.

This plague is for India a grievous calamity; none the less grievous because it is borne with that wonderful fortitude and patience so characteristic of the people of Hindustan, nor is it limited to the physical pain and mental grief in each home, great as they are. Scarcity of labour and loss of trade are beginning to be felt in the provinces worst affected, and it is not surprising that in the Indian papers fears are expressed that if there is no abatement of the disease, portions of the country may have to face "the possibility of large areas of land untilled, of trade and commerce decaying, because the population has died or fled carrying the disease to districts hitherto unaffected[1]." In fact if the plague continues its ravages, as it has every appearance of doing, it will more slowly but as surely produce the same conditions in India as it did in times past in Europe in the earlier pandemics. A statement like this will come as a surprise to most people, for in the newspapers in England there appear weekly bulletins from Hongkong and the Mauritius giving the number of deaths from plague in the colonies in the plague season. The figures never mount up to more than a hundred deaths a week at the most and seldom to half that number. The impression produced by these bulletins is that they represent the total extent of plague in the English dominions, and the statement that in the epidemic season plague carries off its victims in India at the rate of thirty or forty thousand a week is received with incredulity. When it is found, however, to be true, most of those who hear it are appalled at the condition of affairs affecting our greatest dependency, for whose welfare England is responsible and anxious to do everything in its power to maintain in a state of happiness and prosperity.

Adverse critics are to be met with who view the ravages of plague as a blessing rather than as an evil to be overcome by every means possible, whose contention is that plagues are necessary and are Nature's methods of keeping down an enormous population that would otherwise perish by hunger. It is an easy-going doctrine and saves trouble to those unaffected. It is the reproduction in a more subtle form of an old doctrine held many centuries ago, and which makes strange reading for those imbued with the trend of thought of the 20th century. In the seventh century, according to the records of the Church of Mayo[2], two

[1] Leading article entitled "Plague administration," *Pioneer Mail*, June 17th, 1904.
[2] *A History of Epidemic Pestilences.* By Edward Bascombe, M.D., 1851.

kings of Erin summoned the principal clergy and laity to a council at Temora, in consequence of a general dearth, the land not being sufficient to support the increasing population. The chiefs (*majores populi*) decreed that a fast should be observed both by clergy and laity so that they might with one accord *solicit God to prayer to remove by some species of pestilence the burthensome multitudes of the inferior people,* "Omnes majores petebant ut nimia multitudo vulgi per infirmitatem aliquam tolleretur, quia numerositas populi erat occasio famis." St Gerald and his associates suggested that it would be more conformable to the Divine Nature and not more difficult to multiply the fruits of the earth than to destroy its inhabitants. An amendment was accordingly moved "to supplicate the Almighty not to reduce the number of the men till it answered the quantity of corn usually produced, but to increase the produce of the land so that it might satisfy the wants of the people." However, the nobles and clergy, headed by St Fechin, bore down the opposition and called for a pestilence on the lower orders of the people. According to the records a pestilence was given, which included in its ravages the authors of the petition, the two kings who had summoned the convention, with St Fechin, the king of Ulster and Munster and a third of the nobles concerned. Another and similar account of this incident is given in the doings of the Saints of Ireland[1].

Other critics, bearing in mind the opposition and hostility with which the preventive measures introduced by the Government of India in the early days of the epidemic were met by the people, emphasise the political dangers which are likely to arise from any action and which justify the present policy of leaving things alone and only assisting when aid is desired. The force of this argument must always be given due weight when dealing with the people of India, whose mode of thought is different from that of the West. But while admitting this, the fact must not be lost sight of that hostility was largely engendered by the methods adopted, owing firstly to the absence of an organised sanitary service and the consequent employment of agencies for the inspection of houses, repugnant to the feelings of the people, and secondly because of a lack of knowledge of the channels by which the disease spreads and the consequent futility of the methods adopted at much cost and effort for the prevention of the disease. The lack of an organised sanitary service and the lack of knowledge still

---

[1] *Acta Sanctorum Hiberniae.* Tom. i. p. 601. Lovanii, 1645.

remain, and if hope is to come to India it must be by their removal. It cannot be beyond the power of statesmanship to seek means for averting and ameliorating the sufferings of India, and yet to do so successfully without raising dangers to the well-being of the community or of the Government. Even those who see necessity for caution in the methods of working to save the people from dying of plague in the epidemic season, would probably not object to active measures of prevention during the period of quiescence of the disease, when there is no alarm or tendency to panic. These anticipatory measures could easily be carried out without friction if suitable machinery were there. Elsewhere[1] I have shown the nakedness of India in sanitary organisation, and its inability under present conditions to defend itself against epidemics of any kind. It has no thoroughly trained and fully equipped sanitary army made up mostly of its own people familiar with the ways of its inhabitants. It is now over ten years since this defenceless state was shown to exist, and a scheme sketched out for the organisation of a service for the prevention of disease. Is it too much to suggest that some portion of the large annual surpluses of money, which India is now obtaining by its fiscal policy, shall be devoted to this important object? The maintenance of a well-trained native sanitary service to protect the people of India dying from preventable disease is as feasible, and from a humane point of view as important, as the maintenance of a well-organised native army to protect the country against an external enemy. It is to be hoped that for the sake of India an organised Public Health Service commensurate with the requirements of the country will be created.

The formation and development of a trained sanitary service, with which qualified women should be associated, will not be sufficient to meet the conditions now existing. There is urgent need for systematic and scientific study of the disease. More requires to be known concerning the mode of spread of the disease in India, and of the conditions which favour its continuance during the non-epidemic periods. On a proper understanding of these depend many of the preventive measures. If rats, insects, fleas, and infected clothes are the chief factors in the dissemination of the disease, there is little need, unless it be for pneumonic

[1] "The Need of a Sanitary Service for India." By W. J. Simpson, M.D. *Transactions of the First Indian Medical Congress,* 1894, and *Indian Medical Gazette,* Dec. 1895.

"Plague in India." *British Medical Journal,* 1898.

"An Address on Preventive Work in the Tropics to the Royal Institute of Public Health." By W. J. Simpson, M.D. *Lancet,* 1904.

plague, of resorting to isolation in hospital and segregation camps, which is opposed to the feelings of Hindus and Mahommedans alike. If contaminated food is an important factor in the production of plague, measures to secure purity should be introduced. But all these have to be proved for India. Seven years of golden opportunities have passed unutilised. If the first 18 months in which scientific study and research partly carried out by a scientific committee in India and partly by foreign commissions be excepted, no real and sustained efforts commensurate with the great issues at stake have been made to get to understand the disease and the manner in which it spreads, and no facts of practical value for the prevention of plague have come from India. It seems to have been considered a waste of money to spend 20,000 or 30,000 pounds in studying the disease and its prevention, though twice or three times that amount is but a small fraction of the vast sums spent for the most part uselessly on administrative and executive methods, which, effective enough, perhaps, in a country with a fully equipped sanitary service and when rigorously carried out at the commencement, have proved to be in India with its conditions of no avail.

For preventive work much more light is needed on a subject involved in obscurity, and this can only be obtained by scientific research which shall be regular and systematic in its nature and which shall be closely associated with a skilled and special organisation devoted to plague administration and which shall not be confined to laboratory experiments. Plague requires scientific investigation outside as well as inside the laboratory. Research and administration in this matter need to go hand in hand. Each if worked on its own lines without reference to the other will accomplish but little, and that little is not likely to be of much practical value. In a disease such as plague the efforts of a sanitary service are only likely to be successful when directed into the proper channels by its close association with scientific research both in the laboratory and in the locality affected.

It is unnecessary to dwell on the danger of the disease spreading to other countries or of the serious risk attendant on plague being allowed to spread without understanding the methods by which this happens. An optimistic opinion prevails that the disease will not spread and soon die out in India. This view has been strenuously held from the first and the continuance of the plague with its three million deaths has been a source of disappointment in this respect. Doubtless if held long enough this view will ultimately prove true, but it may not be in this generation. This dying out and failure to spread are not in accordance with the history of plague in the past when it has acquired such dimensions as those existing in India, and there is nothing so far as may be judged in the present condition of the world for it to act differently now than formerly. On the contrary, with war in the East, with grave economical and political disturbances existing at present and with unusual seasons, the conditions which in earlier times favoured the prevalence of plague do not appear to be altogether wanting for its expansion in the present age. Whether history will repeat itself or not or whether the risk of extension to neighbouring countries is great or small remains for the future to decide. No one can prognosticate one way or the other. But amidst this uncertainty there is one thing absolutely certain, and it is that owing to this invasion of plague the condition of the people of India in the worst affected provinces is most deplorable. It not only claims the deepest sympathy, but also in the interests of humanity imperatively demands the closest attention and the adoption of suitable and adequate remedial measures for its amelioration and for combating the spread and ravages of the disease.

In conclusion a pleasant duty devolves on me to acknowledge with grateful thanks the kindly assistance given me in writing this book. My acknowledgements are due to the Syndics of the Cambridge University Press for the facilities they have afforded me in its publication. They are also due to Dr Norman Moore and Dr Joseph Frank Payne for assistance and advice; also to Mr W. M. Haffkine, C.I.E., for his microscopical specimens of involution forms of plague bacilli. It is impossible to over-estimate the splendid services which have been rendered to India by Mr Haffkine by his discoveries of a cholera and plague prophylactic, and by his work carried out in India amidst great difficulties in connection therewith. Such services can never be forgotten. My thanks are also due to Dr Choksy of Bombay and Dr Gregory of Cape Town for the photographs representing plague patients, also to the Colonial and India Office for access to official records; to the Local Government Board for Dr Thomson's translation of the Paris Convention, and to the Controller of His Majesty's Government for permission to reproduce that translation.

W. J. SIMPSON.

KING'S COLLEGE, LONDON,
March. 1905.

CONTENTS.

PART I.

HISTORY AND DISTRIBUTION OF PLAGUE.

CHAPTER I.

CHAPTER II.

CHAPTER III.

The present pandemic originated in Yunnan, one of the Western Provinces of China.—Topographical description of Yunnan.—Trade routes from Yunnan.—Condition of Yunnan in 1871 as observed by M. Rocher.—M. Rocher's account of plague in Yunnan.—Epidemic preceded by sickness and mortality among rats.—Dr Lowry of Pakhoi gives first medical account of plague in Southern China at Pakhoi.—Plague first appeared at Pakhoi in 1867.—Trade route from Pakhoi to Yunnanfu.—Plague endemic in Pakhoi from 1867 to 1884.—Plague not extinct in adjoining prefecture to that of Pakhoi.—Plague at Mengtze, 1874 to 1893. Plague at Nanningfu and Kwaium in 1893.—Plague at Canton in 1894.—Canton connected with the chief towns and districts of Kwangsi and Kwantung.—Plague in Canton in January, 1894.—Hongkong the largest and most important European possession near Canton.—Plague discovered in Hongkong in May, 1894.—The plague bacillus discovered in Hongkong by Dr S. Kitasato and later by Dr Yersin.—Plague in Macao in April, 1895.—Canton and Hongkong become centres of distribution of plague.—Plague at Bombay in 1896.—Commencement characterised by mildness and slow extension.—Opposition to the adoption of preventive measures.—Progress of the disease associated with the migration of rats.—Height of the first Bombay epidemic in Feb., 1897.—Extension of the disease to the Bombay Presidency and to other provinces in India—Slow diffusion of the plague.—Severity of epidemics at Dharwar and Poona.—Extension of the plague to other Presidencies.—Gradually increasing mortality from the plague in India.—Extension of the plague from India and China to other parts of the world.—Distribution of plague in different parts of the world.—An endemic centre in Uganda.

PART II.

EPIDEMIOLOGY OF PLAGUE.

CHAPTER IV.

Earlier views on the nature of infection.—Discovery of the plague bacillus and the evidence as to its causal relationship.—Morphological and staining characteristics of the plague bacillus.—Cultural characteristics.—Involution forms.—Characteristic growth in bouillon.—Formation of stalactites.—Kitasato's plague bacillus.—The vitality of the plague bacillus.—In different media.—Effect of cold.—Effect of heat.—Effect of sun.—Effect of drying.—Variation in virulence.—Effect of the plague bacillus in animals.

CHAPTER V.

Rats and mice susceptible to natural plague infection.—Relationship between certain epizootics and epidemics of plague a current belief for many centuries.—Observations of epizootics associated with plague epidemics.— Plague-stricken rats, their appearance and behaviour.—Cats affected with plague.—Other animals affected with plague.—Result of experiments to produce plague in animals.—Experiments by German Commission.—Experiments on animals by Austrian Commission.—Haffkine's experiments.—Wilm's experiments.—Experiments on a large scale carried out in Hongkong in 1902. —Plague in man possibly not infrequently caused by food contaminated with plague infection.—Plague in animals under conditions of natural infection.

CHAPTER VI.

Some questions related to spontaneity.—Origin of plague long attributed to putrefaction of dead bodies, or to great physical disturbances.—Pariset's theory. —Creighton supports Pariset's views.—Mortality of rats from plague not against Pariset's theory.—Origin of plague attributed to great calamities, cosmic and telluric.—The Black Death preceded by great disturbances in the balance of nature.—Creighton places the origin of the Black Death on the borders of the Euxine or Black Sea.—Considerations showing the difficulty and even the impossibility of now locating the origin of the 14th century pandemic.—Volcanic eruptions are recorded to have rendered plants and herbage poisonous.—Great multiplication of disease germs associated with lean or famine years.—Exceptional meteorological conditions preceded the epidemic of plague in Hongkong.—Scarcity preceded plague in India.—Abnormal season preceded epidemic of plague in Hongkong.—Unusual season preceded epidemic of plague in Cape Town.—Conclusion.

CHAPTER VII.

Variation in diffusive powers.—Self-limiting plagues.—The existing pandemic possesses comparatively small diffusive powers.—The danger of existing pandemic.—Plague epidemics and seasonal influences.

Plague epidemics occur at particular seasons of the year.—Temperature affects the endemicity of plague.—Season a composite force.—Mr Baldwin Latham's analysis of the influence of climatic factors on plague.—The varying condition of the soil and its fluctuating temperature likely to have an effect on microbic and insect life.—The temperature of the air itself not directly influential.—At the end of the plague season infected articles lose their infectivity, but may regain it the following season.—Instances.—The same observation has been made in regard to small-pox and vaccine.—Seasonal periodicity of plague, and seasonal breeding period of the rat.

CHAPTER VIII.

Variation in virulence.—Mild epidemic of plague at Astrakhan and Vet-lianka.—The Vetlianka outbreak suddenly acquires great virulence.—Early malignity of the Avignon epidemic of 1348, with its pneumonic symptoms followed by a less malignant type.

Different types with varying degrees of virulence may be seen running concurrently or following one another in the same epidemic.—Four different types of plague in the Pali epidemic of 1836.—Five degrees of severity noted in the Marseilles epidemic of 1720.—Three degrees of severity observed in the Russian epidemic of 1771.—An Aura Pestilentiae noticed in the Egyptian epidemic of 1834–35.—Three degrees of severity in the Egyptian epidemic of 1834–35.—Sporadic cases of mild plague may precede severe epidemics of plague, or they may bridge over the intervals of epidemics.—The import of glandular swellings before and after plague prevalence.—Presence and absence of certain symptoms in different epidemics.—Extraordinary and coloured sweats in the plague of London.—Plague may increase in virulence if it appears in the same locality in successive years.

Variation in the virulence of the disease dependent on conditions to which the microbe and those attacked are exposed.—Natural immunity.—Plague commits its greatest ravages on people subjected to depressing influences.

White people have a fairly uniform mortality from plague wherever they may be attacked.—Susceptible races may become less susceptible out of their own country.—Susceptibility may vary in the same race in different localities.—Variety of type is seen in all infectious diseases.

CHAPTER IX.

Discrimination between recrudescence and endemicity.—Endemic centres.—Kurdistan.—Kumaon and Garhwal.—Characteristics of the outbreaks.—Poverty of the inhabitants, exceptionally insanitary houses and close association of animals and men.—Dr Francis' description of the houses.—Dr Planch's description of the houses.—Conditions in Yunnan.—Conditions in Assyr.—Fostering conditions of plague prevalence similar in exotic localities to those in endemic centres.—Paris in the 17th century.—Oporto in the 19th century.—Canton in the 19th and 20th centuries.—Hongkong in the 19th and 20th centuries.—Bombay in 1896.—The chawls of Bombay.—The crowded buildings in Mandvi.—The Jains and their indifference to death.—A scene in a Bombay building.—Mortality in the Bombay outbreak of 1896–97 small owing to preventive measures.—The three conditions in city of Bombay observed by experts.—Notes of a morning's inspection in Bombay.—Cape Town.—Plague chiefly a disease of the poor.—A Chinese village.—Macao.—Conclusion.

CHAPTER X.

CHAPTER XI.

PART III.

PLAGUE IN THE INDIVIDUAL.

CHAPTER XII.

sera prepared by Yersin, Roux, Calmette, and Borrel.—Amoy.—Bombay.—
Karad.—Karachi.—Oporto.—Glasgow.—Cape Town.—Natal.—Hongkong.—
Brisbane.—Observations on Lustig's serum.—Observations on Prof. Terni's and
Bondi's serum.—Observations on Kitasato's serum.—Dosage of serum.—Antiseptic treatment.—Carbolic acid.—Cyllin.—General treatment.—Nursing.—
Hygienic conditions.—Medicines.—Local treatment of buboes.—Treatment
of carbuncles.—Treatment during convalescence.—Prophylactic measures in
an infected house.—Use of disinfectants.—Protective inoculation.—Personal
hygiene.—Hygiene of the house.

PART IV.

MEASURES FOR PREVENTION AND SUPPRESSION OF PLAGUE.

CHAPTER XVII.

Two periods to be considered.—Preventive measures depend on the views
which are held concerning the cause of the disease.—Trespass offerings.—
Removal from plague-stricken locality.—Fumigation of the dwellings and
attention to diet.—Prayers and processions.—Resignation and fatalism.—
Disposal of the dead.—Isolation of the rich.—First preventive measures of an
organised nature in Venice in 1348.—First governmental measures in 1374.—
Lazaretto established by the Venetians in 1403.—A council of health and
quarantine established in 1485 in Venice.—The Venetian system of quarantine.—
Preventive measures against extension of plague to other countries.—Measures
in Austria and Germany in 16th century.—Educational tracts and pamphlets
in 16th century.—Measures in London in 16th century.—First government
orders issued in London in Henry VIII's reign.—Orders more severe in the
reign of Elizabeth.—Severity of measures in Aberdeen.—Enlightened policy in
Edinburgh.—First quarantine station for London established in 1664.—
Special plague officials appointed in every parish in London.—Regulations in
London against the plague in the 17th century.—Hodges opposed to the shutting
up the sick and the well in the same house.—Dr Mead's views in 1720.—
Advocacy of the establishment of hospitals and quarantine stations.—Evacuation of infected houses.—Passport system for those wishing to leave infected
towns.—First Quarantine Act passed in reign of George IV.—International
preventive measures introduced in 1831 and 1838.—Disappearance of plague
from Turkey and Egypt attributed to these international measures.—Other
causes also at work.—Failure of measures to prevent spread of strong invading
epidemics, and the possible cause.—International conferences of European
Powers to consider measures of mutual protection against epidemic disease
from the East.—New basis for maritime preventive measures adopted at the
Vienna Conference, 1874.—Quarantine and sanitary cordons brought into
requisition in the Russian outbreak of plague in 1879.

LIST OF ILLUSTRATIONS.

MAPS.

PART I.

HISTORY AND DISTRIBUTION OF PLAGUE.

CHAPTER I.

PLAGUE FROM THE EARLY CENTURIES TO THE NINETEENTH CENTURY.

PLAGUE in the modern acceptation of the term is a specific and
infectious disease affecting man and some of the lower
Definition. animals, and possessing certain definite and well-marked
symptoms which are always more or less present in every outbreak.
These symptoms in man are fever, severe headache, giddiness, congested
eyes, extreme mental depression, stammering, incoordination of the
voluntary muscles when called on to act, staggering gait and bodily
weakness, accompanied by painful swellings, with effusions into the
surrounding tissues, in the groin, armpit, neck, or other regions of the
lymphatic glandular system, and with an occasional eruption on the skin
of so-called carbuncles or pustules. They end in death in a large percentage of cases in the course of three to five days, or even in a shorter
period. The swellings or buboes which are so characteristic of the
disease, and which contain a special micro-organism recognised by its
bipolar staining, may be absent in a varying proportion of cases. In
the pneumonic variety of plague, which primarily attacks the lungs,
there are no buboes, or only a late development of them as secondary
manifestations of the disease. In the fulminating or septicaemic plague,
which is another rapidly fatal variety, there are seldom any buboes to
be detected. Plague may be therefore with buboes or without buboes.
This fact has always rendered the diagnosis of plague very difficult and
uncertain in the early stages of an epidemic, though as the epidemic
develops the types without buboes may be recognised clinically,
especially the pneumonic type with its fever, spitting of blood and great

1

prostration.   Even the laity who have seen much of plague are able to distinguish this form in its most severe manifestations.   Since the discovery of the plague bacillus both the pneumonic and septicaemic types can be as readily recognised as the bubonic by the tests which bacteriology has recently placed in the hands of the physician.   The sputum of the one type and the blood of the other contain the plague bacillus.

Accompanying or preceding plague in man there is usually an outbreak among the lower animals, particularly among rodents such as rats and mice.   In these the same micro-organism is to be found as in man and is the causal agent of the disease.   This causal agent is transportable from place to place, carried by infected persons or animals or by articles soiled by the infection, and may thus set up in a fresh centre plague which may manifest itself in a sporadic epidemic or pandemic form and may assume a mild or virulent type.

It is not in the above restricted sense of a specific disease that ancient writers on epidemics and epizootics use the term plague.   With them it implies something more general and is applied to any pestilence in man or beast with a high mortality.   Dysenteries, famine fevers, the fevers of armies, typhus fever, small-pox, and other fatal maladies in man are included in the older designation of plague as well as the disease which is now being dealt with.   Under these circumstances it is almost impossible to determine which of the pestilences that prevailed in the Assyrian, Macedonian, Egyptian, Roman, and Grecian empires were due to true plague and which were due to those other diseases which went under the same general designation.

That plague in the specific sense understood in the present day did exist, especially in Mesopotamia, there can hardly be any doubt.   Occasionally it is recorded that the Assyrian kings were deterred from visiting certain places because of the prevalence of plague.   The historian seldom describes the symptoms of any pestilence which he mentions, being content with relating that an epidemic raged at a certain time and describing its effects on the inhabitants.   To assume that most of the epidemics thus referred to were plague is to give an exaggerated notion of the prevalence of the disease in the different centuries, while to recognise as plague only those epidemics in which the disease is unmistakeable from the description of its symptoms would be to give a very inadequate conception of its prevalence and importance.

A middle course is probably the safest, with the qualification that plague epidemics of a severe type were not nearly so numerous as is generally supposed.   The long interval between the appearance of plague in Europe and its present threatening aspect, or between its occurrence in India in the 18th century and its serious prevalence now in that country during the past eight years is merely a repetition of its behaviour in earlier times. The disease appears to come in cycles between which the intervals are of considerable duration. Papon[1], who has collected a chronological list of great pestilences, gives 41 epidemics of plague as occurring in the course of 1500 years before the Christian era, among the empires and nations the shores of whose countries bordered on the Mediterranean sea; 109 during the first 1500 years of the Christian era, and 45 from the year 1500 to 1720, when plague ravaged Marseilles, Aix, and Toulon.

Plague as stated manifests itself in the sporadic, epidemic, and pandemic forms, and it is only severe epidemics or pandemics which receive the attention of the historian. Even in modern times severe epidemics in one part of the world escape attention in another part, and it is not to be expected that under the conditions of the early period of the world's history, mention should be made by the nations bordering on the Mediterranean of epidemics in remote and unexplored places. With all the advantages of modern life, with its rapid communication and telegraphic news, how little is known or heard of the plague prevailing in China at the present day or of the plague in India which for some months this year caused some 5000 deaths a day. If India were not a dependency of Great Britain we should hear still less. The details are in the archives of the Government of India.

However uncertain may be the nature of the majority of pestilences The antiquity of plague. of a bygone age it is certain that plague is a disease of great antiquity, for occasionally in some of the oldest records the description is sufficiently explicit to remove all doubt as to the disease being plague.

The Levant and the countries adjoining have been the centres of plague for at least 3000 years, the first notice of the disease being in Syria. Plague is mentioned in the Bible as occurring centuries before the Christian era in the land of the Philistines, having broken out in Canaan[2] during military operations against the Israelites. The inhabitants of the cities of Ashdod, Gath, and Ekron as well as those of Beth-shemesh were attacked with " emerods " or tumours in their secret parts, the pestilence causing a deadly destruction. It is related that in Beth-shemesh over 50,000 persons died.

[1] *De la Peste, ou époques mémorables de ce Fléau.* Par J. P. Papon.
[2] 1 Samuel, chaps. v. and vi.

Even at that distant date the disease was observed to be accompanied by an epizootic among mice, for it is recorded that in order that the plague might be stayed the Philistines made propitiatory offerings to the Lord of Israel, of golden images of their tumours and golden images of their mice that marred the land.

On another occasion the retreat from Pelusium of Sennacherib's army is attributed to a pestilence in which field mice are stated to have played an important part, and in commemoration of the event, according to Herodotus, a stone statue of Sethon stands in the Temple of Venus with a mouse in his hand, with the following inscription, "Whoever looks on me let him revere the gods."

There are earlier references in which the Israelites are threatened with the botch of Egypt and with emerods, the disease being apparently well known. Hippocrates gives no description of the disease. He however states that "all fevers complicated with buboes are bad except ephemerals," which may possibly be considered as evidence that he was acquainted with plague.

With the exception of the biblical record there is no known trustworthy account of the disease until we come down to the works of Oribasius in the 4th century A.D. in the reign of the Emperor Julian. In this collection of ancient authors there is a fragment on plague by Rufus of Ephesus, who lived in the time of the Emperor Trajan and wrote at the beginning of the 2nd century B.C. He not only refers to the plague of his own time, but also to that described by writers who lived at least a century before him. Rufus says, "[1]The buboes that one calls pestilential are very acute and often cause death. It is especially in Lybia, Egypt, and Syria that they are seen to occur. Dionysius Curtius the Humpback has referred to these buboes. Dioscorides and Posidonius have referred to them at length in their treatise on the plague which in their time raged in Lybia, and they have said that it was accompanied by an acute fever, intense pain, perturbation of the whole body, delirium, eruption of large buboes hard and without suppuration, developing not only in the usual places but also in the popliteal space and elbow, although in general such inflammations do not form in these places." A treatise on plague written in the 3rd or 4th century B.C. indicates a fairly ancient history.

The identity of the disease thus described with plague admits of no doubt, while to complete the picture Rufus further states that " one can

Plague in Syria, Egypt, and Lybia.

---

[1] *Œuvres de Oribase, Bussemaker et Daremberg*, livre XLIV. c. xvii. p. 608.

foresee a plague which approaches by paying attention to the bad condition which the seasons present; to the manner of living less profitable for health, and to the death of animals which precedes its invasion."

The evidence is sufficient to establish the fact that plague is of great antiquity and that it prevailed in Lybia, Egypt, and Syria at an early period of the world's history when these countries on the southern and eastern shores of the Mediterranean played a leading part in the civilisation of the day and their towns were important centres of commerce. Plague has always been more or less connected with great commercial centres.

At intervals down to most recent times Lybia, Egypt, and Syria have been the scenes of plague prevalence. Situated in a unique position, at one time centres of powerful empires and always the gateways between the East and the West, it was there the commerce of the world converged during the ancient and middle ages. The marts of the ancients and of the middle ages centered here. It was immaterial what nation wielded the sceptre of commercial supremacy, the land and sea routes by which the produce from Asia and Africa was brought remained the same. For thousands of years the Arabs were the principal carriers of merchandise to and from the shores of the Mediterranean. They brought the rich produce of the East on camels and in caravans over the old caravan routes to Tyre and Sidon, to Pelusium, to Alexandria, to Syria, and to Constantinople, the great marts of which were the binding links between the East and the West. It was there that the merchants exchanged the produce of the West for the produce of the East, and it was there that the commerce of the cities of Africa and Europe met that of the cities of Asia. In times of peace the highways were thronged with caravans and merchants, but in times of war they were the roads traversed by invading armies.

The first well-authenticated pandemic of plague is recorded to have originated at Pelusium in Egypt in the year 542 B.C. **The first recorded pandemic.** Pelusium was in those days a large commercial entrepot to which the merchandise from Aethiopia, Mesopotamia, and the East was brought and there exchanged for the merchandise of the West.

In a busy and crowded mart of this kind where merchants from every commercial nation of the time were gathered together for barter, conditions were favourable not only to the formation of a dangerous focus and to the extension of the disease, but also to the disease attracting more attention than its occurrence in some obscure village or town. Pelusium was fixed upon by the historian as the starting-point of the epidemic, but plague was more or less prevalent in Lybia, Egypt, and Syria for centuries, and possibly in Aethiopia an endemic centre. One author distinctly states that it arose in Aethiopia.

Plague seldom arises in the town in which it assumes such dimensions as to attract more than local attention. The pandemic of the present day is generally traced back to Hongkong and Canton, two commercial cities, one of which is generally supposed to be its source, whereas it will be seen later on that the actual origin was from the Chinese endemic centre of Yunnan. As a general rule the distributing centres are mistaken for the source.

The disease was slow in travelling in those days, as it is in these. It took two years to reach Constantinople from Pelusium. Procopius of Caesarea in his history of the Persian war gives a vivid account of the epidemic which attacked Constantinople. For accuracy and faithfulness in detail it might without difficulty even after 1400 years apply to some of those towns which have been severely affected in the present day. Transcribed the account is as follows:

"[1]About the same time arose a pestilence which all but entirely

Account of the plague at Constantinople by Procopius.

destroyed the whole human race and, as it happens, men of over-confidence in their own ability referred its origin to things which pour down secretly from the heavens, and, indeed, those who profess a skilfulness in these matters do often love with marvellous vain speaking to mention causes for them absolutely incomprehensible by the human mind, and to devise certain strange arguments concerning nature, knowing full well that they are saying no word of truth but quite content if they can deceive the average man by their contentions. But, of a truth, no cause for this pestilence can be given or imagined except God. For it did not make its attack in one quarter of the world or against any one race of men, or at any certain time of the year, whence any specious reasons for its cause might be given. Spreading throughout the whole world it attacked people of every race however far removed from one another, sparing neither age nor sex. For whether they differed from one another in dwelling-places or in manner of living, or in their pursuits or any respect whatsoever, so long as the plague prevailed the difference availed them not. Some it attacked in summer, others in winter, some at one time, others at another. Let the sophist discuss the matter, let the

---

[1] Procopius, *De Bello Persico*, lib. II. cap. xxii. et xxiii.

meteorologist take his view each in his own way, but I am going to relate where this pestilence began and in what manner it destroyed mortals.

"It arose in Egypt, with the inhabitants of Pelusium, then dividing, it spread one way through Alexandria and the rest of Egypt, the other into Palestine which borders on Egypt, and then travelled over the world, always advancing with a progress marked by certain definite spaces of time. For it seemed to advance by a certain law and to demand a certain space of time in every country, discharging its venom against no one on the way casually, but spreading on this side and on that to the uttermost ends of the world, as if it feared lest incautiously it should pass by any corner or recess upon earth. It spared neither island nor cave nor mountain top where men dwelt. If it passed over any place, only slightly or mildly touching the inhabitants, it returned there after- wards, leaving untouched the neighbours against whom it had spent its rage before, and it did not depart from there before it made up the full measure of the dead in proportion to the amount of destruction which it had brought on its neighbours. Always beginning at the sea coast it spread into the interior. In the second year it reached Byzantium about the middle of the spring, where, as it happened, I was staying. Such was its origin.

"Many persons saw visions of spirits arrayed in human shapes. Who- soever came across these visions fancied that they were struck in this or that part of the body by some man who met them, and as soon as they had met the spectre they were smitten with the plague. And in the beginning those whom ghosts of this sort met, tried to avert them by imploring the most holy names and by unceasing expiations, as long as each of them could. But it was all in vain; for many died even in the temples into which they had fled for refuge. Others, shutting themselves up within their chambers, would not listen even to friends, and although the doors were broken in, pretended they could hear nothing, fearing evidently that they were being called out by one of the demons. Some did not catch the disease in that way, but when a vision presented itself in the form of a dream, suffered the same as those awake or seemed to hear a voice which proclaimed to them that they were enrolled in the ranks of the dead. Many, seeing no vision, either when awake or asleep, as a warning of the future, the disease attacked generally in the following way. On a sudden they became feverish, some immediately on awakening, others while walking, others while doing one thing, others another. There was no change in their colour and the body did not burn as if attacked by fever; no inflammation was apparent, but from morning until evening the fever was so mild that neither the patient nor the physician who felt the pulse had any suspicion of danger; and none of those who caught the plague thought of death. But, in some cases, on the same day, in others on the next, in others in a few days after there arose a bubo, not merely on what is called the groin, but under the armpit; in some cases the bubo appeared behind the ears and in other parts.

"What I have mentioned happened in pretty much the same way to all who contracted the disease. As to the ensuing symptoms, I cannot say whether the difference between them arose from a difference of constitution or from the mere will of the Author of the plague. Some were stricken with a heavy lethargy, others with raving madness, but each and all suffered what was in keeping with these results. Those who were weighed down with lethargy always seemed to be asleep, forgetful of their usual avocations. If there was anyone present to look after them they would take food at times: those who had no one to attend to them perished for want of food. But the delirious, unable to sleep and thinking everyone ready to murder them, were struck with terror and shrieking horribly tried to flee away. Those who attended upon them, distracted by the trouble, suffered terribly, so that people pitied the nurse as much as the patient, not because the nurses caught the disease by coming near the patient, for neither the physician nor layman caught the disease by touching the sick, for many who attended upon or buried others, contrary to general expectation, remained unharmed at their post, and many without running any risk were seized and died very soon, but because they were so terribly fatigued. For they had to put back the sufferers who threw themselves out of bed and rolled upon the floor, or had to drag them back and restrain them by force when they wished to throw themselves out of window, when they found water they burned to throw themselves into it, not from a desire to drink, for men threw themselves into the sea, but moved by their delirium. Nor was the struggle in the matter of food less, they would not take it if they could help it.

"With some of those who were not suffering from lethargy or delirium the bubo disappeared and agonies greater than they could bear took away their life. Some one may conjecture that the same thing happened to all the rest, but since they were not conscious they felt but little the sense of pain which their delirium took away from them.

"The physicians being in darkness as to these attacks of plague and thinking that the fountain-head of it was to be found in the buboes

determined to examine the bodies of those who died of it; they therefore opened several of them and found a growth of foul carbuncles.

"The malignant violence of the disease killed some at once, others
after many days; with some, all over the body black pustules, as large
as a bean broke out. These could not survive even for a single day,
but in the same hour as the pustules appeared they breathed their
last. Many dropped down dead from a sudden vomiting of blood.

"This I can truly and sincerely affirm, that the most celebrated
physicians predicted the death of several who, soon after, contrary to
the general opinion, recovered, and on the other hand predicted the
recovery of many who were on the point of death.

"So in the matter of this plague, no cause was reached by man's
reason. In every case the result was something out of the usual. A
bath did one patient good; it did another just as much harm. Of
those who were left destitute of all help many died and many escaped
without it. In a word no one had discovered any way by which either
by precaution one might avoid the plague, or when the plague had
once been caught might avoid death. That one man should fall sick
was unexplainable; that one should escape seemed a mere matter of
chance. If a pregnant woman caught the plague death was sure and
certain. Some miscarrying, others fairly delivered perished forthwith.
Yet it is said that three women in labour survived, though the children
perished; on the other hand, in one case, the mother died but the child
lived.

"Those with whom the bubo swelled and filled with pus recovered
from the plague because the violence of the carbuncle had grown less
and passed into pus, and experience teaches us that this is a sign of
recovering health. Those with whom the bubo remained unchanged
the sufferings mentioned above came upon. With some of them the
thigh became completely dried, and so however much the bubo swelled
it gathered no pus. There were some who escaped with a defect in the
tongue, so that as long as they lived they stammered or stuttered in
such a way that they could not be understood.

"The plague lasted four months in Byzantium; it was at its height
for something like three. At the beginning only a few more persons
died than ordinarily, but afterwards as the evil increased, the number
of the dead reached 5000 a day and subsequently 10,000 and even more
than that. In the early days of the plague a man buried his own
people and cast the corpses either stealthily or perforce into graves
belonging to others; but afterwards everything was in utter confusion.

For slaves were left deprived of their masters, and citizens who had previously been in the highest consideration found themselves destitute of the services of their domestics, some of whom were suffering from the plague, while others had succumbed to it. Many houses were left absolutely empty; and it came to pass that many people from want of relatives or servants lay unburied for several days.

"To deal with this the Emperor as was fit and proper charged Theodorus with the business and supplied him with soldiers and money from the Treasury. Theodorus was in charge of the 'Emperor's answers,' laying before him the quests of petitioners and conveying to them the Emperor's answers. The Romans call this officer in Latin *Referendarius*. Those whose houses had not been made entirely desolate buried their friends and relations themselves. Theodorus, paying out the Emperor's money and adding sums of his own, saw to the burial of the dead belonging to the needy. When all the burial-places which were in existence were filled with dead bodies they buried the dead bodies wherever they could round the city, and other buriers pressed under the numbers of the dying, ascended the towers of the Sycean walls. Removing the roofs of these towers they cast their dead into them indiscriminately and packing them wherever they could, when they had filled all of them almost full they placed the roofs upon them again. The awful stench from these dead spreading over the city at all times, but especially when the wind blew from the direction of the towers, became daily more harmful and distressing to the citizens.

"All rites connected with the burial of the dead were neglected. The corpses were not carried out with the usual funeral procession or funeral hymn, it was thought enough to carry the dead to the sea shore and cast them out there, and these they heaped up in piles upon barges to be carried out whither hazard would take them. At that time, too, the various factions into which the people had been divided, laying aside their natural hatred attended to the funerals of their dead in common and even buried those with whom they had no communion, and moreover those who had been given over to profligacy and who delighted in wickedness and unbridled licentiousness of life, began strenuously to practise piety, not because they had unlearned wickedness and acquired self-control and had become all of a sudden lovers of virtue (for the evils which either by nature or long-continued habits or tradition have become ingrained in man, cannot easily be altered unless some spirit of holiness has breathed into them), but because in most cases they were appalled by the calamities before their eyes and thinking that their own death was imminent, they were assuredly forced by extreme necessity and had to learn self-restraint from the awful crisis. In consequence of this, as soon as ever they recovered from the sickness and had made up their mind that they were quite out of danger, as though the plague had departed far from them, their disposition fell back again into evil, and becoming much more dissolute than of old, they surpassed themselves in wickedness and debauchery of every kind, so that one might say with truth that the plague, whether by accident or design, had held a searching examination and spared the basest of the base.

"At that time it was hard to find any one at business in Byzantium: those who were in good health remained at home and either attended to the sick or mourned their dead. Most people who met in the streets were bearing a corpse. All business had ceased: all the craftsmen had deserted their crafts and the work they had in hand. The result was a dreadful famine, which raged without limit, in a city which was accustomed to all good things in profusion. To have even bread or anything else enough was difficult, and was thought to be a good thing, and so untimely death came upon certain sufferers owing to lack of food. But to be brief: it was impossible to see any one in a purple cloak at Byzantium, especially when the Emperor fell sick, for he had a swollen bubo; but, in a royal city supreme throughout the whole Roman Empire, all dressed as private, kept at home; such are the particulars of the plague as it appeared in Byzantium and in other parts of the Roman Empire. It attacked Persia too and all the countries of the East."

There has been little or no change in the nature of the disease from the time of its earliest description. Perhaps the mental phenomena or the eruption of pustules or some other symptom may be more prominent in one epidemic than another, but the similarity of symptoms and general behaviour of the disease are remarkably constant. There is the same sudden onset and the same appearance of the bubo on the day of attack, or the next day, or a few days later; the drowsiness in some, the madness in others, the desire to wander and the difficulty of keeping some patients in bed characterise the disease now as formerly: the large size and suppuration of the bubo indicating a milder attack, and the reverse a severe and fatal illness; the deceptive appearance of the patient rendering prognosis difficult, and the comparative immunity of physicians and attendants are observations which apply equally well to the disease of to-day as it did then.

Other writers besides Procopius refer to the pandemic. From these

we learn it continued for some 52 years, visiting different places. It reappeared in Constantinople a second time in 558. Agathias describing its second visit says: "[1]In the same year, *i.e.* 558 A.D., at the beginning of spring the plague again fell upon the city and destroyed innumerable multitudes; it had never really ceased from the time when in the fifth year of the reign of Justinian it had first visited our world. Passing frequently between whiles from one place to another, and polluting one place after another, and so granting, as it were, a truce to those left alone, it then returned to Byzantium, deceived, as I think, before and having departed from these sooner than it should. Anyhow, many persons fell down dead as though struck by a violent apoplexy: but those who held out the best died at last on the fifth day. The symptoms in this plague were pretty much the same as those in the former. For they had buboes and fevers, fevers continuous and not quotidian or daily fevers merely, and never ceasing in the slightest degree, but stopping only on the death of the person whom they had attacked. Some people without any feverishness or any pain, going about their daily work, sometimes at home and sometimes abroad fell down, and at once became lifeless, as if they had taken death as a chance turn up. People of all ages perished indiscriminately, but especially the young and vigorous and in the flower of youth; and of them the males, for the females were not affected so much."

Evagrius, a citizen of Antioch, writing of the starting-point of this pandemic states that it began in Aethiopia. He himself was attacked when a child at school. His account supplements that of Procopius, being of later date, although it is evident from the context that he was not acquainted with the writings of Procopius on the subject.

Evagrius says: "[2]Now I am about to declare a certain historie which

was not found until this day, it is of a certain pestilent disease which plagued mankind the space of two and fiftie years and prevailed so much that it destroyed in maner the whole world. For it is reported that this contagious disease lighted upon *Antioch* two years after the Persians had taken the

---

[1] *Corpus Scriptorum Historiae Byzantinae Niebuhrii. Agathiae Scholastici Historiarum* lib. v. cap. x.

[2] The ancient ecclesiastical histories of the first six hundred years after Christ written in the Greek tongue by three learned historiographers, Eusebius, Socrates, and Evagrius. *The ecclesiastical historie of Evagrius Scholasticus*, lib. iv. cap. xxviii, translated out of the Greek tongue by Meredith Harmer, D.D.

citie in some part much like that which *Thucydides* hath described, in other respects farre unlike : it began in Aethiopia even as that which *Thucydides* wrote of and spred itself afterwards throughout the whole world, neither was there almost any one that escaped the infection thereof. It raged so vehemently in some cities that all the inhabitants thereof were despatched : with other towns it dealt most gently and mildly. Neither began it at any certain time of the yeare, neither did it cease and relent after one maner and order, for in some places it entred with winter, in some other places about the end of spring, in certain countries about the midst of somer, in certain others in autumne. In some regions when it had infected some part of one city or other it left the rest untouched. Then might a man have seen very oft where this malady reigned certain families wholly despatched, at another time one or two rooted out and all the city besides not once visited. Moreover (as we have marked diligently) the families which escaped this yeare were alone and none others despatched the next yeare, and that which is most of all to be marvelled at, if any which inhabited the infected cities fled into other countries where the sickness was not, they onely were visited, although they removed (hoping that way to save their lives) out of yë contagion into yë cleare. This Calamitie during the terme and compass of these years which they call revolutions passed through both towns and country, but the greatest mortality of all fell upon mankind the second yeare of the revolution which comprise the term of 15 yeares : so that I myself which write this history (for it will not be amiss to interlace this, that the consequents may agree with the premises) while as yet I frequented the schooles, was then troubled with an impostume or swelling about the privy members or secret parts of the body, and despatched diversely and sundry kinds of wayes it fell out to my grief and sorrow that God took from me many of my children, my wife also with divers of my kinsfolks, whereof some dwelled in the citie and some in the country. Sych were my adventures and such were my calamities which the course of those lamentable times distributed unto me. When I wrote this I was 58 yeares old. Not two yeares before, this sickness had been four times in *Antioch* and when as at length the fourth revolution or compasse was paste besides my aforesaid children God took away from me a daughter and a nephew of mine. This disease was compound and mixt with many other maladies. It took some men first in the head, made their eyes as red as blood and puffed up their cheeks : afterwards it fell at their throte, and whomsoever it took, it despatched him out of the way. It began with some with a fire and voiding of all that was within them, in some others with swellings about the secret parts of the body, and thereof arose burning fires so that they died thereof within two or three days of the furthest in such sort and of so perfect a remembrance as if they had not been sick at all, others died mad, and carbuncles that arose out of the flesh killed many. It fell out oftentimes that they which had this disease and escaped the first and the second time died thereof afterwards. The order and maner that men came by this disease was so diverse, that it cannot with pen be expressed. Some had it by keeping company and lying together: some others onely by touching and frequenting the infected houses: some again took it in the market. Many of them which fled out of the contagious cities, and were not visited themselves infected where they came. Others which kept company with the sick and touched not onely the sicke but the dead also were not at all. Other some who gladly would have died for the sorrow they conceived because their children and deare friends were departed, and therefore thrust themselves among the sick could not have their will, the sickness did as it were fly away from them. This pestilent disease, as I said before, reigned throughout the whole world the space of two and fiftie yeares and exceeded all the diseases that ever had been before *Philostratus* wondered at the plague which was in his time because it continued fifteen yeares. But the things that are to come are uncertain and unknown unto men and they tend to the end which God hath appointed, who knoweth both their causes and what shall become of them." It will be noticed that Evagrius refers to a diphtheritic or tonsillar form of plague, to a bubonic form, and to a carbuncular.

The information as far as it goes concerning this pandemic is very definite. Procopius, Agathias, and Evagrius agree in the **Information scanty concerning other countries attacked.** disease being not only very destructive but also very wide spread. Probably the remarks as to its passing over the whole world apply less to Europe than to Asia and Africa, with which authors were better acquainted. But beyond the outbreak they describe there is hardly any information as to other localities attacked; nor is it to be found in other authors. As regards Europe this silence may be explained by the conditions of affairs at this time. Rome had fallen. The dissolution which had overtaken the western portion of the Roman empire, overwhelming it with chaos, ruin, and destruction, was followed by an age in which culture and leisure were almost unknown. Ignorance and strife were not favourable to literature, nor to the record of historical events. Whatever was accomplished in this direction was done by some of the clergy in their ecclesiastical chronicles. There, mixed up with accounts of religious ceremonies and of the doings of kings, nobles, and bishops, may occasionally be found allusions to the pandemic. They are however mere echoes and traces of the disease infrequent in their occurrence, which while affording evidence as to its virulence leave us none the wiser as to its course or extent in the countries attacked.

In his ecclesiastical history of the Franks and in his other works Gregory, Bishop of Tours, mentions several times the ravages of plague.

References to the pandemic by Gregory, Bishop of Tours.

(*a*) In 546 the "Lues inguinaria" devastates Germany.

(*b*) In 552 it rages in different countries, and depopulates particularly the province of Arles.

(*c*) In 563 it is in Auvergne, after an inundation, and attacks Clermont, where the mortality was so great that it was impossible to count those that died. Coffins and biers failed, and ten and even more than ten persons were buried in the same trench. On a particular Sunday 300 corpses were counted in the basilica of St Peter. Death was sudden. There arose in the groin and armpit a swelling resembling a serpent, and the poison so promptly affected the sick that they died in the course of two or three days. After Clermont, Lyons, Bourges, Chalons, and Dijon were cruelly ravaged by the plague. Instances of heroism and of abject fear are not wanting in the narrative. While many fled for fear of the plague, Cato the priest remained burying the dead, saying mass for each victim, and died of plague performing these rites. In contrast to this Cautin the bishop removed from place to place to avoid the plague, and returning when it was thought to be safe, was nevertheless attacked and died.

(*d*) In 582 the disease is in Narbonne and evidently of a most virulent type: "Audivimus enim eo anno in Narbonensem urbem inguinarium morbum graviter desaevire ita ut nullum esset spatium cum homo correptus fuisset ab eo."

(*e*) In 584 its ravages in the town of Albi are such that the majority of the inhabitants died, and only a small number of citizens were left.

(*f*) In 588 it attacks Marseilles and spreads from thence northwards. It is this year imported from Spain by a ship bringing

(*a*) Ex libro *de Gloria Confessorum*, cap. lxxix.

(*b*) *Recueil des Historiens des Gaules et de la France.* Martin Bouquet. Tom II. 1739. *Sancti Georgii Florentii Gregorii Episcopi Turonensis Historiae Ecclesiasticae Francorum*, lib. IV. cap. v.   (*c*) *Ibid.* lib. IV. cap. xxxi.   (*d*) *Ibid.* lib. VI. cap. xiv.

(*e*) *Ibid.* lib. VII. cap. i.   (*f*) *Ibid.* lib. IX. cap. xxi. et xxii.

merchandise to Marseilles some of the purchasers of which appear to have been attacked, one family of eight being destroyed. It is noted that the disease was not communicated at once to the different houses but remained some time inactive and then suddenly broke out. It is further remarked that afterwards Marseilles suffered epidemically several times from the same plague.

(*g*) In 590 it is in Rome following close upon an inundation of that city from the Tiber.

(*h*) In 591 it invades the province of Marseilles and while a famine desolates the towns of Angers, of Nantes, and of Mans "Vivariensem Avennicamque urbem graviter lues inguinaria devastavit."

There is an account by Paulus Diaconus of plague in the province of Liguria in 565 in the time of Narses: "[1]At these times, especially in the province of Liguria, a very great plague broke out. For on a sudden there appeared about houses and doors and furniture and clothes certain marks, which, the more one wished to wipe them out, the more and more appeared. But after the end of a year there began to grow on the groin and other of the more tender parts small glands in the shape of a walnut or a date; these were soon followed by the heat of a fever so intolerable that the sufferer died within three days. If anyone got over the period of three days there was some hope for him. There was mourning everywhere, everywhere tears. For, as the common rumour declared that the plague might be escaped by flight, houses were left deserted by their inhabitants, the dogs alone guarding them: the cattle were left alone in the fields, no shepherd watching them. You might see one day towns or camps filled with crowds of men, and on the next day, as all took to flight, everything in dead silence. Children fled, leaving their parents' corpses unburied. Parents forgetting the bowels of compassion left their children suffering from the fever. If by chance any of the old feelings of affection moved a man to bury a relation, he himself was left with no one to bury him and perished in doing his duty, and while he performed the funeral rites for the corpse his own corpse was left without any burial rites. You might see the time reduced to the silence of old. No voice in the country, no whistling of the shepherds, no attacks of wild beasts upon the flocks. The cornfields passing the time of reaping untouched were awaiting for the reaper. The vine had lost its leaves, its grapes were bright, but it remained unspoiled. As

Account by Paulus Diaconus.

(*g*) *Loc. cit.* lib. x. cap. i.   (*h*) *Ibid.* lib. x. cap. xxiii.
[1] *Rerum Italicarum Scriptores*, Muratorii tom. i. 1723.
De Gestis Langobardorum Pauli Diaconi, lib. ii. cap. iv.

winter drew nigh, in the hours of night as well as of the day, the trumpet of warring hosts was heard and the roar of armies resounded in the ears of many. There were no signs of the footsteps of passers by, no executioner was to be seen and yet the bodies of the dead were more than the eyes could bear. Country districts had been turned into sepulchres and the dwelling-places of men had become a place of refuge for wild beasts. These evils within the borders of Italy alone fell only upon the Romans as far as the territories of the Boii and the Alamanni."

A period of 52 years brings us to the end of the 6th century. The **Plague in Ireland.** Buide Connaile, which proved so fatal in Ireland from 543 to 548, is ascribed by some to plague. Ireland was at that time in constant communication with Italy, and it is supposed that the infection was imported by some of the ecclesiastics who visited Rome. Certainly it is about the middle of the 6th century the Irish Chronicles record that Tara, which till that time was the residence of the chief king, was abandoned. Diarmait MacCearbhaill, the king, left it and never returned, and it was never inhabited again. The royal burgh appears to have been abandoned because nearly everyone had died there, and the place came to be regarded with such dread that even its fine position, far-extending view, and rich pastures could not induce future kings to return to it. A hundred years later, in 663, plague again ravaged Ireland, and in 664 was epidemic in England. Dr Norman Moore[1] favours the view that the plague in 664 was brought to England from Ireland and not from the Continent. It is a moot point whether St Etheldreda died of tuberculosis or of plague. She had a swelling in her neck, which was opened by her physician[2] three days before her death. In favour of plague there is the fact that pestilence prevailed at the time.

No more is heard of plague in Europe till at least a century later, but if we return to the lands in which it prevailed inter- **Plague from the 7th century until the Crusades.** mittently if not continuously for centuries there are sufficient records to show that although it appears to have died out in Europe it continued to exist in its old haunts. The most valuable document in this connection is "Kremer's[3] great epidemics from Arabian sources," which shows Syria and the Euphrates valley to have been during the Saracenic period the scenes of repeated plague.

---

[1] *A Lecture on the History of Medicine as illustrated in English Literature*, by Norman Moore, M.D. [2] *Bede's Eccles. Hist.* lib. IV. cap. xix.

[3] *Ueber die grossen Seuchen des Orients, nach arabischen Quellen*, A. v. Kremer, 1880.

2

Plague epidemics broke out at Ctesiphon in 628 during the reign of Shyrujih, one of the Persian kings of the Sassanidae dynasty. It extended to the Mahommedan dominions, the foundations of which were then being rapidly laid by Mahomet. This was the first outbreak of plague in Islamic history. The next was in 638. It broke out in Palestine at the village of Emmaus, in Galilee, and spread over the whole of Syria. In the same year it appeared in Bassora, carried there by a portion of the Arabian army, which had lost from it in Syria 25,000 men. Among other historical persons who died in this epidemic was Abu Obaidah Ibn Garrah. Two commanders-in-chief died of the disease, the third resolved to adopt preventive measures and distributed his troops in the highlands and desert, whereupon the plague was extinguished.

Besides many local outbreaks there were during the 7th century three great epidemics in Syria and four in Irak. The disorganised condition of these countries brought about by the wars of conquests and the conflicts between the Byzantians and Arabs rendered them highly susceptible to the devastations of plague. Only twice in this century does the plague pass beyond its endemic centres. Once in 686 it spreads into Egypt and there becomes epidemic, and again in 697 it attacks Constantinople. In the 8th century it was epidemic in Egypt in 704, and for the first half of the century in Syria about every ten years. So regular was its annual recurrences at Damascus during the reign of the Caliphs of the Ommiades dynasty that it became a custom for them to withdraw to the desert at the season when plague began to appear. Irak also suffered from at least six severe epidemics during the first 75 years, Bagdad being attacked with plague in 763, the year after it was built. There was a wide-spread epidemic both in Irak and Syria in 745, and it is likely that the destructive plague which prevailed in Sicily and Calabria in 746—748 and spread to Constantinople in 749 was an incursion into Europe from the endemic centre. According to Nicephorus Byzantinus this plague continued in Constantinople for a year and nearly exterminated the population.

Paulus Diaconus describing this epidemic in Constantinople says: "[1]In the same year the plague beginning in Sicily and Calabria, like some devouring fire, came to Hellas and the Aegean Islands, through the whole fourteenth indiction, scourging the impious Constantine, and restraining him from the madness which he aroused against the holy churches and their holy and venerable images. He, however, as

---

[1] *Rerum Italicarum Scriptores*, Muratorii tom. i. lib. xxii.

Pharaoh of old, remained uncorrected. But this plague of the bubo, spreading in all directions, in the fifteenth indiction[1] reached the royal city. Moreover in the spring-time of the first indiction the plague spread, and in the summer it raged so furiously that even houses that were not attacked were closed and no one remained except such as were bound to bury the dead.

"And so of necessity many plans were devised : boards were laid upon animals and thus the dead placed thereon were taken to burial. Similarly others were piled in waggons and carried out. But when all the cemeteries not only in the city but in the suburbs were full, all the reservoirs without water, and the pools and the vineyards, and the private gardens inside the old fortifications were dug up to ensure the burial of the dead ; and despite all this there was scarcely room to bury the dead."

With the accession of the Abbasides and the transference of the capital of the Caliphs to Bagdad and the prosperity which it brought to the country under their sway, plague appears to have become quiescent for some 50 years in Bagdad. Political capital was made of the cessation of plague with the commencement of the Abbasidic dynasty. An Abbasidic statesman in a public speech in Damascus said it was to be regarded as a particular sign of the mercy of God that plague ceased when that dynasty began. But one of those present, a faithful adherent of the fallen dynasty, answered : " God is too merciful to afflict a nation simultaneously with two such scourges as the plague and the Abbasides."

This quiescence in the valley of the Euphrates for some 50 years seems to have formed a part of a general retrocession and decline of the disease after its intermittent activity for 52 years in Europe, Asia, and Africa. Subsequent to this pandemic there were only three devastating epidemics in Egypt, one in 622, another in 686 and a third in 719, after which Egypt remained free of plague until 1010, nearly 300 years. Europe also, with the exception of the visitation of Constantinople in 697 and that of Sicily, Calabria, and Constantinople in 749, remained free from plague for at least 400 years, and Syria for 200 years. While appearing in epidemic form at long intervals during the 9th and 10th centuries in Irak and Persia it was not until the 11th

General retrocession and quiescence of plague in Europe, Egypt, and Syria for several centuries.

---

[1] *Indiction.* The fiscal period of 15 years instituted by Constantine in 313 and reckoned from the 1st of September 312, which became the usual means of dating ordinary events and continued as such down through the Middle Ages.

century that the disease began to show a renewed activity and spread into Syria, Egypt, and Europe. The recrudescence was coincident with a decline in the empire of the Caliphs and a rise in the power of the Turks. The struggle of the contending powers seems to have produced conditions favourable to the virulence of the plague in its endemic centres, while the movements of the different armies were favourable to its extension in those countries brought into contact with them.

The conquests of the Sultans of Ghazna are distinguished by a great plague in India in 1032, which spread over Persia, Mesopotamia, Asia Minor to the neighbourhood of Constantinople, and it is probable that it is this same epidemic which appears in Germany and Western Europe in 1034. Germany in those days comprised the larger part of Europe, including modern Germany, Poland, Austria, Lorraine, Burgundy, and Upper Italy. In 1056 over a million and a half of the inhabitants in the district of Samarcand and Bokhara died of plague.

As in the East so in Europe, the 11th century was characterised by the occurrence of several devastating epidemics of plague.

Plague at the time of the Crusades and after. The worst in Europe was in 1094, two years previous to the commencement of the Crusades. There can be no doubt that plague appeared in Europe before the Crusades, although this has been considered by some the period of its earliest introduction. The return of the Crusaders from the Holy Land, often bringing the disease with them, directed more attention to the mortality which it caused in several parts of Europe. With the Crusades in the 12th and 13th centuries plague assumes a more prominent form in Europe and becomes more frequent and violent in Egypt. In 1167 the victorious army of Frederick the Red Beard is almost exterminated by it in Italy, while in 1270 plague in Tunis decimates the army of Louis XI, who, with his son, died of the disease, while the Crown Prince Philippe was attacked and recovered. Plague was particularly severe in Europe in 1294. Between then and 1346 it prevailed six times in different countries in Europe. But while in Europe and Egypt the plague manifests itself with greater persistency and is characterised by increasing virulence and wider diffusive powers, it exhibits in Irak and Syria towards the close of the 13th century a decline, there being no epidemics of any great magnitude. The depopulated condition of these countries brought about by the loss of life caused by the wars of the Crusaders, by the invasion of the Mongols, and by a series of destructive earthquakes followed by famine, epidemics, epizootics and plague, afforded small opportunity for further devastating plagues. The whole of this region seems to have been in the latter part of the 12th century and the early portion of the 13th in the vortex of violent disturbances of the ordinary course of both natural and social laws.

Quiescence of plague in its old centres did not prevent the gradually

The second recorded pandemic, later called the Black Death.

increasing force and diffusiveness of the plague which began in the 11th century, culminating in the 14th century in an epidemic or pandemic the like of which for destructiveness there are no historical records. The starting-point of this epidemic is not known. The Russian records place it in India; the Grecian in Scythia; the English in the country east of the Indians and Turks; the Arabians in the States of the Great Khan of Tartary and in the land of darkness; and the Italians in Cathay.

The very unsettled condition of the whole of Asia at the time of this epidemic and its being practically a *terra incognita* are probably explanations of the vagueness of contemporary writers on this point. Kublai Khan's empire, extending from Hungary on one side to the coast of China on the other, had been divided among the Mogul Tartar chiefs who fought among themselves for supremacy. It was under these circumstances that the great plague of the 14th century appeared. India, China, Tartary, Central Asia, and Russia had come into closer contact with Persia and Mesopotamia, not by commerce, but by the march of armies. That there was a wide diffusion in some of these countries before it reached Europe can be gleaned from several authors, but how long it lasted is unknown. Galfridi Le Baker de Swynebroke

Constantinople one of the gateways by which the pandemic entered Europe.

sets it down at seven years. One of the gateways by which it appears to have entered Europe was by Constantinople, attacking that city in 1347, the infection having been carried from the Crimea and the Volga, where the disease was then raging. Nicephorus Gregoras thus describes it:

"Now about this time a deadly and pestilential disease swooped down upon the world. It began with the Scythians and at Lake Maeotis and the mouth of the Don, in the very beginning of the spring and continued through all that year, passing from place to place and devastating, in this wise, only the sea coasts, town and country alike, as well our territories as all those which stretch without a break as far as Cadiz and the Pillars of Hercules. But when the second year came it passed also on to the Islands of the Aegean. Then it attacked the Rhodians and the people of Cyprus also, and all that inhabit all the other islands. The disease affected alike men and women, rich and poor, young and old; to put the matter in a word it spared neither rank nor age. Many houses were stripped entirely of their inhabitants in one day, or sometimes in two, since no one was able to render the sufferers help, no one either of the neighbours or of those who were connected by blood or any relationship. Nor was it mankind alone that the plague thus harassed as with a scourge, but all other animals which dwelt with or associated with human beings who took the disease, dogs, and horses and fowls as well. and even the mice that lived within the walls of their houses. The symptoms of the plague which declared themselves signs foreboding a sudden death were the following: A swelling about the upper parts of the thighs and the arms, and accompanying it an effluxion of blood. This in some cases on the very same day carried off from the present life, whether sitting or walking, those who had been stricken by it. Andronicus, among others, the younger of the king's sons, died of it."

There is nothing in this description to indicate that the plague was of a different type from that which had previously prevailed except perhaps its virulence. The Arabian author Ibn Wardy traces the course of the plague in a more definite manner than Nicephorus Gregoras. He relates that it first made its appearance in "the land of darkness[1]," that it then penetrated to China and India, turned thence to the land of Usbekir and to Transoxiania, reached Persia, depopulated Central Asia, Crimea, and Byzantium, then Cyprus and the Islands. The epidemic then appeared in Egypt, depopulated Cairo and Alexandria, and even reached Upper Egypt, and crept in a westerly direction along the African coast to Barca. On the other side the epidemic from Egypt reached the ports of Gaza and Ascalon, invaded Syria, and travelling coastwards and inland, attacked Jerusalem, Damascus, Antioch, and Aleppo, and most of the intervening towns, also those of Asia Minor. Ibn Batuta was in Damascus in 1348 on his return journey from China, and he describes the havoc which the plague caused in that city at the time of his visit.

It is possible that the great epidemic of the 14th century had its origin in its old endemic centres in Mesopotamia and Kurdistan, and

The course of the pandemic as described by an Arabian author.

---

[1] The kingdom of Kiptchak, whose capital was Surai, was held by Arab writers to be the northern limit of the habitable world, and as stated by Yule (*The Book of Marco Polo the Venetian*, by Col. Henry Yule, C.B., vol. i. p. 6) in his *Marco Polo*, Bolghar was the capital of the region sometimes called Great Bulgaria, by Abulfeda Immer Bulgaria, and stood a few miles from the left bank of the Volga in latitude about 54° 54′ and 90 miles below Kazan. The old Arab writers regarded it as nearly the limit of the habitable world and told wonders of the cold, the brief summer nights, and the fossil ivory that was found in its vicinity.

that in its general extension north, east, south and west it reached the Volga by routes similar to those which it has taken in more modern times.   There was intercourse between Persia and southern Russia, and when it was not by commerce it was frequently by the march of armies in the time of war.   Marco Polo relates that while his father and uncle were staying with Barca Khan at Bolghar there broke out a war between Barca and Alan the Lord of the Tartars of the Levant, and great hosts were mustered on either side.   But in the end Barca the Lord of the Tartars of the Ponent was defeated, though on both sides there was great slaughter.

It would serve no useful purpose to follow up this pandemic into **Pandemic distinguished by its rapid spread and destructiveness.** the different countries, provinces and towns in Asia, Africa, and Europe which it successively ravaged.   In the course of three years it passed over the whole of Europe and was unique in the enormous destruction of life which it caused, it being estimated that quite a fourth of the population perished.   This great mortality was not because the plague caused in any one place more deaths than many of the previous or later epidemics of the same disease, but because of its widespread nature. Never before had it shown such diffusive qualities, or attacked so many countries one after the other.   Hecker[1] gives the mortality of some European towns which he has specially collected.   It is as follows:

Towns	Deaths from Plague	Towns	Deaths from Plague
Florence	60,000	Strasburg	16,000
Venice	100,000	Lübeck	9,000
Marseilles (in one month)	16,000	Basle	14,000
		Erfurt	16,000
Siena	70,000	Weimar	5,000
Paris	50,000	Limburg	2,500
St Denys	14,000	London	100,000
Avignon	60,000	Norwich	51,100

A special interest attaches to the epidemic at Avignon as an account **Guy de Chauliac's description of the plague at Avignon.** of it is given by a medical man, Guy de Chauliac, which is very exceptional for these early plagues.   Guy de Chauliac says: "[2]The plague commenced with us in January, it continued seven months during which time it appeared in

[1] *The Epidemics of the Middle Ages*, by J. F. C. Hecker, M.D., translated by B. G. Babington, M.D., F.R.S.

[2] *La Grande Chirurgie de Maistre Guy de Chauliac*, par M. S. Mingelon Saule, Traité II. cap. v.

two forms. During the first two months, it was accompanied with a continuous fever and with a coughing of blood. All who were attacked died in three days. During the other months the continuous fever was accompanied with tumours and boils, which appeared in the external parts of the body chiefly in the armpits and in the groin. Those who were thus attacked died in five days. The disease was so severe and so contagious, especially that which was attended by coughing of blood, that it was contracted not only by visiting and living together with the sick, but by being in their presence, so that people died without service or attendants, men were buried without priests and without religious rites, the father abandoned the son and the son approached not the father; charity was dead and every hope lost."[1]

Few parts of Europe seem to have escaped. The epidemic reached England in the latter part of 1348, and is thus described by Le Baker de Swynebroke: "[2]In the year of Christ 1349[3], in the 23rd year of the King's reign, a general plague

Le Baker de Swynebroke's account of the epidemic in England.

spreading from the East of the Indians and Turks, infecting a half of our habitable world, ravaged with such havoc Saracens, Turks, Syrians, people of Palestine and then the Greeks that, compelled by terror, they determined to accept the faith and sacraments of Christ, hearing that the Christians on our side the sea were not afraid of the death that came upon them more frequently than was wont. At length the dreadful calamity passing in succession the parts beyond the Alps and from there to the west of France and Germany in the 7th year after its outbreak arrived in Europe. And at first it carried off almost all the inhabitants of the seaports in Dorset, and then those living inland, and from there it raged so dreadfully through Devon and Somerset as far as Bristol that the men of Gloucester refused those of Bristol entrance to their country, everyone thinking that the breath of

---

[1] "In connection with this epidemic it is interesting to note that the country people in France dwelt mostly in one-storied huts having mud or clay walls and thatched roofs. Windows were the exception. Over the door was usually an opening for air and light, which also served as an outlet for the smoke from the brushwood fire. The sleeping-places were dark, airless recesses, in which the people having divested themselves of all clothing rested upon straw mattresses or sometimes on feather beds. Bathing was common and much used, especially among the lower classes, and even small villages had their public bath places." (*The Great Pestilence*, A.D. 1348-9, by Francis Aidan Gasquet, D.D., 1893.)

[2] *Chronicon Galfridi Le Baker de Swynebroke*, edited by Edward Maunde Thompson, 1889.

[3] Le Baker de Swynebroke counted the year from Michaelmas, so that the early part of 1349 with him was actually the latter part of 1348.

those who lived amongst people who died of plague was infectious. But at last it attacked Gloucester, yea and Oxford and London, and finally the whole of England so violently that scarcely one in ten of either sex was left alive. As the graveyards did not suffice fields were chosen for the burial of the dead. The Bishop of London bought the croft in London called 'No man's land,' and the Lord Walter de Magne that which is called 'The New Church Hau,' where he founded a house of persons in religion to bury the dead. All pleas in the King's Bench and common pleas of necessity were stopped. Very few nobles died of it. Among them were Lord John of Montgomerie, Captain of Calais, and the Lord of Clistele; they died in Calais and were buried in London in the Church of the Carmelite Brothers of Blessed Mary. A countless number of common people and a host of monks and nuns and clerics as well, known to God alone, passed away. It was the young and strong that the plague chiefly attacked. The old and feeble it commonly spared. Scarcely anyone dared to touch the sick; the healthy fled from relics of the dead, precious then and now, as if they were infectious. One day men were as happy as could be, and on the morrow they were found dead.

"Abscesses suddenly breaking out in different parts of the body tortured them; they were so hard and dry that when they were cut hardly any humour flowed from them: many persons got over them by means of incision or by long patience. Others had small black pustules spread all over the skin, and of these very few, nay rather scarcely one recovered. This great pestilence, which began at Bristol on the feast of the Assumption of the glorious Virgin and in London about the feast of St Michael, raged for a whole year in England so terribly that it cleared many country villages entirely of every human being.

"While this great calamity was devastating England, the Scots rejoicing thought that they would obtain all they wished against the English, and at the time blaspheming were wont from sheer wantonness to perjure themselves 'by the vile death of the English.' But sorrow following on the heels of joy, the sword of the anger of God departing from the English drove the Scots to frenzy through leprosy no less than it had done the English through abscesses and pustules. In the following year it ravaged the Welsh as well as the English: and at last, setting sail, so to speak, for Ireland it laid low the English living there in great numbers, but scarcely touched at all the pure Irish who lived amongst the mountains and on higher ground until the year of Christ 1357, when it unexpectedly and terribly destroyed them also everywhere."[1] The important features in this plague visitation were its rapid and wide diffusion, its comparatively short duration, the virulence of the cases with pustules, the large proportion of cases affecting the lungs with spitting of blood, and the great contagiousness of the pneumonic form. Apart from its attacking the lungs the virulence and diffusiveness of the disease in its other manifestations seem to have been very marked. Diffusiveness may characterise one epidemic and virulence another, but in this epidemic both qualities were united in an exceptionally high degree.

This destructive epidemic of the 14th century formed the climax of that expanding activity of plague which began in the 11th century and which continued at intervals to manifest itself in a widespread manner until the end of the 17th century. In the 15th, 16th, and 17th centuries there were frequent outbursts and epidemics in Europe, Asia, and Africa more or less limited in their extent.

Plague in the 15th, 16th and 17th centuries.

Heberden[2], who ascribes the prevalence of plague to the physical and political miseries of the nations of Europe during these centuries, gives a list of some of the more important places on the Continent attacked with plague in the course of this period. Dresden was attacked with plague in the years 1504–5, 1511–12, 1521, 1535–36, 1547, 1563–64, 1571–72, 1585–86, 1591–92, 1607, 1627–28, 1632–3–4–5–6–7.

"In 1502 the disease was at Brussels; 1517 at Verona; 1525 in Germany; 1531 and 1534 in France; 1539 in Switzerland; 1542 at Breslau; 1550 at Basel; between 1550 and 1553 it spread itself successively over almost all the habitable world; 1559 it was in Holland; 1563 it was in Germany, and again in 1566; 1564 in Savoy; 1566 and 1568 at Milan; 1568 at Paris; 1572 at Basel; 1575 at Milan; 1576 at Venice; 1580 at Marseilles; 1593 it was in Holland and the Low Countries; 1596 and 1597 in Germany; 1603 it was again in Holland, also in 1609, and in the latter part of the year in Denmark; 1618 at Bergen; 1619 in Denmark; 1622 at Amsterdam, where it continued for eight years; 1623 it was at Montpellier; 1625 at Leyden,

---

[1] The effect in England of this severe visitation of plague was as in other countries the disorganisation of the social system which required many years for its recovery and reconstruction. For instance it was not until 200 years later that tillage was revived in England to a similar extent. This improvement began in the time of Elizabeth (*The Growth of English Industry in Modern Times*, lib. II. p. 100, by W. Cunningham, D.D., 1903).

[2] *Observations on the increase and decrease of different diseases, and particularly of the plague.* By Wm. Heberden, Jun., M.D., F.R.S.

in Denmark, and in Germany; 1628 it was at Lyons; 1629 and 1630 at Montpellier; 1631 at Dijon; in 1630 it was besides in Denmark and at Christiania in Norway; and at Parma, Verona and other parts of Italy; from 1633 to 1637 it was in the Netherlands, and in the latter year at Prague; in 1649 more than 200,000 persons are said to have perished by this disease in the southern provinces of Spain; 1649 and 1650 it prevailed at Marseilles; 1650 it was also in Ireland; 1652 at Cracow; 1653 in Poland and Prussia; 1654 at Copenhagen; 1655 at Amsterdam; and in the course of the same year and the three following it was in many places in the south of Europe; 1660 it was in Scotland; 1663 and 1664 at Amsterdam and Hamburg; 1668 in Flanders; 1670 in Italy; 1679 at Vienna; 1680 at Leipsic; 1684 in Norway; 1685 at Leghorn. In 1622 the mortality by the plague at Amsterdam (at that time equal to about one-third of London) was 4000; in 1623, 6000; in 1624, 12,000; 1625, 6800; in 1626, 4400; 1627, 4000; in 1628, 4500. Felix Platerus, physician at Basel, in Switzerland, about 1580, gives an account of seven pestilential fevers which afflicted that country in the space of 70 years. Thomas Bartholin mentions five that raged in Denmark in his time (1660), and Forestus relates that in his time (1570) the plague was frequent at Cologne and Paris; and refers the cause to the multitude of the inhabitants and the nastiness of the streets.

"By another account Paris is said to have been infected eight times between the years 1480 and 1590; in 1607 two hospitals of reserve, St Louis and St Anne, were erected on purpose to receive patients in time of plague or other great calamities. They were opened on account of the plague in 1619, 1631, 1638, 1662 and 1668, since which that disease has been unknown there. We are informed that about the same time Paris was paved and the streets were widened, and the city began to be kept cleaner."

During this period plague also prevailed frequently in Britain. The most important outbreaks are described by Creighton in his history of epidemics of Britain. Many of them are ascribed to importation from the Continent. There is little doubt that the eastern coast was more frequently affected than any other part of the country. Whether the endemicity was kept up by communications with Holland cannot now be determined, but it is not an unlikely explanation.

Plague in London in the 16th and 17th centuries. London itself was never long free from plague, though severe epidemics were infrequent. Some valuable notes on the occurrence of plague collected by Mr Baldwin Latham make this clear. In the course of 136 years plague deaths were recorded in London in no fewer than 84 years, but only six of these years were characterised by severe epidemics. The six years and the number of plague deaths recorded are:—

Year		Number of Plague Deaths
1563	...	23,000
1592–93	...	22,167, according to Creighton 15,003
1603	...	36,269
1625	...	35,417
1636	...	10,400
1665	...	68,596

Notes of the Occurrence of Plague in London and some other places in England since the year 1543, and returns of plague mortality in London, collected by Mr Baldwin Latham, M.I.C.E., from various sources, and mainly from the annual Records of Weddings, Christenings, and Burials, kept in pursuance of orders passed by Thomas Cromwell, Lord Privy Seal, in September, 1538[1].

1543   Plague in London. Lanquette's Chronicle.

1548   Pestilence in London. Stow's Annals.

1551   Sweating sickness in London. Lanquette's Chronicle and Fabian's Chronicle.

1552   Plague prevalent. History of the weather.

1558   Plague in King's Lynn. Richards' King's Lynn.

1562   Plague caused 20,136 deaths. Bills of Mortality, London. Brought by soldiers from the Continent. History of the weather.

1562–3 City and Suburbs of London: Burials 23,630—Plague burials 20,136. Maitland's London, page 736.

1563   23,000 persons died in London of plague between 6th April and last day of November. Lanquette's Chronicle.

1564   Plague not fully ceased in London. Stow's Annals.

1569   Plague in London. Stow's Annals.

1574   Plague in the City. Maitland's London.

1575   Plague in King's Lynn. Mackerell's King's Lynn.

1581–2 Between 28th Dec., 1581, and 27th Dec., 1582, died of plague in London, 6,930. Maitland's London.

1587   Plague raged in King's Lynn. Richards' King's Lynn. Burials in Leeds tripled by the plague. Annals of Yorkshire. Plague rife,—said to be due to famine. History of the weather.

1588   Plague raged in King's Lynn. Richards' King's Lynn.

1589   Plague in Newcastle-on-Tyne. Newcastle Record.

1592*   Plague in London. From March to December, 25,886 persons died, of whom 11,503 died of plague. Graunt.

---

[1] *The Recent Epidemics of Plague in Bombay.* Paper read before the Geographical Society of Manchester, the 19th May, 1898. By H. M. Birdwood, C.S.I., LL.D.
    * Excessive drought.

1593   Plague in London. 17,844 died, of whom 10,662 died of plague, and the christenings were 4,021.

1594* No record for London. Very healthy at Croydon, also in County parish. (Referred to by Graunt.)

1595   No record for London. Great dearth in England. No record for London until 1603.

1603   Burials for London and Liberties, 42,042. Plague burials, 36,269.

1604   Burials, London, 5,219; Plague burials, 896. Plague raged in many country places.

1605	Burials, London, ...	6,391	Plague,	444
1606	„ ...	7,920	„	2,124
1607	„ ...	8,022	„	2,352
1608	„ ...	9,020	„	2,262
1609	„ ...	11,785	„	4,240
1610	„ ...	9,087	„	1,803
1611	„ ...	7,343	„	627
1612†	„ ...	7,842	„	64
1613	„ ...	7,519	„	16
1614	„ ...	7,389	„	22
1615	„ ...	7,887	„	37
1616	„ ...	8,072	„	9
1617	„ ...	8,286	„	6
1618	„ ...	9,614	„	18
1619	„ ...	8,008	„	9
1620	„ ...	9,712	„	21
1621	„ ...	8,123	„	11
1622	„ ...	8,959	„	16
1623	„ ...	11,112	„	17
1624	„ ...	12,210	„	11
1625	„ ...	54,265	„	35,417
„	Burials within walls,	14,340	„	9,197
1626	Burials, London,	7,535	„	134
1627	„ ...	7,715	„	4
1628	„ ...	7,743	„	3
1629	„ ...	8,814	„	*nil*
1630	„ ...	10,554	„	1,317
1631	„ ...	8,358	„	274
1632	„ ...	9,439	„	8
1633	„ ...	8,428	„	*nil*
1634	„ ...	10,865	„	1
1635	„ ...	10,865	„	*nil*
1636‡	„ ...	23,359	„	10,400
1637§	„ ...	11,763	„	3,082
1638	„ ...	13,624	„	363
1639	„ ...	9,862	„	314

* Wet year.   † Tempests, Oct., Nov., and Dec. Drought.
‡ Great drought.   § Summer hot and droughty.

1640	Burials, London, ...	12,771	Plague,	1,450
1641	„	... 18,291	„	3,067
1642	„	... 12,167	„	1,824
1643	„	... 13,202	„	996
1644	„	... 10,933	„	1,492
1645	„	... 11,479	„	1,871
1646	„	... 13,532	„	2,436
1647	„	... 14,059	„	3,597
1648	„	... 9,996	„	611
1649*	„	... 10,532	„	67
1650	„	... 8,581	„	15
1651	„	... 10,773	„	23
1652	„	... 12,539	„	16
1653	„	... 9,083	„	6
1654	„	... 13,126	„	16
1655	„	... 11,409	„	9
1656	„	... 13,752	„	6
1657	„	... 12,434	„	4
1658	„	... 14,993	„	14
1659	„	... 14,756	„	36
1660†	„	... 15,118	„	14
1661	„	... 19,771	„	20
1662	„	... 16,554	„	12
1663	„	... 15,356	„	9
1664	„	... 18,297	„	6
1665‡	„	... 97,306	„	68,596
1666	„	... 12,738	„	1,998
1667	„	... 15,842	„	35
1668	„	... 17,278	„	14
1669	„	... 19,432	„	3
1670	„	... 20,198	„	*nil*
1671	„	... 15,729	„	5
1672	„	... 18,230	„	5
1673	„	... 17,504	„	5
1674	„	... 21,201	„	3
1675	„	... 17,244	„	1
1676	„	... 18,732	„	2
1677	„	... 19,067	„	2
1678	„	... 20,678	„	5
1679	„	... 21,730	„	2
1680	„	... 21,053	„	*nil*

There are no further records of the plague.

Many of the epidemics on the Continent were recrudescences of former outbreaks in the same locality or were caused by the infection brought from neighbouring States. They were manifestations of a

* Commonwealth commenced.   † Charles II.   ‡ Hot and dry.

disease which had become more or less endemic in some portion of the
country in which they appeared, but in addition to these
there were apparently now and again great epidemic
waves spreading in every direction from the old endemic
areas then in possession of the Turks and the Tartars.
Some conditions which have not yet been recognised

Recrudes-
cences and
epidemic
waves from
old endemic
centres.

imparted to the disease an exceptional amount of diffusibility and
infectivity which enabled it to advance irresistibly along the ordinary
trade routes of travel and to become epidemic in most places it visited.
Plague is not the only disease which has displayed these characters.
Cholera and influenza in their visitations during the 19th century
comported themselves in a similar manner. The epidemics of plague
gradually became less frequent even in those places most exposed to its
invasion. There were eleven epidemics in Marseilles in the 16th century,
only two in the 17th century and only one in the 18th century. In
these subsequent visitations the all-pervading destruction which distinguished the 1348 pandemic was absent, though at times some
circumscribed areas would suffer from as virulent if not a more virulent
type of plague. This was the case in 1437 in Cairo, which was almost
depopulated; in 1576 in Venice, which lost 70,000 of its inhabitants; and
in the same year in Moscow, which lost 200,000 of its inhabitants; in 1656
in Naples, which lost 300,000 of its inhabitants; and in Rome, which lost
in the same year 145,000. Genoa also lost 60,000. There died in
London of plague in 1665 nearly 70,000 persons.

Unless maintained by fresh importations from the East the endemic
areas in Europe never seem to have long retained their endemicity.
There were many facilities for fresh importations.

From the 10th to the 16th century the Venetians possessed almost
a monopoly in the commerce between the East and the
West, their only rivals being other Italian States, such

Plague and
commerce.

as Genoa and Florence. Italy, more particularly Venice, was practically
the gateway through which the produce of India, China, and Persia
passed into Europe. The merchandise was brought overland in caravans
to the shores of the Mediterranean or Black Sea, and thence by ships to
the Italian State, which was the great distributing centre for Europe.
On their way through Mesopotamia and neighbouring countries the
caravans passed through endemic areas of plague. The great trade
routes from Venice to the north-west of Europe, to the Baltic and to the
North Sea, were not by sea but by land through central Germany. The
Hanseatic League, that great confederacy of towns for the furtherance

and protection of trade on the north, was the connecting link between Venice and the north. It carried on an immense trade with Venice. The great commercial cities of Bremen, Dantzic, Lübeck, Hamburg, Cracow, Ratisbon, Augsburg, Nuremburg, Frankfort, and other towns were connected by these land routes; and periodical fairs were held in them to which merchants flocked from all parts, bringing their goods and exchanging them for others. They afforded facilities if plague were present for its extension. During this period plague appears to have prevailed periodically and with great persistence in Europe, being maintained by fresh incursions of the disease from the East brought in the train of armies or of commerce. Venice alone in the course of six centuries from 900 to 1500 suffered from 63 epidemics of plague. The Venetians were the first to learn that there was a connection between merchants and merchandise coming from or passing through countries affected with plague and the conveyance of that disease to healthy localities, and for self-protection they were the first to practise against ships from Alexandria and the Levant preventive measures in the form of quarantine, which was based on the medical doctrines of the day. Venice established a Lazaretto in 1403 on the island of Ste Marie of Nazareth, and was followed in 1467 by Genoa and by Marseilles in 1526, both towns having considerable commerce with the East. The effect of the introduction of quarantine in these three ports was however small compared to that which followed the decline of the Venetian trade in consequence of the discovery of America and of the sea route to the East Indies round the Cape of Good Hope.

These two great discoveries at the end of the 15th and the beginning of the 16th century were gradually to effect a great change in commerce, one of which was the transference of a commerce which was exclusively overland or coasting to a sea commerce, and the other was to change the routes of international commerce so as to deprive the Italian States of the monopoly which they had possessed for several centuries. Venice, the principal mart of the products of the Orient, was not long in discovering the injurious effect likely to arise from the discovery of the Portuguese, and in the 16th century its Government made advances to the Portuguese with the object of buying everything brought by the Portuguese from the East. These proposals were rejected. Trade, however, seldom becomes suddenly diverted from its customary routes, and though much of the commerce of the East was shifted to Lisbon, a great deal remained in the Mediterranean, shared by Italy and France; and it was only at the beginning of the

17th century, when Venice lost its power in the Levant, and when the Netherlands and England began to take the place of Portugal and Spain, by which the commercial activities of Europe with the East were transferred to the ports in the North Sea, that the roads northwards from Venice and Marseilles became no longer the routes by which the produce of the East was carried to northern towns. The Hanseatic League came to an end about 1641. The Thirty Years' War, from 1618 to 1648, which had been the means of spreading plague largely in Europe, had practically destroyed the mercantile intercommunications between the North and the South, and at the same time had destroyed the League.

France, which was the only other country having direct dealings with the Levant through Marseilles, was in a state of misery and disorganisation during the first half of the 17th century, and was afflicted not only with plague, but also with famine. Its commerce with the Levant and North Africa was brought to its lowest point on account of piracy in the Mediterranean and the unfriendly attitude of the Turk. A new route to Persia through the Caspian Sea, Astrakhan, Novgorod and Narva, was accordingly opened out in 1630, by which for a considerable time the produce of Persia and the East was conveyed to France.

With the altered circumstances there were fewer facilities for the importation of plague, and after the great outbreaks

Remarkable cessation of plague in Western Europe at the end of the 17th century. between the fifties and eighties in the 17th century, of which the plague of London in 1666 with its 70,000 deaths formed a part, plague rapidly disappeared from the whole of Western Europe. The last epidemic in Ireland was in 1650, in Denmark 1654, in Sweden 1657, in Italy 1657, in the Netherlands and Belgium 1664–66, in England 1666, in Switzerland 1667–68, in France 1667–68, in Western Germany 1667–68, in Spain 1677–81 and in Eastern and Southern Germany in 1679–81. The cessation of plague in all these countries in so short a time is a remarkable epidemiological fact. There may have been and probably were other powerful causes at work, particularly in connection with the natural history of the epidemic, which tended towards its exhaustion and decline, but there is also the important fact that difficulties arose in opportunities of renewal of the disease by fresh invasions. The abandonment of the Mediterranean as the centre of commerce for Europe, the shutting up of the Levant as the high road for the conveyance of the produce of the East to the West, and the transfer of commercial activity to Amsterdam and London, whose connections with the Far East were by sea and not by land, and consequently the avoidance of the former intimate connection with endemic centres, were changes which came into operation in the early part of the 17th century; and it appears that it is in these great changes in the commercial relations of Western Central Europe that the explanation of the rapid disappearance of plague from Europe is to be sought, once the influence of war in Central Europe and famine in France was over, rather than in any great social change effected at that period.

Under these circumstances, quarantine, as practised in the Mediterranean ports, became easier in its application and more effective in its results. Plague continued at intervals in the neighbourhood of the new overland route, and in those countries with which Turkey was at war, for more than another century, but it spread very little out of the beaten track.

During the 18th and the early part of the 19th century plague **Plague in the** continued to prevail in Turkey, Asia Minor, Syria and **18th century.** Egypt, and from there the disease occasionally extended to those countries immediately bordering on their territories or to ports in very intimate intercourse with them. In 1709 it was in Russia and it is estimated that over 150,000 persons died in the epidemic. In 1719 it prevailed in Transylvania, Hungary and Poland, and again in Hungary, Moravia and Austria from 1738–1744. Its extension beyond the countries mentioned was rare. Sometimes the spreading of the disease was connected with commerce and sometimes with war.

The plague of Marseilles in 1720 was imported from Tripoli in Syria by a merchant vessel which had lost six of its crew on the voyage from the disease. From Marseilles the plague spread to Toulon, and in the two towns nearly 90,000 persons died.

The plague in Messina in 1743 was brought by a merchant vessel from the Morea. The captain put in at Misselonghi in the Gulf of Lepanto and there renewing a clean bill of health deceived the health authorities as regards the original port which the vessel started from. He moreover accounted for a death on board by attributing it to an accident in which one of the sailors fell overboard. The captain died on the 24th March, four days after the arrival of the ship, and one of the sailors three days after the captain. The landed goods and the vessel were burnt and the rest of the crew placed in the Lazaretto. These measures allayed all alarm. In the meantime a fisherman had received from the captain some infected goods and had taken them home. The plague first appeared in this quarter of the town. But so slow was its progress that on the 15th of May a thanksgiving service was held for deliverance from this terrible malady. One physician persisted in stating that a number of his patients were suffering from plague, but his announcement was so unwelcome that he narrowly escaped with his life. From the 15th to the 31st of May between three and four hundred people perished, and yet on the 31st of May at a Council held at the Governor's palace twenty-three of the physicians solemnly declared that the disease was not the plague. Notwithstanding this the deaths rose early in June to one hundred a day, and then the Government becoming alarmed issued orders for the necessary regulations: "[1]A panic terror seized at once the people and the city was in a manner abandoned, except by the magistrates of the health and senate, who kept firm in the discharge of their duty, and only one of each magistracy survived. But none of these orders were executed, the common people could not be kept under any government, so that many who had shut themselves up in their houses, began to think of providing themselves by force of money not only with the common necessaries for their sustenance as flour, rice, oil, etc., but also firearms and powder to be able to make defence against the fury of the populace, who would have assuredly committed violence had they not perished so very suddenly by the distemper which swept away the greater part in a few days. The principal mortality did not continue above 20 days, that is from the 12th of June to the beginning of July."

Cyprus in the years 1759 and 1760 suffered from a severe epidemic of plague, Nicosia losing 25,000 of its inhabitants. The disease was first introduced by infected Turkish sailors shipwrecked not far from Limsol, and later by merchant vessels from Damietta. It lasted two years, spread over the greater part of the island and destroyed 70,000 of its inhabitants.

The plague of Moscow in 1771, on the other hand, was the result of war. It occurred when Catherine was at war with the Turks, the Russian troops becoming infected as early as September 1769 by Turkish prisoners of war. The infected troops returning to Jassy spread plague among the inhabitants and later carried it to Moscow, which lost over 60,000 of its population. The disease was unrecognised at first and was called malignant epidemic fever, not an uncommon mistake in the early days of a plague epidemic. At the commencement its progress was slow. The infection was introduced in October 1770, but it was not until March 1771 that the disease assumed

---

[1] *A Treatise of the Plague*, p. 516. By Patrick Russell, M.D., F.R.S., 1791.

threatening proportions and the people became alarmed. According to Dr Athanasius Shafonski, who writes an account of the epidemic and is quoted by Dr F. C. Clemow[1], there were in April 778 deaths, in May 878, in June 1099, in July 1708, in August 7268, in September 21,401, in October 17,561, in November 5235, and in December 805. The plague continued throughout 1772, and it was not until December that Moscow was officially declared to be free from plague. On its rapid development in Moscow it invaded the provinces of the south and west and destroyed 300,000 of the inhabitants.

At the close of the 18th century when plague was affecting the French army in Egypt, West Barbary suffered severely from plague. It is not known how the disease originated. Some ascribed it to infected merchandise imported into Fas from the East; others attributed it to the locusts which had infested West Barbary during the seven preceding years. It was a most destructive and wide-spread epidemic and is estimated to have destroyed two-thirds of the population of the empire. Morocco lost 50,000 of its inhabitants, Fas 65,000, Mogodor 4500, and Saffy 5000. Many villages had nearly the whole of their inhabitants swept away. Deabet, a village near Mogodor, lost 100 persons out of 133 in twenty days, though it remained free for over a month from disease whilst Mogodor was suffering, notwithstanding daily communication. The narrator records the following: "[2]Travelling through the province of Haba shortly after the plague had exhausted itself I saw many uninhabited ruins, which I had before witnessed as flourishing villages. On making inquiry concerning the population of the dismal remains I was informed that in one village which contained 600 inhabitants four persons only had escaped the ravage. Other villages which had contained four or five hundred had only seven or eight survivors left to relate the calamities they had suffered. Families which had retired to the country to avoid the infection on returning to town when all infection had apparently ceased were generally attacked and died. A singular instance of this kind happened at Mogodor where after the mortality had subsided a corps of troops arrived from the city of Zerodant in the province of Suse where the plague had been raging, and had subsided; these troops after remaining three days at Mogodor

Plague in West Barbary.

---

[1] "Plague epidemics in Russia." By Frank C. Clemow, M.D., *Indian Medical Gazette*, Sept. and Oct. 1898.

[2] *An account of Timbuctoo and Hausa Territories in the interior of Africa, by El Hajee Abd. Salam Shabeeny with notes critical and explanatory.* By James Grey Jackson, Resident for upwards of 16 years in South and West Barbary in a diplomatic and commercial capacity, 1820.

were attacked with the disease and it raged exclusively among them for about a month, during which it carried off two-thirds of their original number, one hundred men; during this interval the other inhabitants of the town were exempt from the disorder, though these troops were not confined to any particular quarter, many of them having had apartments in the houses of the inhabitants of the town." This epidemic of plague in 1799 in West Barbary had only been rivalled in violence by the pandemic in the 14th century when two-thirds of the population perished.

As plague prevalence lessened the origin of plague epidemics in healthy localities became easier to trace and resolved itself, in the case of Europe, into importation of the infection from infected localities. Recrudescences in the same locality might recur year after year for a longer or shorter period, but with this exception plague was an exotic which could seldom maintain itself in one place except by fresh invasions brought about by the movement of troops or the activity of commerce.

In the early part of the 19th century plague still lingered in Turkey, Plague in the Asia Minor, Syria and Egypt. In 1803 Constantinople 19th century. lost 150,000 of its inhabitants from the disease. There was a lull again until 1812–13 when the same city lost another 100,000. Only twice in the century did plague extend beyond these limits, once in 1812–15 and again in 1828–29. On both occasions it spread to the frontiers of Austria and of Russia, becoming epidemic in Odessa, the Crimea, Wallachia, Moldavia and Transylvania. In the former years it reached Malta and Noja.

In 1829 it was epidemic in Greece after an absence of a century, having been imported by Egyptian troops. Finally it was epidemic in Constantinople in 1831 and again in 1841 and in Egypt in 1844. Then as in the West at the end of the 17th, so in the East towards the middle

Disappear- of the 19th century a repetition of the phenomenon which
ance of has been more than once noticed in the history of plague
plague from occurred. In the course of five years, from 1839 to
Turkey and 1844, plague disappears entirely from its old haunts in
Egypt in the South-Eastern Europe, the Levantine countries and Egypt.
middle of
the 19th In 1846 the Russian Government and in 1849 the Austrian
century. Government sent commissions to Egypt to enquire as to the disappearance of plague from that country. Both commissions failed to discover a single case of plague.

The cessation of plague in the Levantine regions in the middle of the 19th century was a remarkable phase in the natural history of the disease, but it was not more remarkable than that which occurred in the

8th century and which was followed by a prolonged period of quiescence. Measured by the standard of great epidemics plague has been since 1844 quiescent in the Levantine regions some 60 years, but that quiescence is short compared with the duration of the former lull.

Notwithstanding the disappearance of plague from Turkey, Egypt, Syria and Asia Minor, the disease exhibited at intervals a leisurely activity in Arabia, Mesopotamia, Persia and the coast of Tripoli. In 1853, nine years after the disappearance of plague in Egypt, an outbreak of the disease was heard of in Assyr, a mountainous district of Western Arabia in Northern Yemen. This is an isolated region in which epidemics of plague are known to have occurred in 1826, in 1832 and in 1844, since which time there have been almost annual recurrences. These epidemics are limited to the high Assyr plateau. Probably endemicity of plague in this plateau is even of more ancient date. According to Kremer a virulent outbreak of plague is mentioned in this region as far back as 1157. Since 1853 there have been severe outbreaks in Assyr in 1874, 1879, 1887, and 1889. In 1858 the disease once more reappeared at Benghazi on the coast of Tripoli after an absence of 15 years, and again in 1874. The events preceding the plague in Benghazi were three or four years of unusual drought followed by famine and an epizootic among cattle. It was at a time of the utmost misery that plague broke out in an Arab camp. Plague was also heard of as prevailing in epidemic form in 1863 in Persian Kurdistan, and further south in the same district in 1870, 1871, the villages being situated some 6000 to 7000 feet above the level of the sea. Later investigations indicate that this highland region has been, like Assyr, an endemic centre of plague for many years. Tholozan counted 15 epidemics between 1865 and 1875.

Recrudescence of plague in Arabia, Mesopotamia, Persia and Benghazi.

To the south of Kurdistan in Mesopotamia in the plains of the Euphrates and Tigris plague is recorded as having been prevalent in one district in 1867, in another in 1873–75, in a third including Bagdad in 1873–75, and again in 1880–81, a fourth in 1884–85, and a fifth in 1891–92. Tholozan considers Mesopotamia or Irak Arabi to be a secondary plague centre, being of opinion that the plague is imported from the mountainous districts of Turkish and Persian Kurdistan along the Euphrates. This would agree with what is known of the topographical features of the endemic centres in India and China, both of which, Kumaon and Garhwal in India and Yunnan in China, are at a high altitude. To the east of Kurdistan plague appeared in Astrabad in 1876–77, in Resht in 1877, and at the mouth of the Volga in

1878–79. Astrakhan at the mouth of the Volga is a great resort at certain seasons of the year for Persian fishermen, so that diseases prevalent in Persia are soon apt to find their way by this route to this part of Russia. This outbreak in the province of Astrakhan, being the first in Europe since its disappearance from Turkey in 1841, gave rise to much alarm and particularly so on account of its destructive character in the village of Vetlianka, where in less than two months it caused 350 deaths in a population of 1700 inhabitants. It attacked six other small and adjacent communities on the banks of the Volga and destroyed

Plague in the Province of Astrakhan. altogether about 420 persons. The disease began early in October and at the commencement manifested itself in a mild form. The patients suffered from fever, slight but debilitating. They had abscesses of the lymphatic glands, either in the groin or in the armpit, which suppurated freely, and the duration of the sickness was from 10 to 20 days. The disease gradually became more virulent, and at the height of the epidemic from December the 9th to the 21st the mortality reached 100 % of those attacked[1].

The early stages of this epidemic with its mild form of plague were similar to a bubonic or glandular malady which had prevailed the year before in the city of Astrakhan and its suburbs, where some 200 of the inhabitants were affected and only one died. The outbreak in Vetlianka was the last appearance of plague in Europe for 17 years[2].

[1] "On the progress of Levantine plague in 1878–79," by Mr Netten Radcliffe. *Medical Supplement to the Ninth Annual Report of the Local Government Board*, 1879–80.

[2] Though the plague had disappeared from Europe Dr Bruce Low (*Twenty-eighth Annual Report of the Local Government Board*, 1898–99. *Medical Supplement*. "On the diffusion of bubonic plague from 1879 to 1898," by Dr Bruce Low) in a brief summary shows that from 1879 to 1896 not a single year passed without the development of plague in at least one country, and in later years the disease was present in several countries at one and the same time.

"In 1880 plague was reported to be present in Mesopotamia.
,, 1881 it was present in Mesopotamia, Persia and China.
,, 1882 in Persia and China.
,, 1883 in China.
,, 1884 in China and in India (as " Mahamari ").
,, 1885 in Persia.
,, 1886 in India (as "Mahamari") ⎱ Mahamari in the
,, 1887 in India (as "Mahamari") ⎰ districts of Kumaon
,, 1888 in India (as "Mahamari") and Garhwal.
,, 1889 in Arabia, Persia and China.
,, 1890 in Arabia, Persia and China.
,, 1891 in Arabia, China and India (as " Mahamari ").
,, 1892 in Mesopotamia, Persia, China, Russia and ? Tripoli.
,, 1893 in Arabia, China, Russia and India (as " Mahamari ").
,, 1894 in Arabia, China and India (as " Mahamari ").
,, 1895 in Arabia and China.
,, 1896 in Arabia, Asia Minor, China, Japan, Russia and India."

CHAPTER II.

PLAGUE IN INDIA.

THE English established factories at Surat, Ahmedabad, Bombay
Plague in India. and Agra, at the beginning of the 17th century, and until
that time and even later the history of plague in India
is veiled in obscurity. That plague did prevail in India in or before
the 11th or 12th century is certain, for in some of the Puranas which
are at least 800 years old there are references to the disease and
instructions to the Hindus as to the precautions to be taken in the
event of its appearance. One of these is that whenever a mortality
among the rats of a house is observed the inhabitants are to leave.

It has already been stated that according to the Arabian chronicles
India was severely visited by plague in 1031, and that this epidemic
spread to the vicinity of Constantinople. It has also been stated that
Russian authors ascribed the origin of the great pandemic of the
14th century to the advance of an epidemic from India. There is
evidence of extensive pestilences in India in the 14th, 15th and
16th centuries. References to these are to be found in the history
of the Mahommedan wars. Doctors George and John Thomson[1] in
their treatise on plague mention the years 1345, 1399, 1438, 1574 and
1597 as plague years in India. Nathan[2], taking his information from
the *Bombay Gazetteer*, in the article on Ahmedabad, mentions two references which may point to the existence of plague in the west of India
in the 14th and 15th centuries. The first is from Ibn Batuta, who
notices that Muhammad Tughlik's army in Ma'bar (1325–51) mostly
perished of pestilence, and that at the end of the century (1399), after
Timur left, the districts through which he passed were visited by pestilence. The second relates to the year 1443 when in Malwa the plague

---

[1] *A Treatise on Plague.* By Major George S. Thomson, I.M.S., and Dr John
Thomson. 1901.

[2] *The Plague in India*, 1896, 1897. R. Nathan.

caused such loss of life in Sultan Ahmad I.'s army that, leaving many of the dead unburied, he returned to Gujarat.

The connection established between Northern India and the endemic areas of plague in Central Asia, Persia, and Irak by the Mongols would facilitate the spread of plague into India in these early periods.

In the first decade of the 17th century plague appears to have broken out in the Punjaub and spread over different parts of India, lasting about eight years. Its commencement seems to have been connected with disease in Kandahar in which the land was overrun with mice[1].

Plague in the early part of the 17th century.

The Emperor Jehangir writing of this epidemic in his memoirs says, "[2]In this year (1615 A.D.), or rather in the tenth year of my reign, plague (waba) broke out in many parts of Hindústán. It first appeared in the districts of the Punjaub and gradually came to Lahore. It destroyed the lives of many Mahommedans and Hindús. It spread through Sirhind and the Doab to Delhi and its dependent districts, and reduced them and the villages to a miserable condition. Now it has wholly subsided." Nawab Mu'tamad Khan referring to the same event in the *Ikbál-náma*[3] mentions its precedence by a mouse mortality. "When it was about to break out a mouse would rush out of its hole as if mad, and striking itself against the door and the walls of the house, would expire. If immediately after this signal the occupants left the house and went away to the jungle, their lives were saved; if otherwise the inhabitants of the whole village would be swept away by the hand of death." Mu'tamad Khan also adds more information concerning the epidemic than that found in the memoirs of the Emperor Jehangir. Thus, "If any person touches the dead, or even the clothes of the dead man, he also could not survive the fatal contact. The effect of the epidemic was comparatively more severe upon the Hindús. In Lahore its ravages were so great that in one house ten or even twenty persons would die, and their surviving neighbours annoyed by the stench would be compelled to desert their habitations. Houses full of the dead were left locked, and no person dared to go near them through fear of his life. It was also very severe in Kashmir where its effects were so great that (as an instance) a *darwesh* who had performed the last sad offices of washing the corpse of a friend, the very next day

Plague in the Punjaub.

[1] *Bombay Gazetteer*, Vol. IV. c. xii. p. 218.

[2] "The History of India as told by its own Historians." *The posthumous papers of the late Sir H. M. Eliot, K.C.B.* Edited and continued by Professor John Dowson, Vol. VI. p. 346. 1875.

[3] *Ibid.* p. 406.

shared the same fate. A cow which had fed upon the grass on which the body of the man was washed also died. The dogs also which ate the flesh of the cow fell dead upon the spot. In Hindústán no place was free from this visitation which continued to devastate the country for a space of eight years."

The following note kindly supplied to the author by Mr W. Foster of the India Office refers to the plague epidemic in Ahmedabad in 1617 and 1618.

"[1]The city Amadawar[2] (at our being there with the King[3]) was

Plague in Ahmedabad. visited with this Pestilence in the month of May, and our family was not exempted from that most uncomfortable visitation; for within the space of nine dayes seven persons that were English of our family were taken away by it; and none of those that dyed laid sick above twenty houres, and the major part well and sick and dead in twelve houres, as our Surgeon (who was there all the Physician we had) and he led the way, falling sick at mid-day and the following mid-night dead. And there was three more that followed him, one immediately after the other, who made as much hast to the grave as he had done......All those that dyed in our family of this pestilence had their bodyes set all on fire by it, as soon as they were first visited, and when they were dying or dead, broad spots of a black and blew colour appeared on their brests; and their flesh was made so extreme hot by their most high distemper that we who survived could scarce endure to keep our hands upon it. It was a most sad time, a fiery trial indeed...... All our family (my Lord Ambassadour[4] only excepted) were visited with this sickness and we all, who through God's help and goodness outlived it, had many great blisters, fild with a thick yellow watry substance that arose upon many Parts of our bodyes, which, when they brake, did even burn and corrode our skins, as it ran down upon them!"

Information is also obtained from other sources of this epidemic in Hindustan. In the account of the Embassy of Sir Thomas Roe to the Court of the Great Mogul 1615–19 it is stated[5]: "I received news of a great plauge at Agra so that I judgd it dangerous to send up the goodes into an infected place from whence no Comodytye could be suffered to passe."

---

[1] *A Voyage to East India.* By the Rev. Edward Terry, Chaplain to Sir Thomas Roe, published 1655, p. 242.

[2] The old way of spelling Ahmedabad.

[3] Dec. 1617 to Sept. 1618.   [4] Sir Thomas Roe.

[5] Page 307.

Joseph Salbank in one of his letters[1] mentions in 1616 that plague had existed at Agra for three months, and that there was sometimes a daily mortality of 1000 persons. Lahore is also mentioned as being affected, in another letter. The plague continued in Agra for at least four years. The plague[2] is referred to as increasing in Agra early in 1619.

Plague in Agra.

The Emperor Jehangir's autobiography[3] contains the following account of the plague at Agra: "At this time those who were loyal represented that the disease of the plague (taun) was prevalent in the city of Agra, so that in a day 100 people[4], more or less, were dying of it. Under the armpits, or in the groin, or below the throat a lump comes and they die. This is the third year that it has raged in the cold weather and disappeared in the commencement of the hot season. It is a strange thing that in these three years the infection has spread to all the towns and villages in the neighbourhood of Agra, and there has been no trace of it in Fattehpur (Sikri) and as far as for two and a half *koss* from Amanabad to Fattehpur. The people of that place have forsaken their own homes and gone to other villages."

The following extract from the Emperor's journal relates to an occurrence which is particularly interesting as an observation on the intimate relationship between rat plague, cat plague and human plague. To-day similar instances might readily be quoted in which the plague mouse or rat in a house infects the cat and afterwards plague breaks out in the house. "The daughter of the deceased Asaf Khan who is in the house of Khan-i-Azam, told me a strange and wonderful tale. I made particular enquiries into its truth and write it on account of its strangeness. She said that one day in the court-yard of her house she saw a mouse falling and rising in a distracted manner. It was running about in every direction after the manner of drunkards, and did not know where to go. She said to one of her female slaves, 'Take it by the tail and throw it before the cat.' The cat, delighted, jumped up from its place and seized it in its mouth, but immediately dropped it and showed aversion to it. By degrees an expression of grief and pain showed itself in its face. The next day it was nearly

[1] *Letters received by the East India Company*, Vol. VI. p. 198. Edited by William Foster, B.A., 1902.

[2] *Letters from Surat to East India Company*, March 12, 1619.

[3] "Plague an old Indian disease." By Alex. Rogers. *The Indian Magazine and Review*, January, 1898.

[4] There is a great difference between the estimates of the number of daily deaths given by Salbank and the Emperor Jehangir. The latter is more likely to be correct.

dead, when it entered into her mind to give it a little treacle. When its mouth was open its palate and tongue appeared nearly black. It passed three days in a state of misery, and on the fourth day came to its senses. After this the grain of the plague (danah or bubo) appeared in one of the female slaves and from excess of temperature and increase of pain she had no rest. Her colour became changed; it was yellowish inclining to black and the fever was high. The next day she was free of fever and died. Seven or eight people in the house died in the same way, and some were ill. On the day I went to the garden from that halting place, those who were ill in the garden died and in that place the bubo did not appear again. Briefly in the space of eight or nine days 17 people became travellers on the road to annihilation. She also said: 'Those on whom the boil appeared, if they asked another person for water to drink or to bathe in, these also caught the infection and at last it came to such a pass that through extensive suspicion no one would pass near them'."

Plague is again recorded as prevalent in India from 1684 to 1702.

Plague at the end of the 17th century. It attacked Surat in 1684 and Bombay in 1689. Surat was at that time a town of greater commercial importance than Bombay. It possessed all the unwholesome conditions which have been observed to favour the prevalence of virulence of plague. Crowded and unclean, the streets were narrow and in places covered with excrement of man and beast. Fryer, who visited Surat some time before the outbreak, wonders that a city whose people make the streets a dung-hill should never have been visited by the plague. The disease when it was imported in 1684 continued for six years without interruption, varying in intensity at different seasons of the year. Subsiding during the rainy season, viz. from June to September, the epidemic broke out with fresh fierceness in October and, again abating the greater part of the cold and hot seasons, raged with renewed fury towards the end of May.

In 1684 the disease was in the army of the Emperor Aurangzebe. The following details of the prevalence of plague about this time collected from different records are given by Sir James Campbell in the fourth volume of the *Bombay Gazetteer*.

"[1]This outbreak, apparently the true plague taun and waba, raged for several years over a great part of western India. At Ahmedabad, where it lasted for seven or eight years, its visible marks were swellings as big as a grape or banana behind the ears, under the arms and in the

[1] Gemelli Careri in *Churchill's Voyages*, IV. p. 191.

groin, and redness round the pupils of the eyes. In 1689 it broke out with great violence at Bijapur[1]. All attacked with it gave up hope! It had been in the Deccan for several years. Near Goa in 1684 it attacked Sultan Mosam's army and carried off 500 men a day[2]; raged in Surat for six years (1684-90)[3], reduced (1690) the Bombay garrison to 35 soldiers[4]; was so violent that it not only took away all means of preparing a good end, but in a few hours in Surat, Daman and Thana carried off whole cityfuls of people[5], and at Tátha in Sind (1696) killed 80,000 souls[6]. In Surat Europeans were observed to enjoy a remarkable immunity, but when Bombay was attacked in 1690 they suffered as much if not more than the natives, for it is recorded that of 800 Europeans only 50 were left, of whom six were civilians, six commissioned officers, and not quite 40 English soldiers. Bombay, which was one of the pleasantest places in India, was brought to be one of the most dismal deserts."

After the epidemic in the 17th century plague seems to have Plague in the disappeared from India as completely and as rapidly as it 19th century. did from Western Europe, for it is not until 110 years later at the beginning of the 19th century that a small part of Cutch, Káthiáwár, Gujarat and Sindh were again affected with the disease, which continued from 1812 to 1821. It was at the close of a famine that plague appeared in Cutch. "[7]The famine of 1811 and 1812 was, at the close of 1812, followed in Cutch by an outbreak of pestilence so deadly that it was said to have destroyed half the ryots in the country. At the same time a 'contagion raged at Ahmedabad with a fury that can scarcely be believed.' Every house sickened, whole families were carried off and many a funeral party coming back to the house of mourning found that, in their absence, another member of the family had sickened and died. So thinned were some castes that their women had to help to carry the dead. All the fuel was burned, and though houses were pulled down to supply logs many bodies had to be left half consumed. Half of the people of Ahmedabad, perhaps about 50,000 souls, are said to have perished. In Ahmedabad Musalmáns and Hindus suffered alike. But in other parts it was noticed that among Musalmáns the disease was less fatal. Of the symptoms of this sickness no details are recorded. But there seems every reason to suppose that it was the same disease, that lulling for two years, in

---

[1] *Muntakhubu I Lubab :* Elliot, VII. p. 337.   [2] *Orme's Hist.* Frag. p. 142.

[3] *Ovington's Voyage to Surat*, p. 347.   [4] *Bruce's Annals*, III. p. 94.

[5] *Churchill*, IX. p. 191.   [6] *Hamilton's New Account*, I. p. 123.

[7] *Bombay Gazetteer*, Vol. IV. p. 220.

May 1815, after one of the heaviest rainfalls on record, broke out afresh with deadly force at Kantakot in east Cutch. In cases of this disease slight fever was followed by great weakness and weariness, and then swellings came in the groin and armpits, suppurating in some cases and in others remaining hard lumps. Few stricken with the disease recovered. Most died between the third and ninth day......It seemed to attack most fiercely the sluggish and vegetable eaters; Rajputs escaped where Brahmans and Vainos rotted off; oil makers were believed to be safe. From Kantakot it spread to other parts of Vagar, causing much loss of life in the early months of 1816. In May 1816 it crossed to Morvi in Káthiáwár." The plague in Káthiáwár was observed by Dr Gilder and Dr Whyte, both of whom reported to the Government on the epidemic. Dr Gilder in describing the symptoms, refers to the two forms of plague observed, the knotty disease and the expectorating disease, obviously the bubonic and pneumonic forms. He also observed that the epidemic confined itself principally to such of the native population as subsisted entirely on vegetable diet, namely, Brahmins, Soonars, Dhurzees and Khoomtees; those using animal food with but few exceptions generally escaped. It is deserving of notice that this epidemic occurred at a time when plague became widely diffused in the Levant, spreading to the Lower Danube, Asia Minor, Armenia, and Northern Africa, and lasting nearly 20 years. In the epidemic of 1812–13, 100,000 persons died of plague in Constantinople.

Nothing more is heard of the disease on the western side of India until 1836 when the Pali plague broke out in Marwar in Rajputana, and lasted until 1838[1]. It is estimated that 100,000 Marwaries perished. The Pali plague was preceded by a great mortality among cattle not only through Marwar but in Mullani and the desert·country to the west, occasioned by a complaint said to be different from the epizootics usually observed. In Pali itself from November 1836 to October 1837 the disease was mild and the deaths were comparatively few, but later it acquired a more virulent form and became more prevalent and fatal. The inhabitants fled from the town. At Taiwali rats died just before the outbreak of plague in that place. Dr Forbes mentions that Mr White reports that " this death of the animal attended or preceded the disease in every town that was attacked in Marwar so that the inhabitants of any house instantly quitted it on seeing a dead rat."

[1] *Thesis on the Nature and History of Plague as observed in the North-West Provinces of India.* 1840. Dr Forbes.

The epidemic, which was limited in its nature, also corresponded in time with a fresh and comparatively limited activity in the Levant, which affected the Turkish dominions in Europe and Asia as well as in Egypt, and it is to be observed that the disappearance of plague in Rajputana coincided with its decline and ultimate disappearance in the Levant. Dr Forbes remarks that "for some years prior to 1832 plague had been steadily advancing from Asia Minor through Mesopotamia, Irak, round the head of the Persian Gulf and along the Persian coast, desolating the cities Dujarbehr, Mosul, Bagdad, Busrah, and Abusbeher, at which place it ceased or was withdrawn from European observation." Pali[1] is the chief mart of Western Rajputana and placed at the intersection of the great commercial roads from Mandavi in Cutch to the Northern States, and from Malwa to Baháwalpur in Sindh. It is in a centre like this that the disease being brought by the merchants would once more come under observation.

Apart from the foregoing epidemics which have at long intervals prevailed in India there is a centre of plague at Garhwal and Kumaon, two adjoining districts situated on the southern slopes of the Himalayas. Here plague was discovered to exist in 1823. There is no information as to how long this centre of plague existed previous to its recognition. It is possible that the plague in Kumaon in 1823 was only a part of that which prevailed in Western India from 1812 to 1821, or that it was introduced even earlier and became established during the plagues of the 14th, 15th, or 17th centuries. Whatever may be the date of its origin, there can be little doubt that Kumaon is now an endemic centre, plague having occurred in limited outbreaks even as recently as 1897. The last outbreak before plague appeared in Bombay in 1896 was in July and September of 1893, and occurred in a valley some 6000 feet high. Fortunately this centre is comparatively an inactive one as regards its powers of diffusion, which is in favour of its being a branch of the parent stock in the Levant, which has lost not only its powers of diffusion but also the power of retaining its hold on countries in which it had prevailed for centuries. An epidemic in Hansi, in the province of Delhi, in 1828–29, and another in Rohilcund, around Bareilly, in 1836–38, probably owed their origin to Kumaon.

The districts of Garhwal and Kumaon endemic centres of plague in India.

---

[1] *Imperial Gazetteer of India*, Vol. XI. p. 1.

CHAPTER III.

THE PRESENT PANDEMIC.

THE centre of interest now passes from Europe, the Levant and India
to the province of Yunnan in China from which the present
pandemic originated. The acquisition of Hongkong by
the British in 1841 and the subsequent opening of the
treaty ports to commerce in 1860 were the first incidents
in the process of breaking down that exclusiveness by
which China had isolated herself from the intrusion of
foreigners. Since then many missionaries, explorers and merchants
have penetrated into the interior of China which until their visit was
for Europeans a *terra incognita*.

The present pandemic originated in Yunnan, one of the Western Provinces of China.

They have given accounts of their experiences, with the result that,
though the interior of China as a whole and its internal affairs are still
veiled from foreigners, yet much more is known concerning important
events occurring there than ever before. A favourite field for explora-
tion was Yunnan, because of its proximity to Burma, Siam, and French
Annam, its reputed richness in minerals, and the possibility of its
becoming a highway to Western and Central China. The sixties and
seventies of the 19th century were remarkable for the number of
intrepid travellers who traversed Yunnan and other parts of China.
Lagrée, Garnier, Cooper, Sprye, Sladen, Dupuis, Rocher, Richth,
Margary, Grosvenor, Baker, Gill, and later Colquhoun and Bourne, all
distinguished themselves as modern pioneers.

It was during one of these explorations that M. Rocher in 1871,
i.e. over thirty years ago, came across plague in the province
of Yunnan. This province is situated at the eastern con-
fines of Burma and Thibet, has Tonking on the south, the
province of Sechuan on the north, and the provinces of
Kweichow and Kwangsi on the east. It is very mountainous, with high
and fertile plateaux, which rise towards the central portion of the province

Topographical description of Yunnan.

to between 6000 and 7000 feet. Talifu and Yunnanfu, two of the chief cities, are situated on the shores of inland lakes and on plateaux, respectively 6400 and 6900 feet in height.

The province of Yunnan, isolated by its position and its physical features, has only a limited intercourse with its neighbours and with the treaty ports. There are trade routes connecting Talifu and Yunnanfu with Burma, Thibet, and the province of Sechuan, but the mountainous character of the country which has to be traversed, and the cost and difficulties of transport, which has to be effected by pack animals, cause them to be little used. Caravans from Thibet pass Li Chiangfu on their way to Ssumao for tea.

The trend of intercourse and trade, so far as it is developed, is Trade routes towards Tonking and the provinces of Kweichow, Kwangsi, from Yunnan. and Kwantung. Following the course of the Red River in Tonking and the West River in Kwangsi and Kwantung, the journey can be undertaken in boats for at least some part of the way. Both the Red River and West River rise within the boundary of Yunnan, and form more or less natural trade outlets for the province. The Red River is navigable from Manhao in Yunnan, and passes through Tonking to Haiphong in the gulf of Tonking. This route, notwithstanding its advantages, has not been a favourite. The West River is navigable from Posé, a small town situated on the borders of Yunnan and Kwangsi, away down to Nanningfu, Wuchowfu, and Canton. Even this route has been seldom used further east than Nanningfu. Almost invariably, until recent years, Yunnan goods, brought down the West River as far as Nanningfu, have, at that point, been taken from the boats and carried across country on pack animals to Pakhoi and more recently to Muiluk. Similarly, goods intended for Yunnan have entered Pakhoi, been conveyed overland to Nanningfu, been there transferred to boats, taken up the river to Posé, and then overland again to the towns of Yunnan.

There is yet another trade route from Yunnan through the Kwangsi province. It is more northerly than that by Posé, Nanningfu, and the West River, which it, however, joins before this waterway enters the province of Kwantung. The route is overland, and in an easterly direction from Yunnan to Kingyuan in Kwangsi. It here meets the river Lieou Kiang, and becomes a water route to Lauchaufu, which is a great distributing centre, goods from the west being sent to Yunnan and Kweichow provinces, and *vice versa*. At Lauchaufu the route branches into two, one going overland in a north-easterly direction to Kweilin, the capital of Kwangsi, and thence by water due south to

Wuchowfu.   The other branch is by river, *via* Tsamchaufu to Wuchowfu.

The province of Yunnan, at the time of M. E. Rocher's visit, was
Condition of Yunnan in 1871 as observed by M. Rocher. in a state of rebellion.   The inhabitants, chiefly Mahommedans, had risen against the Imperial Government, and such was their power that it took some twenty years to subdue them.   The traveller found large tracts of the country devastated or deserted, and everywhere signs of depopulation and of the ravages of warfare, great numbers of the inhabitants having been killed in battle or afterwards massacred.   To the miseries of war and of famine were added those of pestilence, the infection of which was often carried by the rival armies from village to village, and from town to town.   What proportion of the depopulation of Yunnan was due to fighting, and what proportion to famine, massacres, and pestilence, is unknown, but their combined effect was to convert a populous and thriving province into a country with few inhabitants, and one which had to be repeopled by immigrants.

That the pestilence was plague there can be no doubt.   M. Rocher's description of the disease and its association with swellings in the armpit, groin, and neck, allow no other conclusion.   The following is M. Rocher's account of the disease:

"La maladie connue au Yün-nan[1] sous le nom de *yang-tzü* (痒 子),
M. Rocher's account of plague in Yunnan. et qui paraît n'être autre que la peste bubonique, y fait chaque année de nombreuses victimes; elle sévit aussi quelquefois dans le Laos et sur la frontière du Kuei-chou.

"D'après les renseignements que nous avons pu obtenir parmi les notables, cette maladie semble venir de la Birmanie, d'où elle est transmise par les caravanes qui trafiquent entre les deux pays.   On n'est pas d'accord sur l'époque de son apparition dans le Yün-nan: les uns disent (et la plus grande partie de la population est de cet avis) que le centre et l'est de la province n'ont connu le fléau qu'au début de la rébellion; d'autres prétendent qu'il s'est montré dans l'extrême ouest jusqu'à Ta-li-fu, quelques années auparavant.   En supposant que cette dernière hypothèse soit vraie, l'épidémie a dû passer bien légèrement dans ces parages, puisqu'on n'en a pas eu connaissance dans les autres districts.

"Depuis le commencement de la guerre civile, cette terrible maladie s'est déchaînée avec fureur sur la province et continue, encore aujourd'hui que la province est paisible, à y exercer ses ravages.

[1] *Notes sur la peste au Yün-nan, La Province Chinoise du Yün-nan*, par Émile Rocher. Deuxième Partie, p. 279.

"Ce qui ferait croire que cette épidémie n'est due qu'aux miasmes malfaisants qui s'exhalent de la terre, c'est que les petits animaux qui vivent dans les égouts ou sous la terre sont atteints les premiers, les rats par exemple. Dès qu'ils se sentent malades, ils sortent par bandes, font irruption dans l'intérieur des maisons, courent affolés, et, après quelques tours sur eux-mêmes, tombent morts; le plus souvent ils crèvent sous les planchers, ce qui détermine dans les appartements des odeurs infectes, dont on ne découvre que trop tard la cause. Le même phénomène se produit chez tous les autres animaux, grands et petits : les buffles, les bœufs, les moutons et les chèvres sont frappés du même mal, et parfois aussi les oiseaux de basse-cour, mais, parmi ces derniers, la maladie fait moins de victimes. A notre arrivée dans la province, nous refusions d'ajouter foi aux nombreux témoignages des indigènes, en les mettant sur le compte de leur imagination troublée ou de leurs idées superstitieuses; mais quand l'épidémie éclata dans le district même où nous nous trouvions, il nous fut facile de nous convaincre de leur véracité.

" Dès que ces symptômes avant-coureurs se manifestent, la population ne tarde pas à être attaquée à son tour. On prend alors les précautions estimées les plus efficaces pour se garantir du fléau. Presque partout, afin de purifier les maisons, on allume du feu dans toutes les chambres, et dans certains districts on cesse de manger du porc.

" Chez l'homme, la maladie s'annonce par une fièvre violente, accompagnée d'une soif intense; quelques heures après, une tumeur d'un rouge foncé commence à paraître aux aisselles, à l'aine ou au cou; la fièvre s'accentue de plus en plus, et le malade ne tarde pas à perdre connaissance. La tumeur grossit d'habitude jusqu'au second jour et reste ensuite stationnaire. A partir de ce moment, le malade paraît reprendre ses sens, mais il est encore en grand danger; car, si la tumeur, jusqu'alors très dure, devient molle, et si la fièvre ne diminue pas, il est considéré comme perdu; dans le cas contraire, si la tumeur perce en dehors, ce qui arrive rarement, il y a espoir de le sauver; mais, arrivé à ce point, le malade est si affaibli que, bien que la tumeur ait abouti, il meurt d'épuisement.

" Quelques médecins chinois ont essayé d'inciser ces tumeurs; mais, soit que l'opération ait été mal faite ou trop tardivement, bien peu de malades y survivent; quand ils sont à bout de ressources, ils ont recours au musc qu'ils ordonnent à la dernière extrémité et à fortes doses.

" Pendant notre séjour au Yün-nan, nous avons vu un grand nombre de cas, et nous devons dire que la plupart ont eu un dénouement funeste.

Dans les endroits où la peste ne fait que passer, on peut estimer que le nombre de ses victimes est environ de 4 à 6 pour 100 ; tandis que dans d'autres districts, plus rudement éprouvés, la population est complètement décimée, et des familles entières disparaissent les unes après les autres. Dans les parages où l'épidémie sévit avec tant de violence, les habitants n'hésitent pas à abandonner leurs demeures et leurs récoltes sur pied pour aller camper sur les hauteurs où, bien souvent, le fléau les poursuit.

"Ce qui, à notre avis, contribue beaucoup à aggraver cette déplorable situation, c'est que les Chinois, superstitieux comme ils le sont, au lieu d'enterrer les pestiférés, se contentent de les placer dans des bières qu'ils exposent au soleil, soit sur la pente des collines ou en plein champ. Il s'ensuit que les gens qui voyagent ou circulent dans les environs des villages empestés sont à peu près asphyxiés par les odeurs nauséabondes que répandent les cadavres en décomposition.

"Pendant les années 1871, 1872 et 1873, nous avons remarqué que le début de l'épidémie se manifeste toujours au commencement de la plantation du riz, c'est-à-dire de mai à juin ; après cette époque, elle sévit avec vigueur dans les localités qu'elle traverse. Durant l'été, qui est, au Yün-nan, la saison des pluies, elle continue de se propager avec moins d'activité ; toutefois, c'est pour reprendre une intensité nouvelle à l'époque de la moisson, et c'est à partir de ce moment jusqu'à la fin de l'année, qu'elle fait le plus de victimes.

"Un fait étrange, que nous avons observé dans plusieurs endroits au midi et au nord de la province, c'est que l'épidémie, au lieu d'englober tous les lieux habités, villes et villages, qui se trouvent sur sa route, passe à côté sans y toucher, les franchit même, et revient quelques mois après, ou l'année suivante, frapper l'endroit oublié. Voici un autre fait, non moins curieux que le précédent : après s'être déclarée dans presque tous les villages dispersés dans les plaines, l'épidémie éclate sur les montagnes où elle produit de nombreux ravages parmi les aborigènes. D'après ce que nous avons vu par nous-mêmes et la façon irrégulière dont la maladie se présente, elle paraît importée sur les hauteurs par les hommes ou femmes qui vont, à certaines époques de l'année, travailler dans les plaines. C'est surtout, comme nous l'avons dit plus haut, après la plantation du riz ou quand la récolte est terminée que le fléau quitte le pays bas pour aller sévir sur les hauteurs.

"L'esquisse, montrant la marche suivie par la maladie pendant les années 1871, 1872 et 1873, a été dressée d'après des notes officielles fournies par les fonctionnaires des lieux pestiférés et d'après nos propres renseignements."

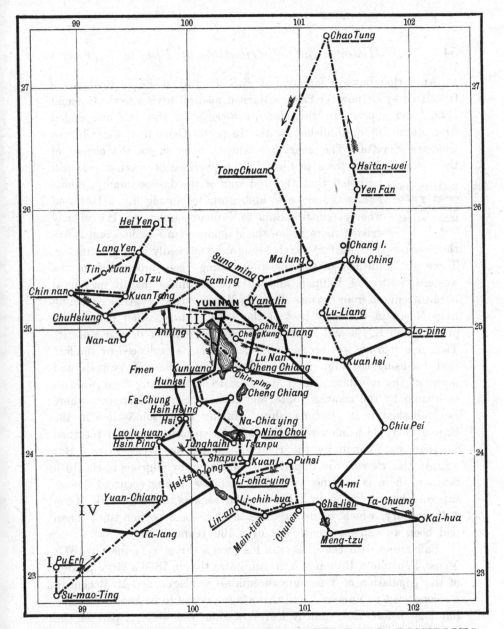

MAP OF YUNNAN FU AND SURROUNDING DISTRICTS.

Showing the Course pursued by the Plague, the Districts wherein it was most fatal
and those through which it merely passed, during 1871, 1872 and 1873.

EXPLANATION.

I   Starting point of the Plague in 1871 and 1872.

–·–·–·   Course pursued by the Epidemic in 1871 and 1872.

II   Place where its advance ceased in 1872.

III   Starting point in 1872 and 1873.

————   Course pursued by the Epidemic in 1872 and 1873.

IV   Place where its advance ceased in 1873.

————   Districts where the Epidemic was notably fatal.

--------   Districts merely visited by the Epidemic.

An earlier but similar account with chart by M. Émile Rocher was translated by Dr, now Sir Patrick Manson, medical adviser to the Colonial Office, and appears in the *Medical Reports* for the half-year ended 31st March, 1878, published by the Inspector-General of the Chinese Customs Service. The chart reproduced here shows the course of the epidemic from town to town in the province of Yunnan. It will be noted that the first sign of the disease in an epidemic form was a sickness and mortality among rats. How and when plague first came to Yunnan is unknown. It evidently existed there before the Mahommedan rebellion, and it was the conditions of warfare which brought it markedly into prominence. There are traditions of the infection having been imported from the western frontier of Yunnan, and M. Rocher thinks that it may have been introduced from Burma. Possibly Mahommedan pilgrims returning from Mecca in the early part of the 19th century, when plague was prevalent in Egypt and Arabia, may have introduced it into Yunnan. That this journey was occasionally undertaken is evidenced by the fact that Ma-hsing, the high priest of the Mahommedans of Yunnan, and leader of the rebellion, visited Mecca in 1839, travelling from Yunnan to Bhamo by the caravan route, and then by boat to Rangoon, where he embarked in a pilgrims' ship. Having spent some time in the Sacred City, Ma-hsing visited Egypt and Constantinople and returned in 1846 to Yunnan by the river of Canton or West River. But against this view of the importation of plague by pilgrims in the 19th century, there is evidence of a fatal sickness having occurred among rats and human beings in Yunnan, as far back as the last decade of the 18th century, which tends to indicate that some portion of Yunnan had been an endemic centre for over 100 years at least.

Epidemic preceded by sickness and mortality among rats.

Baker met with the disease in his travels through Yunnan in 1877. Monsr. Fenoullett, Bishop of Yunnan, states that in 1866 a large portion of the population of Yunnanfu succumbed to plague, and M. Rocher in a second visit to Yunnan found that plague began to be known in 1840, but long before that time it had existed in the western part of the province without prevailing epidemically. The following passage found in Hung Liang-Kih's *Peh-Kiang-Shi-Hwa*[1] bears witness to this, inasmuch as the author, who was born in 1736 and died in 1809, speaks of his contemporary as having died of the pest in Yunnan. " Shi Tau-Nan, the son of Shi Fan, now the Governor of Wang Kiang,

---

[1] *Nature*, Feb. 16, 1899. Note by Mr Kumagusu Minakata.

was notorious for his (poetic) gift and was only 36 years old when he died......Then in Chau-Chau (in Yunnan) it happened that in the daytime strange rats appeared in the houses, and lying down on the ground perished with blood-spitting. There was not a man escaped instantaneous death after being infected with the miasma. Tau-Nan composed thereon a poem entitled 'Death of Rats,' the masterpiece of his; and a few days after he himself died of this *queer rat epidemic.*"

The first medical account of plague in Southern China is given by **Dr Lowry of Pakhoi gives first medical account of plague in Southern China at Pakhoi.** Dr Lowry[1] of Pakhoi in 1882, the year he was first stationed there as Medical Officer to the Customs. His *Notes on an Epidemic Disease observed in Pakhoi in* 1882 are extremely valuable because of the very careful and accurate manner in which the disease is described, and because of the comparisons made between it and the plague of Yunnan and of Northern India. Dr Lowry also observed the mortality in rats which accompanies the disease.

He remarks that " in nearly every house where the disease broke out the rats had been coming out of their holes and dying on the floors." The disease was not new to Pakhoi, nor to Lienchow, a city about 12 miles distant. In 1871, Mr T. E. Cocker, a Deputy Commissioner of Customs at Hongkong, visited Pakhoi, and at the time of his visit there was a severe outbreak of the disease, accompanied by a mortality, not only among rats, but also among pigs and cattle. Mr Scott, Consul General of Canton, saw cases of plague in Pakhoi in 1879. It was then called the "Yunnan sickness" by the Chinese. Mr Netten Radcliffe, of the medical department of the Local Government Board of England, in his memorandum on the progress of Levantine plague in 1878 and 1879 records some important information regarding plague at Pakhoi derived from Surgeon A. R. Lynch's journal for H.M.S. *Mosquito* on the Chinese Station, 1879. It is accompanied by a map showing the presumed route taken by the plague from Pakhoi to Yunnan; and though the map is doubtless correct in showing the localities affected, it is incorrect as to the direction of the route by which the plague spread, which was originally from Yunnan to Pakhoi, and not from Pakhoi to Yunnan.

Dr Lowry states in his notes that "the epidemic which I have observed in this district does not seem to be an old disease, as it occurred for the first time about fifteen years ago, and since that time has occurred

[1] *Imperial Maritime Customs Medical Reports* for the half-year ended 30th September, 1882. 24th issue. 1883.

at certain intervals, the last severe outbreak being in 1877. I am told,
however, that a few cases occur every year, but my short
residence has not given me an opportunity of verifying
this statement." The plague first appeared in Pakhoi in
1867. It is to be noted that this was at a time when the
Mahommedan rebellion in Yunnan was in full force and troops raised in
Hainan and the Pakhoi district were engaged at the seat of war.

Plague first appeared at Pakhoi in 1867.

Pakhoi is not a large town nor an old one The population to-day is
about 20,000, and it dates back only to 1852, when some
Cantonese merchants settled there. It seems to have
thriven fairly well, for it was one of the treaty ports agreed
to be opened to foreign trade in 1860, though the actual opening did
not take place till some years later. Its principal and most direct
connection with Yunnan is to be seen on the map appended. The
route is long and difficult, partly by land and partly by water.

Trade route from Pakhoi to Yunnanfu.

From Pakhoi to Nanningfu the journey had to be accomplished
overland, from Nanningfu to Posé by the West River and from Posé to
Yunnanfu again overland. Cotton goods are the principal staple article
taken from the port of Pakhoi to Yunnanfu, and there they are
exchanged for tin and opium which are brought to the coast.

During the Mahommedan rebellion trade was much disturbed, and
under the peculiar conditions it is less likely that plague was imported
from Yunnan, by the ordinary limited intercourse of traders, into the
Pakhoi district and the island of Hainan, than by the movement of
Chinese troops, many of which, as previously stated, were drawn from
the island of Hainan and from the western prefectures of Kwangsi and
Kwantung close to Yunnan. No doubt there would be many traders
with the troops for the purpose of supply. This latter view of the
manner in which plague spread from Yunnan to Pakhoi appears to
be held by the Chinese, and it is more in accordance with that which is
known concerning the rapid spread of epidemics from one distant
locality to another, namely, that these epidemics of a sudden and rapid
growth are usually associated with large movements of population. An
epidemic of plague occurs in Yunnanfu in 1866, which decimates the
population while they are in the midst of war, and in 1867 Pakhoi,
one of the homes of returning troops from Yunnan, is attacked.

The distance between Yunnanfu and Pakhoi is about 3000 lis, and
it takes about 48 day stages to travel from one to another. What
intervening localities were attacked is unknown, but it is unlikely
they escaped.

Once the disease was established in Pakhoi it seems to have become
endemic for 18 years. There was a severe epidemic in
Plague endemic in Pakhoi from 1867 to 1884. 1877. Every year it recrudesced and prevailed more or
less from March to June until 1884, when from the reports
of the Medical Officer of the Customs it seems to have
ceased until re-infected in 1894. This spontaneous cessation of the
plague is a phenomenon which has not infrequently manifested itself in
small towns, occasionally in large cities, and rarely in commercial towns,
such as Smyrna and other busy entrepôts of trade in close communication
with infected centres.

Although Pakhoi seems to have enjoyed a freedom from plague for
10 years, from 1884 to 1894, the disease was far from being
Plague not extinct in adjoining prefecture to that of Pakhoi. extinct; it not only continued to prevail in the province of
Yunnan and at varying intervals in the neighbouring
towns of the Kweichow, Kwangsi, and Kwantung pro-
vinces, but it was also present in the adjoining prefectures to that
in which Pakhoi is situated. They are localities away from European
contact, and it is only incidentally that plague is discovered to prevail
in them. Distant from the coast ports, from the customs stations, or
from missionary outposts, news becomes exceedingly scanty, infrequent
and unreliable, and occurrences, however important or disastrous they
may be to the localities affected, come but rarely to the ears of
Europeans. It is certain that from 1890 a gradually extending area
of the western parts of Kwangsi and Kwantung was becoming affected
with plague.

Plague prevailed at Lungchow, Posé, Nanningfu and Taipingfu in
1890[1]. It again prevailed at Lungchow in 1893. As soldiers were the
first victims of the outbreak, Dr Simmonds, who was at Lungchow at the
time, was of opinion that the disease was imported into the garrison of
Lungchow from Liencheng, a frontier town on the borders of Yunnan.
There was another epidemic in Lungchow in 1894, which was evidently
a recrudescence of the outbreak of the previous year.

Plague occurred at Kaochao in 1891, and at Ampu, which is east of
Pakhoi, in 1891[2]. It was also prevalent at Mouiluk in 1890 and 1893.
Mouiluk is south of Kaochao and near the French possession of
Kwan-shan-wan. It is about 300 miles south-west of Canton.

[1] *Imperial Maritime Customs Medical Reports* for the year ended 31st March, 1890,
38th and 39th issues, 1894.

[2] *Imperial Maritime Customs Medical Reports* for the year ended 30th September,
1893. 45th and 46th issues, 1895.

If we now go back to the Yunnan province we shall find that as soon as the Customs opened a station at Mengtze, one of the principal towns in the south-east of the province, plague is immediately reported as epidemic there. It is the usual history of plague in China. Nothing

Plague at Mengtze, 1874–1893. is heard of it in a particular locality until that locality is visited by a European. The disease prevailed in Mengtze for many years prior to the advent of the Customs officers, but it was not discovered and described by a European medical man until 1894.

Mengtze is situated in the south-eastern part of Yunnan, in latitude 23° 34′ N., and longitude 103° 36′ E. Like most of the principal towns of Yunnan it is in the middle of a large plateau elevated 4500 feet above sea-level and surrounded by mountains rising from 6000 to 9000 feet above the sea-level. The town is the centre of a large traffic between Yunnan and the province of Kwangsi, as well as between Yunnan and Tonking.

The Imperial Chinese Customs opened a station at Mengtze in 1899, and the European officers on their arrival found plague prevailing. It had recurred every year in Mengtze since 1885, and first appeared there in 1874. There was a severe epidemic in 1892, but according to native reports the epidemic of 1893, which continued during the months of June, July and August, was, compared with previous epidemics, not particularly severe. Dr Michoud[1], in describing the epidemic, remarks that "however, out of an estimated population of 10,000 or 12,000 a thousand people died. Carried outside the dwellings, the victims of plague lay dead or dying unheeded in the streets or set in rows leaning against the city wall." Dr Michoud continues: "In some places whole families disappear. At the beginning of the last epidemic, we were called to the young son of the Chengtai (Chinese General) of Mengtze. The poor boy had just been given over by the native doctors, who, probably from fear of displeasing the father, would not declare the nature of the disease. As we were aware of a case of yang-tzu-ping having already occurred in the Chengtai's yamen—considering, too, the rapid evolution and extreme gravity of every symptom exhibited by the little patient—disregarding, at the same time, the hypothesis of heat-stroke or pernicious intermittent fever, we had no hesitation, in spite of the absence of any external adenitis (and to the great displeasure of the father), in diagnosing yang-tzu-ping. Although willing to do our best,

---

[1] *Imperial Maritime Customs Medical Reports* for the year ended 30th September, 1894, 47th and 48th issues, 1895.

we insisted on the probable failure of any treatment, and urged the necessity for immediate and energetic disinfection in order to ward off further diffusion of the disease. The boy died shortly afterwards. None of the measures advised were taken because the native quacks denied the accuracy of our diagnosis. Doubtless the failure of our treatment had discounted the value of our advice. However that may be, the Chengtai, an old warrior who had spent his whole life in Yunnan, and had passed unscathed through the previous epidemics which decimated the country, was, in a few days after the death of his son, attacked by yang-tzu-ping and speedily perished. Some of his wives, many of his relations and servants, were in succession attacked, all the cases ending fatally. The people that died from yang-tzu-ping in that yamen before the end of that epidemic numbered at least 25."

The epidemic described at Mengtze, following as it did a severe epidemic in 1892, occurred in May, June and July of 1893.

Plague at Nanningfu and Kwaium in 1893.

Two months later the disease is stated to be epidemic in Lungchow and in many towns of the Kwangsi province, such as Nanningfu and Kwaium, the latter of which is not more than 200 miles from Wuchowfu.

It is clear that plague was extensively diffused at that time. It was epidemic in Mengtze in 1893, and for several years previously. It was also epidemic in some of the south-western towns of Kwangsi, especially those situated on the West or Canton River, and it was more or less prevalent in the south-western districts of Kwantung.

Plague at Canton in 1894.

The existence of plague in these places excited no interest beyond the localities affected, and it was not until the disease reached the delta of the West River and attacked Canton, the capital of Kwantung, and an epidemic of exceptional proportions began to devastate the city in the spring of 1894, that the fact that plague in a dangerous form existed in China became generally known to the Europeans living in that country.

Canton is the chief port, as well as the largest and most important city in Southern China. It is the capital of the Kwantung province and contains a population variously estimated at 1½ to 2 millions. Situated in 23° of latitude N., and 113° 14′ longitude, on the banks of the Pearl River, it is some 70 miles from the coast, and in the centre of a district traversed and intersected with waterways, formed by the convergence of several rivers from the north, east, and west. By this network of waterways, Canton is connected with the chief

Canton connected with the chief towns and districts of Kwangsi and Kwantung.

towns and districts in Kwangsi and Kwantung. At the mouth of the Pearl River lies Macao on one side, and the colony of Hongkong on the other.

The inland water communications of Canton extend westward to the borders of Yunnan and Kweichow. The Sikiang or West River, or Canton River as it is sometimes called, is navigable for small steamers as far as Wuchowfu. From there to Nanningfu the passage is more difficult on account of some dangerous rapids, but native boats make it successfully, and ply between the two towns. From Nanningfu to Posé the river is suitable for light draught boats, which are busily engaged in carrying produce to and fro. Posé is on the borders of Yunnan, and the produce reaching it by boat is taken by pack animals overland to Mengtze.

West of Nanningfu a branch of the river leads to Taipingfu and Lungchow. It will be seen from the map that Mengtze and Lungchow, both infected centres of plague, are on the lines of direct communication with Canton. The West River is the natural and most convenient trade route for produce and traffic from Yunnan, Lungchow, and the greater portion of the Kwangsi province, but as previously stated, notwithstanding the advantages of this route, it used not to be favoured by Chinese merchants, who preferred to take their merchandise from Nanningfu overland to Pakhoi, rather than direct to Canton. The reason for this was partly because it was a shorter route to the coast, but mainly because of the numerous likin charges between Nanningfu and Canton, there being no fewer than sixteen likin stations. This was altered in 1891, and the system of traffic introduced, which resulted in a greater use of the West River for the conveyance of produce and passengers both to and from Canton.

Whether plague reached Canton from the infected towns and villages of the south-western part of Kwantung, or direct from Yunnan and Kwangsi by the West River, is unknown. Probably the infection arrived by both channels, but whichever was the first, the original source was Yunnan. Fatshan, a town situated on the delta of the West River and a few miles from Canton, is said to have been infected in 1893. It is the custom of the Chinese to send their dead to be buried in their native village or town, and the infection at Fatshan is attributed by them to bodies of persons who died of plague at Mengtze having been sent to Fatshan for burial in badly fitting coffins. The first cases in Fatshan occurred in families who were connected with Mengtze. It has already been noted that, both at Mengtze and Lungchow, plague occurred among the military stationed at each place, and it is a curious fact that the first case seen in Canton by a European physician was in the family of a soldier.

The first recorded case of plague in Canton[1] occurred on January 16th, 1894, when Dr Mary Niles was called in to see **Plague in Canton in January, 1894.** General Wong's daughter-in-law, who was reported to be suffering from a "boil," and who, when seen, was found to have a very painful swelling in the inguinal region, a temperature of 104·8° with a pulse of 160, and a petechial eruption. The patient recovered, but the bubo, owing to sinuses forming, took a very long time to heal. Out of seven cases seen by Dr Mary Niles up to May 2nd, in no fewer than four purpuric spots appeared before death. In a number of cases met with the illness was of a light character; for instance Dr Niles records a case in which "a lady came in a chair but walked into the office. She looked perfectly well, temperature, pulse and digestion normal. She said she had fever six days before, and the following day when taking a bath discovered a swelling in the inguinal region, of which she had not been previously aware, and which caused her no pain. I examined the bubo and saw for myself." This case is suggestive of other similarly mild cases, and the likelihood of these occurring at an early stage of the outbreak without attracting any special attention. Dr Niles further states: "It has been noticeable to the people that rats in infected houses have died. In the house where the child from the school was visiting when she took the disease thirteen dead rats were swept out one morning...One of the officials, I am told, offered 10 cash for every dead rat brought to him. He had collected 35,000 in one month; 2000 were brought to him in one day."

It was only towards the end of March of 1894 that the disease began to attract attention. Dr Alexander Rennie reports[2] that "a few stray cases occurred in the beginning of March, but it was not until the end of the month that attention was awakened on account of its fatal prevalence in a poor neighbourhood near the south gate of the city, and also in Nan-sheng-li, a quarter occupied by Mahommedans, among whom the mortality was very high. At this time the type of the disease was exceedingly severe—of those attacked quite 80 % dying. Towards the middle of April the cases we saw were of a milder type,

---

[1] Plague in Canton, by Mary Niles, M.D., *The China Missionary Journal*, June, 1894, p. 116.

[2] Report on the plague prevailing in Canton during the spring and summer of 1894, by Alexander Rennie, M.A., M.B., C.M., *Imperial Customs Maritime Report* for the year ended 30th September, 1894, 47th and 48th issues, 1895.

but the disease subsequently became more severe, and extended its boundaries to other parts of the city and also to Honam, the maximum mortality being reached about the middle of May...Rain fell copiously during the month of May and beginning of June, so that many streets were under water; the temperature remained comparatively low. But both these factors seemed to favour the propagation of the disease, as by the beginning of June it was rife in the western suburbs as well as in the surrounding towns and villages. It is impossible to give any correct estimate of the mortality, as no official records of burials are kept. Comparing the estimates obtained from various sources, we believe the mortality from the beginning of the epidemic to the middle of June (the date of writing) to have been about 40,000.

"Although a goodly number of well-to-do people fell victims to the pestilence, the chief sufferers were the poor, over-crowded and badly housed. The people who escaped the scourge in the most marked degree were those living in upper stories and the boating population. With the exception of those put in boats after falling sick, scarcely a case was noted on the river. Many well-to-do people, observing this immunity, removed from their houses and made their homes on the river. Judging from this circumstance, therefore, and also from the fact that rats living in the ground and drains were the first animals to fall victims, we infer that the specific poison emanated from the soil. What the specific poison may be is not determined, but no doubt the insanitary conditions referred to, exaggerated by a prolonged drought, provided a specially suitable nidus for its growth and dissemination.

" The immunity enjoyed by residents on the foreign settlement of Shamien is remarkable, seeing that it is separated only by a creek some 20 yards wide from houses where cases of plague occurred. Not only did foreigners living on the settlement enjoy excellent health, but no case of plague occurred among their servants living on the premises. The rats also, up to the time of writing, remain healthy and lively."

Dr Rennie further states in this report that on the outbreak of the disease occurring in Canton many persons, especially the well-to-do, removed to the country, thus forming fresh foci for its dissemination; and in the same way the outbreak in Hongkong no doubt arose from persons having migrated from Canton to Hongkong while actually suffering from the disease, or during the short incubation period.

Dr Mary Niles also states that " patients went home to the country in passage boats, some died in the boats, and others in their native towns."

Under such circumstances and from such a centre as Canton, which communicates with so many places, the infection was bound to be disseminated.

The largest and most important European possession near Canton is

Hongkong the largest and most important European possession near Canton. Hongkong, situated at a distance of only some 80 miles, with daily river communication with Canton both by steamers and junks. Hongkong, on account of its position at the mouth of the Pearl River, its population being mainly Cantonese, and the great and increasing traffic with Canton, has been suggestively called the suburb of Canton. The extent of intercourse between the two ports may be gathered from the fact that nearly half-a-million of people pass each way to and fro annually, and some 4000 river steamers and 8000 junks annually enter the port of Hongkong from the Canton and West River district, most of them coming from Canton and its neighbourhood.

Under such conditions it is not surprising that whatever affects

Plague discovered in Hongkong in May, 1894. Canton is not long in making itself felt at Hongkong. In 1902 when cholera broke out in Canton there was only an interval of a few weeks before the disease appeared in Hongkong. And so it was with plague in 1894. As soon as the disease was well established in epidemic form in Canton, it was discovered to be present in Hongkong.

Although there is no positive evidence of the first cases of plague coming from Canton, rather than from the other affected areas in its vicinity or from Pakhoi, yet as large numbers of the inhabitants in order to escape plague were fleeing from Canton to Hongkong, the probabilities are greatly in its favour, particularly so when the enormous ordinary traffic is taken into account, together with the circumstance that detection of sick people entering the colony is impossible, because there is no system of enquiry as to sickness, nor is there any inspection of passengers on steamers and junks from Canton or from the West River.

Dr Lowson, in his report on the epidemic of bubonic plague in Hongkong in 1894[1], is of opinion that the disease was imported from Canton rather than from Pakhoi, where it did not prevail until the latter part of the spring, and between which and Hongkong the traffic is insignificant compared with that between Hongkong and Canton. Once introduced into Hongkong, the disease caused the greatest alarm,

[1] The Epidemic of Bubonic Plague in Hongkong, 1894, *Medical Report*, by James A. Lowson, M.B., Medical Officer in charge of Epidemic Hospital, Hongkong, 1895.

but the epidemic, though severe, is not to be compared in intensity with that in Canton, even if the lowest estimate of 40,000 be accepted as the highest number of deaths. Many in Canton have estimated the deaths from plague in that city in 1894 to have been between 80,000 and 100,000. The deaths in Hongkong did not exceed 3000.

It was in the Hongkong epidemic of 1894 that the causal agent of plague, the plague bacillus, was discovered by Dr S.

The plague bacillus discovered in Hongkong by Dr S. Kitasato and later by Dr Yersin. Kitasato of Tokyo, on June 14th. Later Dr Yersin made independently a like discovery in Hongkong. The Hongkong epidemic began in May and ended in August, and its incidence was proportionately more severe on the female portion of the population than on the male. Macao did not suffer epidemically from the disease until April, May and June

Plague in Macao in April, 1895. of 1895. During the winter of 1894 and 1895 there prevailed a fatal epidemic which attacked the respiratory organs, and which was believed to be influenza. It is worth noting that this was at a time before the pneumonic type of plague was recognised as a variety of the disease. The first case of bubonic plague which came under the notice of the Portuguese authorities was an imported case from Hongkong, and to this source is ascribed the origin of the epidemic; but as the case came under the care of the sanitary authorities the next day after arrival, also as there was a high mortality among the Chinese with no means of ascertaining the exact cause of death, and as the epidemic quickly followed the introduction of this single case, which is an unusual occurrence with plague, whose progress at the beginning is generally slow, it is likely that Macao was infected earlier. The epidemic reached its acme in April and May, and disappeared in June, and returned in 1897 and 1898. From the position of Macao and its intercourse with Canton, Pakhoi, Hongkong, and the villages of the delta, it could only be a matter of time for it to be infected by people coming from one or all of these places.

With Canton, Hongkong, Macao and Pakhoi infected with plague,

Canton and Hongkong become centres of distribution of plague. it was not long before the disease became extensively diffused and the whole of the southern coast of China invaded. The accompanying map of Southern China shows the course of plague in its advance from Yunnan, and the distribution of the disease in this region up to the year 1902.

The two most important emporia of China are Canton and Hongkong, and every year but 1895 the disease has recurred in Hongkong and Canton.

Admirably situated for commerce, Canton and Hongkong are the great marts and distributing ports for the produce of Southern China; and Canton sends its merchandise down by the Canton River on large and small native craft to Hongkong, where it is stored in large warehouses until ships arrive to take it away in exchange for the cargoes they bring. Hongkong, though not more than sixty years old, possesses one of the busiest harbours in the world, and has trade connections, not only with the southern ports of China and the neighbouring islands of the Pacific and Chinese Seas, but also with India, Australia, Japan, and America.

It has already been stated that it was from Canton and the province of Kwantung that Hongkong became infected with plague in 1894, and from these sources it continues periodically to receive fresh infection. Plague since 1896 has also become endemic in Hongkong. A great commercial centre continually exposed to fresh infection, and in which plague is endemic, is apt to be dangerous to places with which it is in frequent communication, and it has thus happened that Hongkong, besides being a great distributor of merchandise, has become also an active centre for the distribution of plague. Sea-going ships have conveyed the infection over the seas to India, Australia, Japan and America, and coasting steamers have distributed it to adjacent ports. It has not always been possible to indicate the ship that conveyed the infection or the exact agent by which the infection was carried, whether by man, by animals, by infected clothing, or by infected merchandise; but it is possible to exclude the infection being conveyed in any other way to Japan, Australia, and America, and there is sufficient evidence to leave no doubt as to the infection being carried by shipping having commercial relations with infected ports in Southern China.

Hongkong is separated from most places by the sea, and the infection has not passed overland to China, but has followed the trade routes of the sea.

It is a very remarkable fact that plague has not spread very far inland in China, and that hitherto its chief ravages have been limited comparatively more or less to that portion of the country near the coast. The infection on land has followed chiefly the routes of busiest intercourse. There are no railways in Southern China, and the disease has made no extensive inroads into the interior of the country, except in those districts in which their waterways connect them with infected localities. In the case of the infected provinces of Kwangsi and Kwantung, and Fokien, a range of hills which forms a natural boundary between the north and the south, and which restricts commercial activity between them, also prevents plague from passing northwards. But apart from this natural obstruction it seems to be a characteristic of plague not to spread much beyond the towns and villages on the more frequented roads of trade.

The precise date and manner of the arrival of plague infection at
Plague at Bombay in 1896. Bombay are unknown. There is constant trade intercourse between Bombay and Hongkong, the ships of Hongkong taking the produce of Canton and the provinces of Southern China to Bombay, and the ships of Bombay taking the produce of Western India to Hongkong. The disease may have been introduced by some one infected among the crew of a steamer coming from Hongkong, or by infected rats, or possibly infected cargo. It has happened even as late as 1902 for plague to be imported from Bombay to Hongkong by these ships and for the disease not to be suspected by the captain, and it has also happened for plague-stricken rats to have been conveyed in this way from Bombay to Hongkong. But before plague broke out in Bombay in 1896 there was so little suspicion of the possibility of the disease being conveyed from Hongkong to Bombay direct before attacking intervening ports that no alarm was felt in this direction; nor did there seem grounds for that alertness essential for the discovery of first cases and the protection against importation. Bombay had not been attacked by plague for nearly 200 years, though the disease had prevailed in Gujarat, Cutch, Káthiáwár, Rajputana and Sind from 1812 to 1821, in Kumaon and Garhwal on the slopes of the Himalayas in 1823, 1834, 1847, 1876, 1884 and 1893, and in Marwar, Jodhpur, Rajputana and Pali in 1836 and 1837.

Bombay also remained free of the disease when it was epidemic in Mesopotamia as recently as 1891–92, which is a country much nearer to Bombay than China. With such an experience there was an inclination to think that Bombay was invulnerable to plague; besides, nearly everything concerning plague had been forgotten. By many it was considered an extinct disease so far as modern times were concerned, and at the most could only prevail to a limited extent among filthy and uncivilised people. Its diagnosis, its connection with rats, and its modes of extension needed all to be learnt afresh. Cholera was the epidemic disease of India, and the infection of plague, an unknown disease, was largely judged and measured by what was known of cholera. The possibility of plague infection being spread at times by merchandise and other agents, besides sick persons, was discarded as antiquated and obsolete. It was forgotten that plague itself was antiquated, and that our predecessors with much experience of the disease may have correctly observed many things connected with it. Plague had been absent from Bombay since 1702, or a period of 194 years. These long intervals seem peculiar to the epidemiology of plague. Between the epidemic in London in 1348 and that of 1499, a period of 150 years elapsed. An interval of 70 years occurred between the epidemic of 1720 and the previous great epidemic in Marseilles. Moscow was attacked in 1771, after a period of immunity of 150 years, and Malta when attacked in 1813 had been free from an epidemic of plague for 137 years.

Though it is now evident that plague must have existed as early as March, 1896, in Bombay, the first cases noticed appear to have occurred near the docks on the Port Trust Estates in the Mandvi district in August, 1896, among Moltanies who had dealings with China and among the Lohannas and Banias of the same district. The cases were mistaken for diphtheria and fever. At this time the mortality in the Mandvi district was unusually high, but it was attributed to remittent fever and lung affections. The rats were also dying in numbers, but no particular importance was attached to this phenomenon then. It was not until the 23rd of September, 1896, when Dr A. G. Viegas drew attention to the disease being probably plague, that public anxiety was aroused. The diagnosis of plague was bacteriologically confirmed by W. Haffkine, the Government Bacteriologist, on October 13th. After the first alarm there was a reaction and opinions fluctuated from day to day as to the nature of the disease, now being pessimistic and now optimistic, according to the number of deaths. The majority of citizens were, however, disinclined to believe in the possibility of plague. The mildness of the disease and its slow progress led to its being called glandular fever, or bilious fever, or indeed anything but plague. Haffkine's report, however, dispelled illusions, at least on the part of the thinking public.

Commencement characterised by mildness and slow extension.

For the first month or so after the discovery it was more or less limited to the Mandvi district, and then it commenced to spread. Rats were noticed to be dying in other quarters of the town than the Mandvi district, and wherever this happened cases of plague began to appear. The Health Department set vigorously to work to cleanse and disinfect the infected areas and houses, and to segregate the sick. But the population to be dealt with was a peculiar one. Oriental in its thoughts and habits, superstitious and fanatical, it was particularly sensitive and antagonistic to innovation of any kind. It was used to small and short-lived epidemics of cholera, and knew the measures taken for that disease, and it was persuaded that plague, if it existed, would be equally short-lived.　At first the preventive measures were

Opposition to the adoption of preventive measures.

endured with grumblings, but as the disease continued, and began to look more serious, the policy adopted, western in its conception, suited neither Hindú nor Mahommedan. Hostility and ill-feeling were soon apparent.　People did not and would not understand that the disease was infectious.　One medical man, convinced of the non-infectious nature of the disease, insisted on sleeping in the ward with his patients, and died of plague. Every sanitary measure was opposed.　Denunciations and protests were soon followed by active demonstrations of ill-feeling by stoning of the officers engaged in plague work, attacking of the ambulances, and even storming of the plague hospital　To such a pitch of excitement were the rougher classes of the population aroused, that there were good grounds for fearing a riot and, worse than a riot, there were threatenings of an exodus of the whole conservancy staff and of the dock and mill hands, and possibly of the police themselves.　To allay this state of feeling the notification authorising compulsory removal to hospital was withdrawn three weeks after its first appearance.　This was on the 30th of October.　The difficulties which beset the local authority in its endeavour to stay the progress of the disease were not removed by this concession.　Popular feeling, moved by wild rumours, the offspring of an excited imagination, or evil design, or ignorance, was swayed first in one direction, then in another, but never in sympathy with, or in support of, the sanitary measures devised to check the disease.　And so the plague continued to spread.　The people had lost confidence in medical treatment.　It was not a question of notification of the sick by medical men, but of finding out the sick and dead, and cleansing and disinfecting the house.　The disease spread remarkably slowly, considering the conditions which it met with.

During October and November, the disease seemed to be stationary

Progress of the disease associated with the migration of rats.

as regards the number of deaths recorded, but there was an ominous circumstance; it was infecting new districts, and it was observed as a curious phenomenon that the progression of the disease was intimately associated with the migration of rats.　It was not the localities to which people were fleeing from infected districts that were showing grave infection, but those to which the rats were migrating.　Suddenly, in the beginning of December, the mortality from plague and from general causes rose to twice the height it had attained before. Then the epidemic began in earnest, the mortality rising week by week until the 2nd and 3rd week in February. By this time the crisis was reached, and there was a gradual but fluctuating fall in the weekly mortality from general causes and from plague, until the last week in May, when it descended to the same level as in October and November. Once the epidemic set in, panic seized the inhabitants, and there was a general exodus from Bombay. Homes and shops were closed, and the inhabitants sought safety in flight. Rumour exaggerated the ravages committed by the plague, and it was only when nearly half the population had fled from the city, and the deaths from plague showed marked signs of declining, that the panic began to subside. To this exodus is to be chiefly ascribed the infection of localities outside Bombay.

Height of the first Bombay epidemic in Feb. 1897.

In consequence of the spread of plague beyond the city the Government of Bombay took over the control of plague operation early in March, not only for the city but for the whole Presidency.

Plague committees were formed for every large centre where plague existed. Hospitals were erected, health camps established, and search parties constituted. With this organisation a vigorous policy of segregation of the sick, and removal of the healthy from infected houses and areas to health camps, was carried out. It is difficult to gauge the value of these measures, for they were introduced into Bombay after the crisis was reached and the epidemic was already waning. But, like the preventive measures carried out by the municipality, there can be no doubt that they contributed in no small degree in limiting the ravages of the epidemic. In May and June the disease was distinctly of a milder type, and hopes were entertained that not only the worst period had passed but also that the city of Bombay would soon be free. These hopes were not to be realised, for since its first appearance in 1896 plague has never left Bombay. Every year there have been recrudescences, reaching epidemic proportions in January, February, March and April.

Plague soon began to spread beyond Bombay, both by land and by sea. Poona was affected in December, Karachee in the same month, and as distant parts as Suhkur on the Indus not long after. The infection was carried even as far as Calcutta, where in one quarter occupied by Bombay merchants the rats began to die, and there were a few cases of plague, but the stringent measures there taken, especially against the rats in the infected area, were successful in preventing the disease gaining a lodgement in 1896, and it was not until April,

Extension of the disease to the Bombay Presidency and to other provinces in India.

1898, that plague gained a firm hold in Calcutta, apparently by fresh introduction of infection.

Besides these important centres the malady spread to the adjacent districts of the Bombay Presidency and its Native States, where it prevailed from January to June, causing a large mortality. Each new centre of infection in turn gave rise to others, so that in the middle of 1897, although owing to the decline of the epidemic at that period the deaths from plague were comparatively few, yet there were many centres where the disease had acquired a firm hold.

The maps taken from an account of plague administration in the Bombay Presidency from September 1896 to May 1897, by M. E. Couchman, I.C.S., show the diffusion and spread of the disease from Bombay along the coasts and along the lines of railway and traffic in the interior of the Presidency. It will be observed how many places were infected by June. These localities, in the next epidemic of 1897–98, acted as fresh centres from which more places were infected.

The diffusion of the disease was slow and by no means corre-
Slow diffusion   sponded locally with the flight from Bombay; often long
of the plague.   intervals elapsed between the first recognised imported
case and the first indigenous case, and in many localities imported cases were not followed by indigenous cases, and when indigenous cases occurred some considerable time usually intervened before they assumed epidemic proportions. This slow diffusion is one of the most constant characteristics of plague. The Great Plague of London took six months to travel from St Giles' to Stepney. In 1830 plague existed eight months at Alexandria before passing to Damietta and Mansurah, though traffic was quite uninterrupted. In Bombay the plague remained confined to the dock quarters for a considerable time before it spread to other districts. At Poona over six months elapsed before the disease established itself at Kirkee which was in daily communication with Poona, and only separated from it by a river spanned by a bridge. By September and October of 1897 there was a general rise in plague prevalence in the Bombay Presidency. The southern portion of the Presidency, which had remained more or less free during the first epidemic, became extensively infected, and by June, 1898, the deaths in the second epidemic were double those of the first. 61,000[1] deaths from plague were recorded against 29,000 in the first period. The second epidemic was not only twice as severe as the

---

[1] "The Bombay Plague, being a history of the progress of the Plague in the Bombay Presidency from September 1896 to June 1899." Compiled under the orders of Government, by Capt. J. K. Condon, 1900, Bombay.

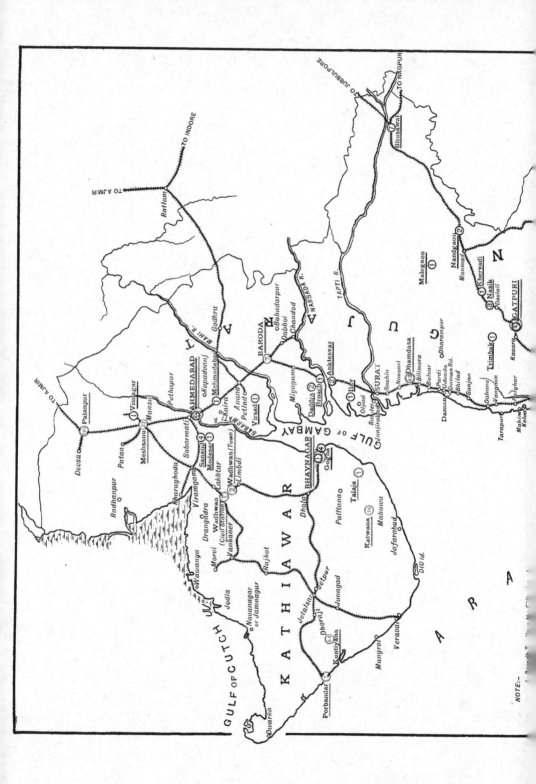

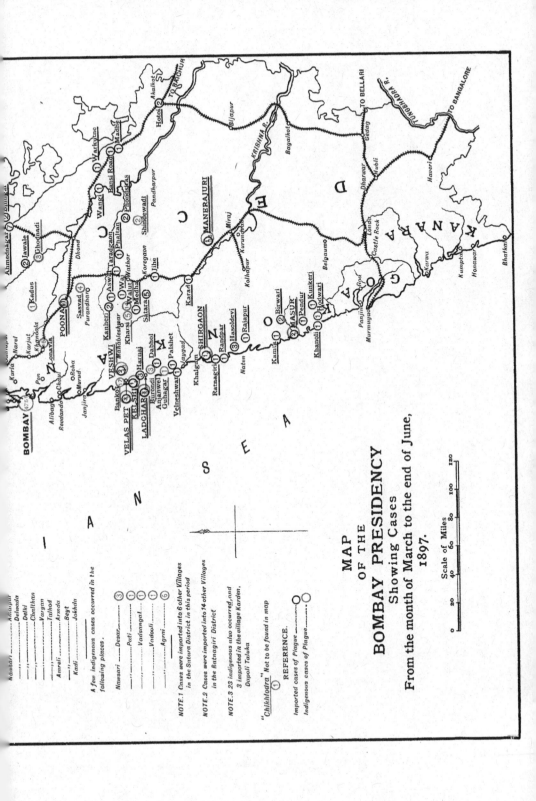

MAP
OF THE
BOMBAY PRESIDENCY
Showing Cases
From the month of March to the end of June,
1897.

Scale of Miles

REFERENCE.

Imported cases of Plague
Indigenous cases of Plague

"Chikhlodra" Not to be found in map

NOTE. 1 Cases were imported into 6 other Villages
in the Satara District in this period

NOTE. 2 Cases were imported into 14 other Villages
in the Ratnagiri District

NOTE. 3 23 indigenous also occurred, and
3 imported in the village Karden.
Dapoli Taluka

A few indigenous cases occurred in the
following places.

Nausari .... Desar
,, ... Pati
,, ... Vadsangal
,, ... Vadaoli
,, ... Agrai

Nausari .... Anhalpur
,, ... Delwada
,, ... Delhi
,, ... Chatlbav
,, ... Vargan
,, ... Talhod
Amreli .... Armda
,, ... Beyt
Kadi .... Jokhda

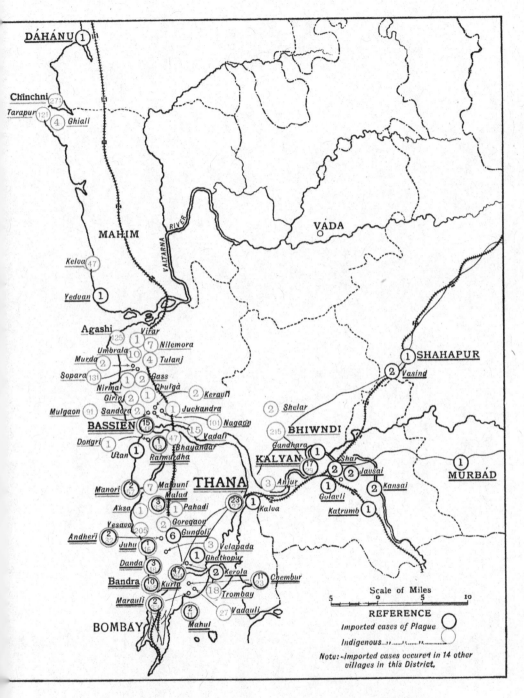

DÁHÁNU ①

Chínchni ㉛
Tarapur ⑫① ④ *Ghiali*

MAHIM

VÁDA

Kelva ㊼

Yedvan ①

Agashi *Vifar*
⑫ ① ⑦ *Nilemora*
Umbrala ⑩
Murda ② ④ *Tulanj*
Sopara ⑬① ① ② *Gass*
Nirmal *Chulga*
Girini ② ① ② *Keravli*
Mulgaon ⑨ *Sandora* ② ① *Juchandra*
BASSIEN ⑮ ⑩① *Nagaon*
⑮ *Vadali*
Dongri ① ① ㊼ *Bhayandar*
Utan ① *Raimurdha* KALYAN
Gandhara
②① SHAHAPUR
② *Vasind*

② *Shelar*
㉑⑤ BHIWNDI

Manori ② ⑦ *Matauni*
㊼ *Malad*
Aksa ① ③① *Pahadi*
Yesava ⑳⑤ ② *Goregaon*
Andheri ② ⑥ *Gundoli*
Juhu ③ *Velapada*
Danda ③ ① *Ghatkopur*
Bandra ⑩ ④ *Kurla* ② *Kerola*
Marauli ② ⑱ *Trombay*
② ㉗ *Vadauli*
BOMBAY *Mahul*

THANA
② ③ *Anjur*
㉓ ① *Kalva*

① *Shar*
⑰ ② ② *Javsai*
① ② *Kansai*
Golavli
Katrumb ①

① MURBÁD

Scale of Miles
5   0   5   10

REFERENCE
Imported cases of Plague   ◯
Indigenous...,,.....,,.....,,.   ◯
Note:- imported cases occured in 14 other
villages in this District.

MAP OF THANA COLLECTORATE IN BOMBAY PRESIDENCY.

Plague cases from month of March to end of June, 1897.

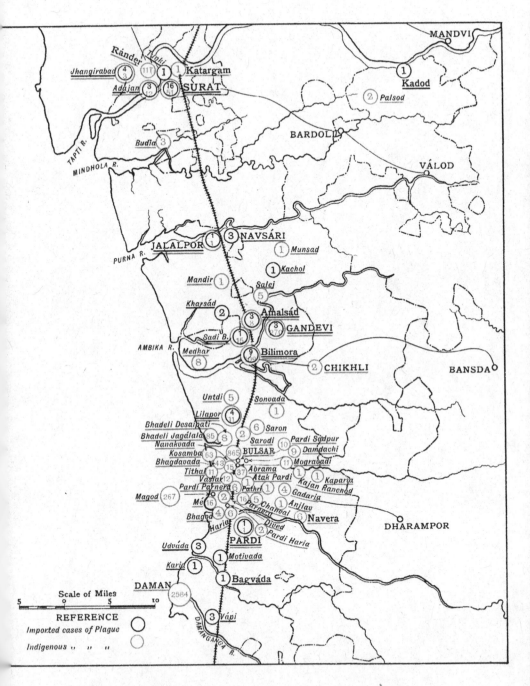

MAP OF SURAT COLLECTORATE IN BOMBAY PRESIDENCY.
Plague cases from month of March to end of June, 1897.

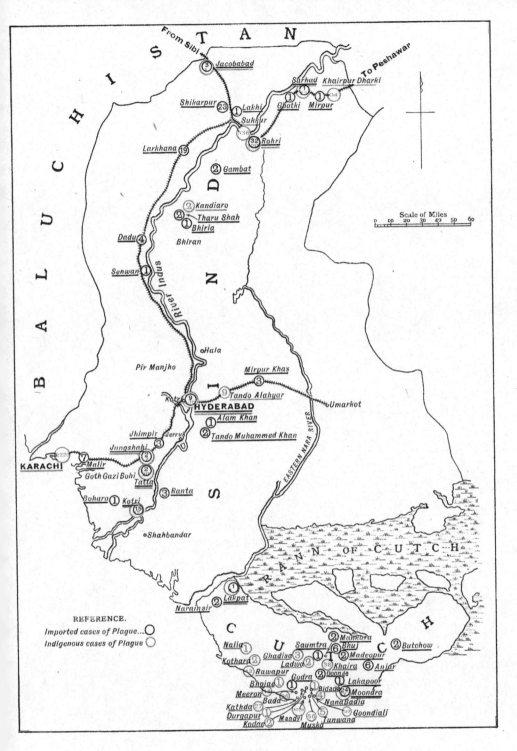

MAP OF SIND IN BOMBAY PRESIDENCY.

Plague cases from month of March to end of June, 1897.

first, but it also established a wider area of infection. In the third
epidemic ending June, 1899, the deaths reached over 115,000. In the
district of Dharwar alone there were in the course of eight
months 30,000 deaths from plague. In the same year
Poona suffered from its third epidemic, which was the
most severe of all. In the course of four months, during
June, July, August and September, it lost nearly 10,000 of its inhabitants, although half its population fled panic-stricken from the city
at the commencement of the epidemic. The normal population of Poona
was 61,000. For a period of over six weeks it lost over 1000 persons
a week from plague. The greatness of the mortality may be gathered
from the fact that if a similar mortality had prevailed in London, the
metropolis would have lost over 10,000 persons a day.

Severity of epidemics at Dharwar and Poona.

Fugitives from Bombay and the Bombay Presidency were not long
in carrying infection to the other provinces of India, and
this notwithstanding certain precautionary measures of
inspection taken on the railways. The development of
the disease in these new localities was slow, and at first
it appeared as if the disease were quite within control, but gradually,
in spite of every endeavour to stay its progress, it has spread throughout the Indian Peninsula, affecting some places but lightly, inflicting
terrible ravages in others, and leaving many untouched.

Extension of the plague to other Presidencies.

The progress of the plague in India has been slow. During the
first three years, as pointed out by the Indian Plague Commission, the
disease was not able to extend and take a hold of the country in such
a way as seriously to affect the ordinary death rate. The Commission
dealing with that period conclude that "[1]although the figures of plague
mortality when taken by themselves are high, it is evident that plague
has not as yet been able to make itself felt as one of the most important
factors that influence the total mortality of India." It is evident that
this stage is past, and that the plague is now a very important factor in
the Indian mortality.

Each year the area of its activity widens; each recurring epidemic
seizes on new districts besides maintaining its hold on the
old, and now at the end of eight years the annual mortality
from plague in India has risen from less than 30,000 in the
first year of its prevalence to little less than a million
per annum in 1903. This represents nearly one-sixth of
the annual mortality of India.

Gradually increasing mortality from the plague in India

[1] *Report of the Indian Plague Commission*, Vol. v. chap. ii. p. 50.

Reported Deaths from Plague in India.

Year	Bombay Presidency	Bengal	Madras	Punjab	United Provinces	Central Provinces	Mysore	Rajputana	Hyderabad	Central India	Other Provinces	Europeans	Grand Total
Sept. 1896 to end of 1897	57,943	—	—	—	—	—	—	·—	—	—	—	22	57,965
Total for 1898	104,881	166	496	1,871	116	103	6,382	118	3,945	—	9	16	118,103
Total for 1899	117,176	3,288	1,817	253	6	522	6,629	23	4,359	—	15	14	134,102
Total for 1900	38,345	37,265	667	525	116	595	13,268	10	805	—	24	7	91,627
Total for 1901	158,080	78,629	3,035	18,877	9,778	9	11,936	191	95	—	1,858	8	282,496
Total for 1902	217,910	32,270	12,343	221,767	41,509	458	28,316	101	8,729	204	10,886	12	574,493
Total for 1903	353,504	65,654	12,250	210,188	77,966	41,201	22,088	2,350	26,901	30,095	11,376	—	853,573
January to end of April 1904	116,420	51,136	9,743	199,999	102,643	31,695	6,598	10,559	13,350	15,994	4,994	2	563,133

Number of Deaths.

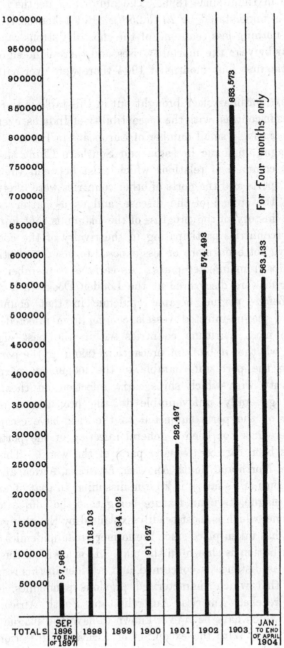

TOTALS | SEP. 1896 TO END OF 1897: 57,965 | 1898: 118,103 | 1899: 134,102 | 1900: 91,627 | 1901: 282,497 | 1902: 574,493 | 1903: 863,573 | JAN. TO END OF APRIL 1904: 563,133 (For Four months only)

The preceding tabular statement gives the annual recorded deaths from plague in India since 1896. The number of deaths is large, but probably it is understated by 20 to 25 %. But taken as it stands the mortality is nothing less than one of the most disastrous calamities for India. Year by year the mortality rises and there is no sign of abatement. In the first four months of 1904 there were over half a million deaths.

A very extraordinary fact brought out in this table is the immunity of Europeans in contrast with the susceptibility of Indians, even allowing for the comparatively small number of Europeans in India.

With plague epidemic in India and Southern China the intimate commercial relations which exist between their infected ports and the ports of other countries were likely to favour the spread of the disease, and as a matter of fact the history of the progress of the plague is that few maritime countries participating in the rivalry of the commerce of the East have not been more or less exposed to plague infection by the arrival of ships from infected ports. As early as September, 1896, two cases of plague were discovered at the London Docks in a vessel that left India before plague became epidemic in that country. This experience of plague-infected vessels coming from infected ports has happened to most maritime countries within the past eight years. Fortunately, whether it be from precautions taken at the port, or from conditions in the port unfavourable to the lodgement of plague, or from the rarity with which ships carry infection on them, or from ships being generally unfavourable to the propagation of plague, the majority of the ports subjected to the risk have escaped. But although there has not been a general infection of the ports, yet the infection has been carried to many parts of the world. They include ports in Asia, North and South America, Australia, Africa, and Europe. It is a distribution, as far as is known, dissimilar to that of any former epidemic of plague, its main feature being that the course followed is a maritime one, which is most readily explained by the change in trade routes which has taken place since the former great epidemics of plague.

The distribution is shown on the map. It is a wide diffusion so far as distance is concerned, and is wider in this respect than that which characterised previous pandemics, for it has reached America, Australia, and South Africa, none of which have been ever known to have had plague imported into them before. With the exception of Africa, the infection appears

Extension of the plague from India and China to other parts of the world.

Distribution of plague in different parts of the world.

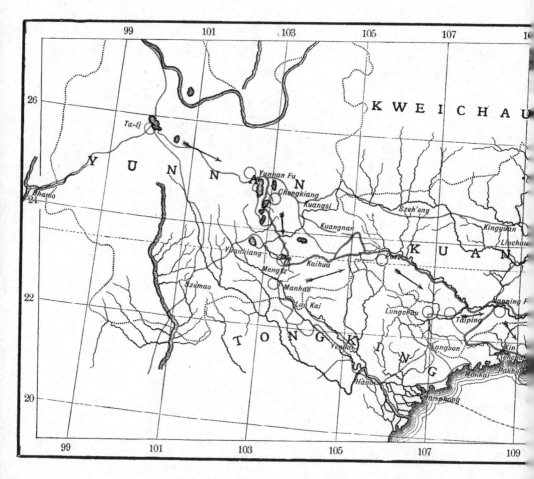

COURSE AND DISTRIBUTION OF PLAGUE

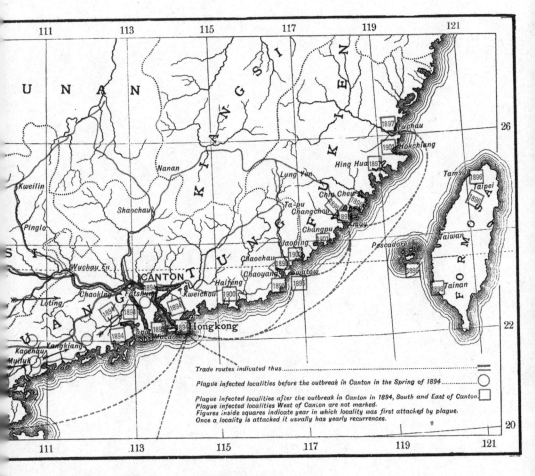

SOUTHERN CHINA BEFORE AND AFTER 1894.

Trade routes indicated thus ....

Plague infected localities before the outbreak in Canton in the Spring of 1894....................

Plague infected localities after the outbreak in Canton in 1894, South and East of Canton.
Plague infected localities West of Canton are not marked.
Figures inside squares indicate year in which locality was first attacked by plague.
Once a locality is attacked it usually has yearly recurrences.

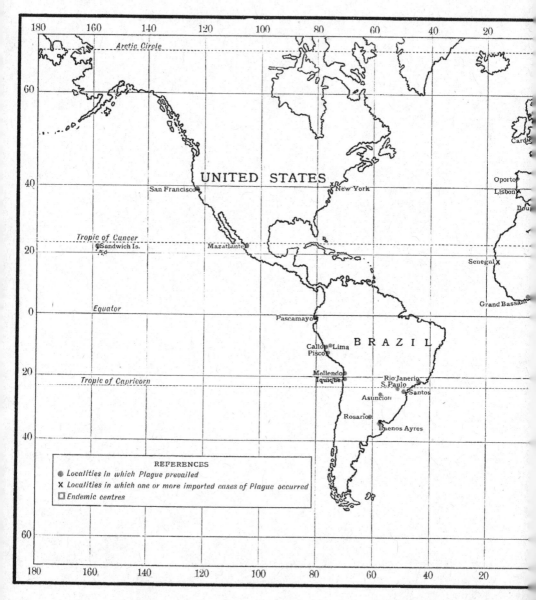

DISTRIBUTION OF PLAGUE

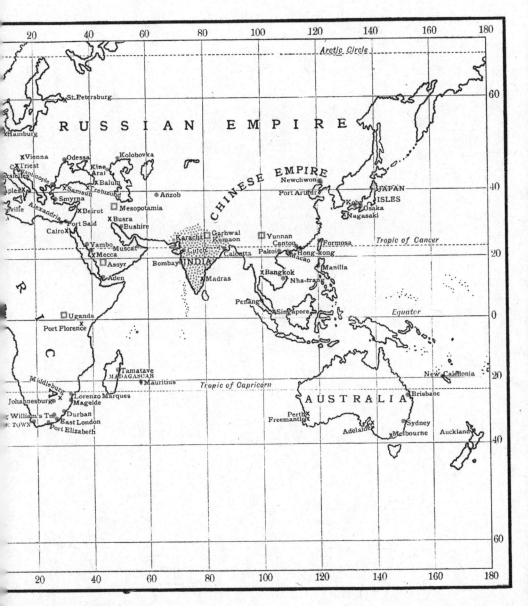

Arctic Circle

St.Petersburg

60

R U S S I A N   E M P I R E

Hamburg

×Vienna   ×Odessa   Kolobovka
C×Triest   Kine
stantinople   Arai
ples×   ×Balum
×Samsun   ×Trebizond   Newchwong   40
Smyrna   Port Arthur   JAPAN
eville   Alexandria   ×Beirut   Mesopotamia   Kobe   ISLES
×Busra   Osaka
Cairo×   Port Said   Bushire   ×Nagasaki
×Yambo   Karachi   Garhwal   Yunnan   Formosa   Tropic of Cancer
×Mecca   Muscat   Kumaon   Canton   20
Assyr   Cutch   Calcutta   Pakoi   Hong-kong
×Aden   Bombay   INDIA   Macao
Madras   ×Bangkok   Manilla
Nha-trang
Penang   Equator
Uganda
×Port Florence   ×Singapore   0

C

Tamatave   New Caledonia
MADAGASCAR   20
Middleburg   ×Mauritius   Tropic of Capricorn
Johannesburg   ×Lorenzo Marques   AUSTRALIA   Brisbane
Mageide   Perth×
William's Tm   ×Durban   Freemantle×
E TOWN   East London   ×Sydney
Port Elizabeth   Adelaide×   Auckland
×Melbourne
40

60

ROM 1894 TO END OF 1904.

mainly to limit itself to the ports, or to localities near these. It is also to be noticed that, notwithstanding the extensive sowing of the seed or germ of plague which has taken place, there has hitherto been no disposition for the disease to become severely epidemic except in India, China, the Mauritius, and in the year 1900 in Cape Town. How long this fortunate condition of affairs will continue it is impossible to say. Plague is slow in its progress and development, and evidently has difficulty in adapting itself to new conditions; it remains not infrequently for years in a more or less quiescent state, and then bursts out in a destructive and expanding epidemic. While, therefore, the ports of a country are infected or liable to infection from communication with infected ports, that country is never free from the danger of suffering from a plague epidemic which may assume large proportions.

A point of great interest in regard to the distribution of plague is

An endemic centre in Uganda.

the discovery in 1897 of an independent plague focus in the district of Kissiba, to the extreme north-west of German East Africa. Enquiries seem to point to the fact that plague has been endemic in Uganda for many years, and that, for the last 30 or 40 years, it has prevailed in sporadic or epidemic form in the provinces of Buddu, Koki, and Nkole. It appears that about 1889, at the time of a severe epidemic of plague in Buddu and Koki, the disease was introduced into the district of Kissiba, where it spread rapidly, and where in 1897 it was definitely proved by Dr Zupitza and Professor Koch to be plague.

PART II.

EPIDEMIOLOGY OF PLAGUE.

CHAPTER IV.

NATURE OF INFECTION.

THE nature of the infection is no longer a matter of surmise. The discovery of the plague bacillus with its well-marked characteristics and powers of inducing the disease in some of the lower animals, especially rodents, when inoculated into them, has put an end to the speculations as to the nature of the virus.

Pestiferous emanations from the soil contaminating the atmosphere **Earlier views** have always been a favourite explanation of the source of **on the nature** the plague virus, the nature of which has been looked upon **of infection.** as consisting of some venomous vapour or gas. Boghurst in his Loimographica on the Plague of London of 1665 records the general opinion, not only of his contemporaries but also of the medical men of many previous centuries, when he says: "My opinion falls in wholly with those who make the earth the seminary and seed plotts of these venomous vapours and pestiferous effluvia which vitiate and corrupt the air and consequently induce the pestilence[1]."

This opinion was not, however, held by all. There was another school which suspected that the infective agent of plague was a living entity and that it was conveyed from person to person by contagion. Athanasius Kircher is an exponent of this view. In 1658 he writes[2]:

---

[1] *Transactions of the Epidemiological Society of London*, Vol. XIII. 1893–94. "Loimographica. An account of the Great Plague of London in the year 1665 by William Boghurst, Apothecary." Edited by Joseph Frank Payne, M.D.

[2] Athanasii Kircheri, E. S. J., *Scrutinium Physico-Medicum Contagiosae Luis, quae Pestis dicitur*. Rome. 1658.

" Plague is in most cases a living being ; for the sick man harassed by pestiferous virulence soon contracts a marvellous putrefaction which we have shown to be most apt to create worms. Now these worms, propagators of the plague, are so small, so light, so subtile, that they elude any grasp of perception and can only be seen under the most powerful microscope. You might call them atoms, but they spring up in such numbers that they cannot be counted ; these worms when they have been conceived and generated from the putrefaction are easily forced out through all the passages and pores of the body, and since they are moved by the slightest movement of the air, just like so many sunbeams, are diffused here and everywhere in such a way that whatsoever they run across, they at once adhere to most tenaciously, insinuating themselves deeply right down to the bottom of the pores...Now all things are liable to catch this pestiferous brood, linen, cloths, clothes, skins, carpets, feathers, bedsteads, ottomans, tables, articles of every sort even to spoons, knives, table-tops, cups, belts, &c. For when this outburst of worms or worm sprouting, even at the smallest breath of air (which can happen either while the sick man upon his bed tossing himself now on this side and now on that, throws the clothes and coverlets now here now there; or while the nurses attending on the sick man make the bed and arrange its coverings that have been cast off, or place, or raise, or turn in any way the patient for the requirements of nature or the working of the medicine), get blown abroad, and a virulent brood just like atoms or particles moved by a breath of wind diffuses itself like smoke in all directions, it needs must be that all things are infected to which it adheres."

On this or a somewhat similar hypothesis did the contagionists explain the infectiveness of plague until the Hongkong epidemic of 1894, when Kitasato and Yersin discovered in the buboes and in the blood of plague patients the bacillus of plague. After reading Kircher's description one is left in doubt as to whether he and the physicians of his time did not actually see the plague microbe. If we except the exaggerated facility with which the worms he speaks of as being visible under the most powerful microscope leave the body and diffuse themselves in the air, the notions as to the nature of the infection and its portability are not unlike those of the present day.

In 1894, on the outbreak of plague at Hongkong, a Japanese commission of which Dr Kitasato was the Chief was despatched to Hongkong and in a short time the discovery was made that in the blood, internal organs, and affected glands of the body a micro-organism was to be

found in all cases of plague.   Later Dr Yersin independently made a
like discovery.   The bacillus thus associated with plague
has been proved to be the causal agent of the disease.
It is always found in the buboes and affected glands of
well-marked cases of plague, in the blood and tissues of
the septicaemic variety of plague, and in the lungs and
sputum of pneumonic plague, and this is the case wherever
plague occurs, whether in China, India, Africa, Australia, America or
Europe.   Moreover if the bacillus is isolated from a plague case and a
pure culture grown on ordinary nutrient media, the disease can be
produced in some of the lower animals which are susceptible, by inoculation, and from the tissues of these animals the microbe can be again
recovered in pure cultures.   Even more convincing than this experimental
evidence is the accidental production of the disease in man in some of the
bacteriological laboratories of Europe where no plague existed other
than that artificially produced in animals in the laboratory by inoculation
with cultures of the plague microbe.   These cultures were in every case
descendants through many generations of cultures of original microbes
obtained from plague cases in India or elsewhere, and brought in culture
tubes to the locality in which the outbreak occurred.   There has never
been any doubt as to the plague in the laboratories being caused from
any other source than the cultures, and the cases have occurred when
no plague existed in Europe.

Discovery of the plague bacillus and the evidence as to its causal relationship.

There have unfortunately been three occurrences of this kind.   The
first was that which happened in Vienna when in October, 1898, more
than a year after the return of the Austrian Plague Commission from
Bombay, the attendant of the Pathological Institution in Vienna, who
was acting as assistant to Albrecht and Ghon and had charge of the
animals experimented on, fell ill with pneumonia which proved on
examination of the sputum to be plague pneumonia.   He died on the
fourth day of illness from well-marked plague.   Dr Mueller and two
nurses who attended the patient were also attacked with pneumonic
plague.   One nurse recovered, but Dr Mueller died on the third day of
illness and the nurse a day or two later.   Prompt measures were taken
to prevent the disease from spreading and no other case occurred in
Vienna then or since.

The second occurred in June, 1903, when Dr Milner Sachs, who was
studying bacteriology in Berlin, infected himself while injecting a rat
with a culture of the bacillus of plague.   He contracted plague, it is
thought, by inhaling particles which were ejected from the syringe in

a spray. He suffered from the pneumonic form. He fell ill on June 2nd and died on June 5th, although he received injections of Roux Yersin's serum. A hospital attendant Marggraf who nursed Dr Sachs was also attacked with pneumonic plague, but he was treated energetically with Yersin's serum at an early stage of his illness and recovered. The precautions taken to prevent spread of the disease were successful. They consisted in isolation of the patients and of those who had come in contact with them, and burning the personal effects and any suspected furniture and goods.

The third accident was in January, 1904, which resulted in the death of the Director of the Laboratory of the Imperial Institute of Experimental Medicine at St Petersburg, who contracted plague whilst engaged in experiments with plague cultures. Two others in the laboratory also contracted plague and died from the same cause. All were treated with plague serum, but without success.

It is curious that all the cases of plague contracted in the laboratory and when dealing with animals have been of the pneumonic type.

The specificity of the plague bacillus is still further evidenced by the appearance of specific protective substances in the blood of individuals convalescent from plague and in the production of these specific protectives in the blood of experimental animals treated with plague bacilli, also by the protection afforded by inoculation with killed plague bacilli against a later natural infection.

Much was done in studying the morphological and cultural characteristics of the plague bacillus and in investigating the behaviour of the micro-organism under known conditions, before the full evidence was obtained which established that the bacillus was the causal agent of the disease. It will now be necessary to enter into the results of these researches. The plague bacillus belongs to the same cocco-bacillus group of Haemorrhagic Septicaemias, such as chicken cholera and rabbit septicaemia, all of which at some period of their existence show when stained a bipolar appearance. The typical plague bacillus is a short thick rod rounded at its extremities and more or less ovoid in form. It measures from ·8 mm. to 2 mm. in length and is usually from ·4 mm. to ·8 mm. in breadth. It is more constant in breadth than in length, though it varies in breadth more than other bacilli. It varies considerably in shape and size, so that in a microscopical specimen, in addition to the typical bacilli, very diverse forms may be seen, including long and slender bacilli together with boat-shaped, dumb-

Morphological and staining characteristics of the plague bacillus.

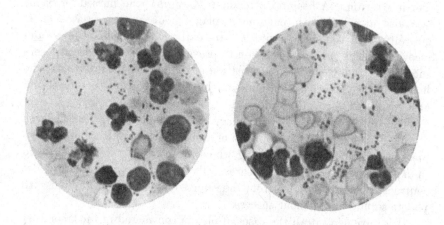

Plague bacilli in contents of Bubo.

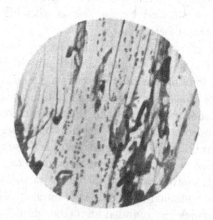

Plague bacilli in Sputum.

bell and spherical micro-organisms resembling cocci and diplococci in their appearance.

This pleomorphism may give rise to difficulty of recognition when plague appears in a locality for the first time and when the decision of the disease has to rest on a single case. Cultures however will solve the difficulty if the stalactite test be applied. For a time the variation in form was mistaken for contaminations and attributed to the presence of bacilli unconnected with plague.

The bacillus is non-motile, the only motion being Brownian and not that of translation; one or two terminal flagella have been observed and described, but they have been seen only by a few. No spores have hitherto been discovered.

The bacillus is easily stained by aqueous solutions of methyl blue, gentian violet, fuchsin, or any of the ordinary basic dyes, but is not stained by Gram's method unless a weakened spirit solution of 50 % is used instead of absolute alcohol for the decoloration process. The bacillus is stained usually more deeply at the extremities than at the centre and thereby acquires a very characteristic bipolar staining. This bipolar staining is more marked in microbes taken from the tissues direct than from cultures, also in the ovoid more than in the longer variety of bacillus. In some cases the unstained portion is not in the centre but at the side or end of the bacillus, and in other cases the ends are not stained. The bipolar staining is well brought out by over-staining in carbol fuchsin for four or five minutes and then decolorising with absolute alcohol, or by treating with acetic acid and then with carbol fuchsin. The bipolar staining is by no means constant in every bacillus, though in a plague specimen it is generally the predominant feature. In some smear preparations from infected tissues nearly all the bacilli show the bipolar staining; in others only a small proportion exhibit this characteristic, and occasionally no bipolar staining is to be observed. In most specimens some of the bacilli show a distinct but unstained capsule, giving the appearance of the bacillus being embedded in a viscous matrix. In preparations from buboes and the haemorrhagic effusions around them the arrangement is generally a few single micro-organisms intermixed with a large proportion of bacilli in pairs, presenting a diplococcal or diplobacillar appearance; and not infrequently several pairs are found together in shorter or longer chains and having the appearance of streptobacilli or streptococci.

Spherical, torula-like, and disc forms may be found in old buboes during life and in affected tissues after death. These swollen and irregularly shaped bacteria do not stain well, and often only a faint outline is to be seen.

In the living plague patient the bacilli are generally very abundant in smear specimens of the contents of the buboes and in the sanguinolent effusion around them, crowds being seen in the microscopic field; they are not infrequently to be seen in the interior of the white blood corpuscles. But while the usual characteristic is the multitude of bacilli in buboes, there are occasions when they are few in number, and they are only detected by inoculating the material from the affected gland into a culture medium. Plague bacilli are very numerous in the sputum of pneumonic cases, which at times literally teems with them. They are also to be seen in the blood of septicaemic cases and in the contents of vesicles and pustules that sometimes appear on the skin. They can be cultured from the blood and urine of living patients suffering from the septicaemic form.

In dead bodies the bacilli are found in the affected buboes and generally in the spleen, liver, lungs, bone marrow, bile, urine, peritoneal fluid, and fluid of the brain. It is this universality of the plague bacillus which is the danger attached to corpses and which renders it imperative that special precautions shall be taken immediately death occurs to prevent the spread of the infection. In septicaemic cases the risk is always pronounced, but even in the bubonic form the bacilli very frequently gain an entrance into the blood stream some time before death and become disseminated in the tissues and in the excretions, so that any dribbling or escape of fluid from the body which frequently takes place will soil the bedding and the floor.

The micro-organism of plague is distinctly aerobic; it grows easily on ordinary culture media such as gelatin, agar agar, broth, blood serum and glycerine agar; it grows also in milk and scantily on potatoes. In isolating the bacillus for diagnostic purposes from the living or dead body the temperature at which the culture medium is maintained is important. Blood heat is not favourable to the growth of the plague bacillus, and if there are other bacilli present, such as the bacillus coli communis, streptococcus pyogenes, or the pneumococcus, these will grow while the plague bacillus will be inhibited. Mistakes may thus easily arise, and the pneumococcus alone or some other microbe be found in a case which is really plague. Plague bacilli grow best at a temperature considerably below blood heat, the most favourable being from 25° C. to 30° C. The first cultures from the body are always slower in growth than sub-cultures. Both

Cultural character-istics.

agar and gelatine plates are used in suspected cases of plague. The growth on most of the media possesses no distinctive features peculiar to plague other than those which are obtained on gelatine, agar agar, and in bouillon. On blood serum it appears in 24 to 48 hours as a moist cream-coloured or yellowish growth. On gelatine it develops in the form of minute, translucent, and raised colonies in the course of 48 to 72 hours, and which have a dew-drop appearance; it may even take as long as four or five days for the colonies to become visible; later the colonies become denser in the centre, of a greyish-white colour and with crenate margins. The colonies differ in their rate and extent of growth, some remaining stationary in size, others becoming considerably larger. Under a lower power of the microscope they have at first the appearance of ground-glass, and later a dense dark granulated centre with notched edges more or less transparent. Deeper colonies in gelatine appear at first as small, rounded refractive granules, white in reflected light and brown in transmitted light. In stab cultures there is, in addition to the granular and later continuous white growth along the tract of the needle, a film on the surface of the gelatine. The bacilli do not liquefy gelatine, but they liquefy blood clots.

On agar agar inoculated with plague material minute, bright, colourless colonies of various sizes and slightly raised develop in less than 48 hours or it may be longer. In a day or two they become small, greyish-white hemispheres with a thin iridescent border. Some of the colonies remain small, but others continue to grow in diameter and some become four or five times the diameter of others. They are generally discrete at first, but on moist agar agar the colonies coalesce and form white and opaque patches. If touched with a platinum needle the culture is found to be of a sticky and viscid nature, adhering in strings to the needle, and allowing individual colonies being moved on the surface of the medium without disintegration.

On dry agar agar slopes when the material has been evenly spread on the surface, minute greyish-white translucent colonies cover the whole surface of the medium, which presents, as a rule, a very characteristic ground-glass appearance by reflected light obtained when the culture is held away from the light and looked at from the back. In a few days there will be seen to be two types of colonies, one of which is of small size, more or less translucent and constituting the majority, the other larger, whiter, more opaque in appearance and gradually changing to a slightly yellowish-brown colour as it increases in size. The latter are the giant colonies, or cannibal colonies described by Haffkine.

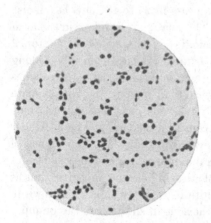

Early stages of involution forms
of plague bacillus (Haffkine).

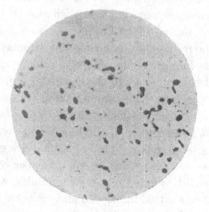

Intermediate involution forms of
plague bacillus (Haffkine).

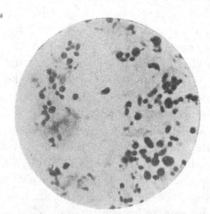

Advanced involution forms of plague bacillus (Haffkine).

Morphologically the two types contain the same kind of bacilli; possibly there are more longer bacilli in the giant colonies and more involution forms. In sub-cultures the colonies appear earlier than in cultures from infected tissues; they have a greater tendency to become confluent and to form a cream-coloured growth with thin translucent and iridescent margins possessing a pronounced crenated appearance. Sub-cultures from the smaller colonies often show a scantier growth than from the larger. Young colonies when examined microscopically are found to be mainly composed of short bacilli which do not attain the average size until the second or third day. Old colonies, especially the giant colonies, may contain a larger proportion of longer bacilli.

The bacilli from cultures stain much more easily than those taken

Involution forms. direct from infected tissues, and there is not the same degree of bipolar staining. Haffkine[1] found that in dry agar agar inoculated with plague material the bacillus may undergo as early as in 24 hours certain involution changes, so that in addition to the short typical bacillus the culture will contain many other forms. These bacillary forms may diverge in a small degree only from the type, or they may become so different as to cause them to have no resemblance to the elements from which they are derived. Some are only enlarged in length and breadth but do not lose their shape nor their staining properties; others become thickened, swollen, filamented and distorted in form, assuming bizarre figures resembling sausages, pears, spindles, clubs, dumb-bells, biscuits, discs and other irregular globular bodies. They stain only very slightly and irregularly and have no bipolar staining. Vacuoles are sometimes observed. The different forms which they assume are to be seen in the accompanying photographs and diagram. These involution forms may develop to such dimensions as to be twenty to thirty times the size of the ordinary young forms. In the same microscopical specimen there will be seen every variety of shape and size ranging from the smallest to the largest. Microbes of other diseases vary in size, but they are usually more or less constant in their diameter. It is not so with the plague bacillus, the diameter of which may show very great differences in different individuals in the same specimen. Similar differences are displayed in their capacity of staining: some stain well and uniformly, others show the bipolar staining, others take on only a pale colouring throughout their substance, others stain at the circumference or only part of the circumference, and others with vacuoles may not stain at all. According to Haffkine this power of producing

[1] *Brit. Medical Journal*, 1897, p. 1461.

involution forms may be lost in the laboratory after sub-culture, and appears to be limited to recent cultures derived from plague cases. The involution forms may not appear on dry agar agar for three or more days. According to Hankin a $2\frac{1}{2}$ to $3\frac{1}{2}$ % of salt added to the agar agar will hasten the production of involution forms. Experiments with salted agar agar on other bacteria do not show the same exaggerated involution forms as are to be observed with plague bacilli. Matzuschita[1] has shown that salted media tend to produce involution forms in bacillus pyocyanus, the lactic acid bacillus, anthrax bacillus, and cholera bacillus.

The involution forms appear in old and dry cultures of agar and in cultures on potatoes. They do not appear in old or fresh bouillon cultures. Any change undergone in bouillon is that of disintegration. The microbes under these circumstances appear to be granular, they however retain their vitality. Involution forms are also to be found occasionally in the tissues of human beings who have died of plague, also in the tissues of lower animals that have been inoculated with plague, and in animals that have died of plague contracted in the natural way and that have been a longer time in dying than usual.

The involution forms are apt to give rise to uncertainty and disputes at a critical stage in the development of a plague epidemic, and a knowledge of them accordingly possesses much importance from a diagnostic point of view. In the early period of the outbreak in Cape Town in 1901 a number of the rats which were dying showed on examination large numbers of bacilli which were larger than the ordinary plague bacillus and of a biscuit shape; mixed up as they were in many instances with typical plague bacilli, they were obviously involution forms of the micro-organism. The first cultures retained the involution character and were fatal to pigeons and guinea-pigs, and harmless to rabbits and a baboon. They however gave when cultivated in broth the stalactite growth referred to later, and subsequently they lost the involution form and approximated to the ordinary type of the plague bacillus.

In bouillon, cultures of the plague bacillus resemble those of "streptococcus pyogenes." The growth begins to be visible on the second day in the form of fine flocculent sticky masses adherent to the sides of the tube and deposited at the bottom of the clear liquid. At times a film may also form on the surface. Microscopically examined the cultures will be found to contain not only bacilli single and in pairs of a coccoid

Characteristic growth in bouillon.

[1] *Zeitschr. für Hygiene*, Vol. xxxv. 1900.

character, but also short and long chains of bacilli composed of five or more elements. These chains have often the appearance of streptococci, but on close examination with a high power will be found to consist of coccoid bacilli. Bacilli from young cultures stain well, and degenerative or granular forms are not found except in old cultures. To Haffkine is due the credit of demonstrating that the bacilli grow in a very characteristic manner in bouillon. A few drops of oil or fat in the form of ghee[1], cocoanut oil, olive oil or linseed oil, added to the bouillon facilitate the characteristic formation, but they are not necessary. Bouillon so treated and sterilised, will if it is inoculated afterwards with the plague bacillus and kept absolutely still and free from any vibrations, show scarcely any signs of change during the first two **Formation of** or three days. Then minute flakes appear underneath the **stalactites.** drops of oil which are floating on the surface of the medium. These flakes, which are colonies of bacilli attached to the drops of oil, grow, in the course of the next 12 to 24 hours, down into the depths of the liquid in the form of stalactites which, scanty at first, in the course of two or three days increase in number and size, and fill up the upper half or sometimes the whole volume of the bouillon.

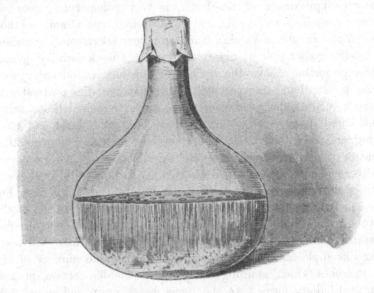

Haffkine's Stalactites.

[1] Ghee is a preparation of clarified butter used by the Hindús as a food and for ceremonial purposes.

If the flask is shaken the stalactites fall in snow-like flakes to the bottom. The fluid again becomes clear, and if the culture is again kept free of agitation small colonies will form afresh underneath the oil globules, and once more a renewed growth of stalactites will take place similar to the first, but slower in growth. By agitation and allowing the flask to remain still the process can be repeated, and a series of fresh stalactite growths can be obtained sometimes for three or four months until the nutritive medium is exhausted. The bouillon will then no longer be suitable for plague bacilli, which will remain alive but will not grow in it. Sometimes when the bouillon is inoculated direct from plague tissues, zoogleic masses of bacilli collect at the sides of the flask and surface of the liquid, but no stalactites are formed. Under these conditions if the flask is gently shaken the stalactites usually appear in 24 to 36 hours.

According to Kitasato[1] there is a bacillus met with in plague cases

Kitasato's plague bacillus. which has not all the marked characters mentioned; but which when found alone resembles in many respects the diplococcus pneumoniae. It is the one to which Kitasato has essentially given his name. Kitasato in describing it points out that Yersin's bacillus is larger than his, does not possess the distinctly diplococcus appearance of the latter, is very polymorphic, does not possess a capsule, is not motile, and is decolorised with Gram's method. Moreover the growth of Yersin's bacillus on agar is extremely luxuriant, and, though rather slow at first, continues for a week forming creamy colonies projecting above the surface of the media, and only young colonies are small and transparent. These characteristics contrast with Kitasato's bacillus, the colonies of which are extremely delicate, transparent, small discs which attain the size of a pin's head and cease growing, and then tend to disappear on the fourth day of incubation, presenting in all respects a close resemblance to the growth of diplococcus pneumoniae. Kitasato's bacillus curdles milk at the end of the second day, renders bouillon uniformly turbid at first, but subsequently forms fine flocculi and sedimentation at the bottom of the test tube. This bacillus is rod-like in shape, rounded at both ends and stains more deeply at the poles. In the glands many of them appear like diplococci, though there is a considerable number of the same microbes which, staining easily in the middle portion, present distinctly bacillary forms. In the lungs, heart, brain and spinal cord they may present an appearance like streptococci. This bacillus stains

[1] "Plague," by Kitasato and Nakagawa, *Twentieth Century Practice of Medicine*, Vol. xv.

with Gram's method, possesses a capsule in the specimens prepared from the blood or tissue fluids of various organs, and also in cultivations in solid serum, is slightly motile and is much more constantly found in the blood during illness and convalescence.

It is to be noted, however, that bacteriologists to whom strains of Kitasato's bacillus have been sent have not found all these marked differences, and have come to the conclusion that Kitasato's and Yersin's bacillus is the same, differing only in unimportant respects as regards morphology and cultural characteristics as are to be observed in other pathogenic bacilli.

Many experiments have been made to determine the power which
The vitality of the plague bacillus. the plague bacillus possesses of maintaining life under unfavourable conditions. The result of these is to show that while the bacillus is very sensitive to drying combined with high temperature, yet when it is protected from these, which must ordinarily be the case under natural conditions, it retains its viability for long periods.

Experimenters differ in the results which they have obtained, but the practical point is to know the longest period that the bacillus survives under certain conditions, and accordingly most importance is to be attached to this, which should always be taken as the safer guide.

Abel[1] found that plague bacilli will live in sterilised, distilled and
In different media. tap water for 20 days. Kasanski found it in water on the 48th day, Wuntz and Bourge in sea water after 47 days. Hankin ascertained that plague bacilli added to grain died out in from 6 to 13 days, Gladin[2] that plague bacilli will live in milk for over 3 months, and on food such as raw and coagulated albumen, turnips, potatoes, plums, apples, cucumbers, and black bread from one to three weeks, Stadler that the bacilli will remain alive in meat pickled for 16 days, Yokote[3] that buried carcases of animals dying of plague retain the bacillus alive for 30 days, Batzaroff[4] that the organs of plague animals, dried in vacuum for 38 days at the temperature of the room, still contain living bacilli, and when the dried pulverised substance, so

---

[1] *Centralblatt für Bakteriologie, Parasitenkunde und Infektionskrankheiten*, 1897. Vol. xxi. Zur Kenntnis der Pestbacillen. Dr Rudolph Abel.

[2] *Ibid.*, 1898. Vol. xxiv. " Die Lebensfahigkeit der Pestbacillen unter verschiedenen physikalischen Bedingungen." G. P. Gladin.

[3] *Ibid.*, 1898. Vol. xxiii. "Ueber die Lebensdauer der Pestbacillen in der beerdigten Tierleiche." Dr L. Yokote.

[4] *Annales de l'Institut Pasteur*, tom. xiii. p. 385. "La Pneumonie pesteuse expérimentale." Dr Batzaroff.

treated, was inserted into the mucous membrane of susceptible animals it caused plague. The same observer noticed that the virulence of the microbe in albuminous tissues decreased very slowly. Faeces containing plague bacilli and left standing at the ordinary temperature for three days infected a guinea-pig with plague. Sputum from a pneumonic case of plague was found to retain its virulence on the 10th day.

While the association of the streptococcus appears to exert a stimulating effect on the virulence of the plague microbe, it has been noticed by a number of observers that the presence of bacillus coli communis, the bacillus subtilis, the staphylococcus and micrococcus prodigiosus appears to exercise a retarding influence.

A gelatine plate with virulent plague bacilli upon it, which was exposed in a dark and damp room, and on which saprophytic organisms of fungi grew, was found by Simonds to have lost its infective properties in two days. On the other hand, Gotschlich found the bacillus alive and virulent in $8\frac{1}{2}$ months old cultures which were partially dry and mouldy.

In broth culture Haffkine found the plague bacillus alive after 18 months. Gabritschewsky kept the bacillus in an agar culture alive stored in a cupboard for two years, also in the pus which was taken from an infected guinea-pig and sealed in a tube. Pure cultures[1] of the plague microbe protected from drying have been known to retain their viability for four years if protected from sunlight and kept in a cool place. Klein[2] has recently reported that the bacillus obtained from the fatal case of plague in the London Docks in 1896 still retains a fair degree of virulence in sub-cultures; such retention of vitality and virulence in sub-cultures has to be distinguished from that obtaining in old and unrenewed cultures.

Even under intense cold the bacilli may thrive: thus Kasansky[3]

Effect of cold. showed that cultures placed outside his laboratory at Kasan during the winter, and which were subjected to temperatures ranging between $2°$ C. and $-31°$ C. below zero for periods of 3, 4, and $5\frac{1}{2}$ months, retained their viability and were only weakened in their virulence. Similarly at St Petersburg bacilli remained alive at temperatures of zero and $-20°$ C.

[1] *Centralbl. f. Bakt.* 1901. Vol. xxix. "Ueber die Lebensdauer von Bacillus pestis hominis in Reinkulturen." N. K. Schultz.

[2] *Medical supplement to the 32nd Report of the Local Government Board for* 1902–1903, p. 402.

[3] *Centralbl. f. Bakt.* 1899. Vol. xxv. "Die Einwirkung der Winterkälte auf die Pestbacillen." Dr M. W. Kasansky.

The capacity of the plague microbe to survive exposure to intense cold is much greater than its power to withstand the effects of intense heat whether moist or dry. In regard to the effect of heat on the plague microbe there is much difference in the results obtained by different observers, the time required for destroying the vitality of the microbe not being constant and differing in some important particulars. The difference in time and the differing results may be due to the different methods employed, and to the probability that in some of the experiments the vessel containing the plague bacilli was not wholly submerged and subjected to the temperature stated. For instance in some experiments a temperature of 80° C. has killed the bacillus in five minutes, in others it has required 15 minutes. Abel observed that with 50° C. more than an hour was required for sterilising cultures. Toptschieff[1], on the other hand, found that from two to four hours were required with a temperature of 50° C. to destroy the vitality of the bacillus. Kitasato killed the bacillus in half-an-hour with a temperature of 60° C. Yersin sterilised cultures of the bacillus by maintaining them at a temperature of 58° C. for an hour, but Albrecht and Ghon after heating cultures for an hour in a water-bath at 55° C. to 60° C. found that all the microbes were not destroyed and that it was possible with the microbes thus subjected to these temperatures to produce plague in animals.

Effect of heat.

According to Haffkine after a quarter of an hour's exposure to a temperature of 45° C. an agar or bouillon culture of plague bacilli is no longer cultivable; and as a matter of routine practice the plague prophylactic is sterilised at a temperature not higher than 55° C. continued for only 15 minutes. The microbes are killed at once when exposed to a temperature of 100° C. moist heat, and this is the temperature to which plague-infected articles should be exposed. Dry heat requires a higher temperature and a longer exposure of the bacillus to be destructive. Dry heat will destroy the vitality of the plague bacillus, as shown by Gladin, in one minute at a temperature of 160° C., in five minutes at 130° to 140° C., and in 20 minutes at a temperature from 100° to 110° C. The effect of the direct rays of the sun is rapidly injurious to the vitality of the plague microbe. In Hongkong and India, where the sun is strong, experiments by Kitasato, Wilm, and the German and Indian Plague Commissions establish the fact that plague bacilli exposed in

Effect of sun.

---

[1] *Ibid.*, 1898. Vol. xxiii. p. 734. "Beitrag zum Einfluss der Temperatur auf die Mikroben der Bubonenpest." F. J. Toptschieff.

thin layers to the direct rays of the sun have their vitality destroyed in the course of a few hours; usually one hour suffices, but it depends on the thickness of the layer. The devitalisation of the microbe takes longer if the bacilli are protected by a covering or by the interstices of woollen or other textile fabrics.

Agar or broth cultures of plague exposed for three hours to direct sunlight in Bombay grew with difficulty when transferred to new culture media, but were only killed after exposure for the whole day.

In temperate climates the effect of direct sunlight is slower in its action, and exposure of cultures for six hours by Albrecht and Ghon had no injurious action on the microbes.

The bacilli are very sensitive to rapid desiccation; plague bacilli on cover-glasses placed in a desiccator containing sulphuric acid or chloride of calcium are destroyed in a few hours. The bacilli are more sensitive to drying at a high temperature than at a low temperature; drying at a **Effect of** temperature of 35° C. will according to Abel's experiments **drying.** kill the bacilli in two to three days, while drying at 16° C. to 20° C. will not destroy them until the 6th and 9th day, and on one occasion the bacilli remained alive till the 14th day.

When Kitasato dried the contents of buboes on cover-glasses and kept them at a temperature of 28° C. to 30° C. the vitality of the bacilli was destroyed by the 4th day. The power of resistance to drying was increased when thread or small pieces of material were impregnated with plague cultures or infectious matter. According to the Indian Plague Commission, laboratory experiments under the ordinary atmospheric conditions of Bombay do not demonstrate any great increase of resistance or any long survival of the microbe when exposed to darkness or diffuse sunlight.

Cotton, silk, wool, linen, glass, blotting-paper and gauze, impregnated with pure cultures of the plague bacillus, with sputum from pneumonic plague, with emulsion of plague organs, or with peritoneal fluid from a plague-infected guinea-pig, were found by the German Commission to be non-infective in eight days, *i.e.* the plague bacilli did not survive more than eight days in these materials under ordinary atmospheric conditions. Moisture under certain circumstances is rapidly injurious to the vitality of the bacillus. Ficker observed that alternate damping of the bacillus during the process of drying hastened its death. By such a process the bacilli were killed in from 20 to 28 hours, whereas by drying only in the desiccator they lived for eight or nine days.

A hot and moist atmosphere will not only cause the death of the bacillus but will destroy its structure. The writer dried and fixed a large number of specimens of bacilli on cover-glasses in Hongkong and kept them in cardboard boxes. By the time they reached England none of the bacilli would stain or could be detected. Their bodies had evidently been macerated, disintegrated and destroyed by the moisture of the air to which they had been subjected. Experiments on silk, wool, cotton, cloth, etc. in Europe have shown that the bacillus may survive 45, 56, 60, and 76 days. The Indian Plague Commission also found the plague bacillus to survive on calico for a period of 70 days.

Experiments in Sydney by Dr Tidswell[1] to ascertain the extra corporeal viability of the plague bacillus on various sterilised materials demonstrated that the plague bacilli died out in periods varying from less than one day to three weeks, the longest being when the culture was mixed with dust, cotton, and straw respectively and slowly dried.

A most interesting observation, and one which is of the highest importance in its bearing on the possible long duration of the survival of plague bacilli, is that which was carried out by Kitasato in Japan when plague was imported into Kobe in 1899. It was suspected that the plague had been introduced by a ship which had arrived at Kobe with a consignment of cotton goods from Bombay: among these cotton goods were some dead rats. It is not known how long the rats had been dead.

Two hundred culture tubes were inoculated with portions of the cotton and in two plague bacilli were grown and isolated.

The virulence of the plague microbes often decreases in some
Variation in   cultures, while in others it apparently not only retains its
virulence.   virulence but increases in intensity. The cause of the
variation is unexplained.

Batzaroff[2] succeeded in increasing the virulence of a broth culture of the plague bacilli, which had lost its power of killing a rat and a guinea-pig even in large doses, by depositing a portion of the culture in the nostril of a guinea-pig. In eight days the guinea-pig died of pneumonic plague. Then, by inoculating a series of guinea-pigs he was able by the third or fourth transmission to raise the virulence of the microbe to the degree of causing death in three days. An atmosphere containing 3 per cent. of carbonic acid gas and 97 per cent. of ordinary air at 80

---

[1] Further observations on the mode of Infection. By Frank Tidswell, M.B. Embodied in the Report of the Board of Health on a second outbreak of Plague at Sydney, 1902. By J. Ashburton Thompson, M.D., President.

[2] *Annales de l'Institut Pasteur.* 1899. Tom. XIII.

to 88° F., also an admixture of 14 per cent. of carbonic acid and 86 per cent. of ordinary air at 92° F., were found by Marsh[1] to enhance the growth and the multiplication of the plague bacillus, and that under this treatment the bacillus increases in virulence and retains its vitality for a long time. From these experiments it is concluded that probably the vitiation of the atmosphere, which is produced when the ventilation of a room occupied by human beings is inadequate, is capable not only of stimulating the reproduction of the plague bacillus but also of increasing its virulence. Other experiments indicated that a deficiency in the amount of oxygen is favourable to the vitality of the plague bacillus. By passage through one species of animal the general result seems to be an increase of virulence for that species, but a diminution of virulence for other species.

Experiments on the duration of the vitality and virulence of the plague microbe, though contradictory in some respects, may be taken as indicating that, though under certain laboratory conditions the microbe is very sensitive to atmospheric and microbic influences when the influence of sunlight and moderately high temperature come into play, yet under other conditions of darkness and low temperature it displays a prolonged power of resistance and retention of virulence.

When cultures or infectious material in the dark can retain their vitality and virulence for two and four years, it is not beyond the bounds of credibility for certain infected articles under favourable conditions to retain their infection for a long time, and that some of the older observations, such as that of a rope used for letting down plague corpses into the grave retaining infection for a long time and causing a fresh outbreak, may not be discarded as impossible.

It has already been stated that the inoculation of susceptible animals with the plague bacillus obtained from pure cultures causes **Effect of the plague bacillus on animals.** certain symptoms ending in death, and that the bacillus is again recovered in pure cultures from the blood and internal organs of the affected animal. The laboratory animals experimented on have been generally rats, mice, guinea-pigs and rabbits. Inoculation of any of these with the plague microbe causes a definite illness in them, followed usually by death in a few days.

A guinea-pig inoculated with the plague microbe or with a portion of the bubo, or the organs of a plague patient, usually becomes drowsy and disinclined for food within 48 hours. After this period it remains

[1] *Report of the Indian Plague Commission*, Vol. III. p. 73, also Vol. v. App. iii. p. 480.

huddled up in its cage with back arched, staring coat and half-closed eyes, unwilling to move even when disturbed, and sometimes breathing in a laboured manner. Towards the end it falls on its side, suffering at intervals from tremors or convulsions, and dies in the course of the fourth or fifth day after inoculation.

The post-mortem appearances show haemorrhagic infiltration with a good deal of effusion at the seat of inoculation, the parts being oedematous for some distance from the point of inoculation. The adjacent glands are congested and swollen, having a sanguinolent effusion around them. The lungs are generally normal, but they may show pneumonic patches, the heart is congested, the blood is fluid and darker in colour than usual, the liver is mottled and congested. There are also small petechial haemorrhages in the lungs, heart, spleen, and kidneys, as well as in the pericardium, peritoneum and parietal pleura. The intestines are not generally much affected. The whole appearance is one of engorgement with dark fluid blood. Plague bacilli are to be found in the blood, liver, and spleen, and may at times be found also in the lungs and kidneys.

Mice and rats inoculated usually show signs of illness within 48 hours and present much the same symptoms as those described as occurring in the guinea-pig. The course of the disease is as a rule more rapid, death occurring on the third day. The post-mortem appearances are similar to those found in the guinea-pig.

The length of illness may vary in the animals inoculated, but death generally occurs in mice in from one to three days, in rats from the second to the fourth day, in guinea-pigs in two to five days, and in rabbits in from four to seven days. A chronic form of plague may occur in rats and guinea-pigs in which the animal does not die, or dies only after several weeks or longer, and then often in an emaciated condition. In this form the affected glands are usually found in a cheesy condition. There are small areas of necrotic tissue in the several internal organs, and the spleen is generally much enlarged. Only few bacilli are to be found, but the tissues containing them, if administered to a healthy rat or guinea-pig, will reproduce the disease.

CHAPTER V.

THE RELATIONSHIP OF EPIZOOTICS TO PLAGUE.

THE results obtained by the experiments on laboratory animals were
Rats and mice of greater import than merely affording evidence that the
susceptible to plague microbe causes a disease in them, and can be again
natural
plague infec- recovered from their tissues. They proved that rats and
tion. mice were susceptible in a high degree to the plague
microbe, and suggested an explanation of the phenomenon which has
been observed from the earliest times, and which has often accompanied
an epidemic of plague, viz. a sickness and mortality among rats and
mice. They directed attention to the rat mortality then accompanying
plague in Hongkong and to the examination of some of the rats, with
the result that the same microbe was discovered in the sick and dead
rats as in human beings affected with plague. Morphologically and
culturally these microbes are not to be distinguished from one another,
and their action on other animals is the same. The epizootic among
rats, which has been observed to prevail in nearly every outbreak
of plague in different countries, during the existing pandemic has been
proved by bacteriological examination to be plague.

That a relation exists between certain epizootics and epidemics of
Relationship plague has been a current belief for many centuries. The
between epizootic was generally looked upon either as a sign of
certain epi- coming plague or as the actual disease attacking animals
zootics and
epidemics of precedent to its affecting human beings. This latter view
plague a is held by the Chinese at the present moment and led,
current belief by those who held it, to the doctrine that plague is a
for many
centuries. soil disease attacking first the animals which burrow in
the ground.

The relationship is not so clear as the many examples cited in
history would indicate, for plague in the early periods was confused

with many other pestilences, and the confusion applied to animal diseases as well. Epizootics occurring at a period when plague prevalence was common at the same season of the year would likely be taken to be connected in some way with plague, but that they were frequently not related to that disease, nor even a sign of a coming plague, may be gathered from the fact that in periods when plague was quiescent or not existing in the country there had been similar wide-spread and fatal epizootics of various kinds, which destroyed immense numbers of cattle, and which were called cattle plagues because of their fatality and the extensive range of their devastation. The designation is retained even to-day for diseases known to have no relation to plague. Rinderpest, for example, is a term which is applied to a number of diseases not yet differentiated and classified, and includes small-pox, haemorrhagic septicaemia, plague, and other infective diseases of animals. In Rhodesia at the present day there prevails a devastating epizootic called tick fever, or red water fever, which is destroying the cattle of the country and which is caused by a sporozoon. Before the microscope came into use for the diagnosis of cattle diseases

Observations of epizootics associated with plague epidemics. this epizootic would not have been differentiated from other infectious diseases of cattle, and consequently the relationship of epizootics to epidemics of plague in any particular case in the past must be doubtful.

With the discovery of the plague bacillus in the rat the relationship of at least one epizootic to plague is established. It is the epizootic most frequently mentioned with plague. The first reference to it is in Syria some 3000 years ago, when the Philistines at war with the Israelites were attacked with plague, and they made golden images of their emerods and of the mice that marred the land[1].

Avicenna recognised a connection in Mesopotamia and refers to the fact that on the approach of plague mice and other animals, which usually live underground, leave their holes and move about in a staggering manner as if they were drunk. The inhabitants of Hindustan were at one time familiar with the connection between rat mortality and plague, for in the *Bhagavata Purana*, written more than 800 years ago, they are instructed to leave their dwellings immediately they notice a mortality among rats.

In the Great Plague of 1348 other animals besides rats are mentioned as having been affected. Nicephorus Gregoras[2] says: "Nor was it

---

[1] 1 Samuel vi. ver. 5.

[2] Nicephori Gregorae *Historiae Byzantinae* lib. XVI. cap. 1.

mankind alone that the plague thus harassed as with a scourge, but all other animals that dwell with or associate with human beings took the disease; dogs and horses and fowls as well, and even the mice that lived within the walls of their houses." This is corroborated by the Emperor Cantacuzine, who stated that even the domestic animals were carried off with plague. A Paduan chronicler[1] says of the epidemic of 1347 that once the sickness entered a dwelling, all were seized by it, even the animals. When Holstein[2] was attacked in 1350 with a grievous bubo plague it raged both in the case of man and in that of cattle.

When the plague reached Avignon[3] it is recorded by Baluze that even the animals in the place, such as dogs, cats and hens, died. In Tournay[4] the mortality was especially great among the chief people and the rich, as well as the poor. Deaths were more numerous about the market-places and in poor narrow streets than in broader and more spacious areas; and whenever one or two people died in any house, at once, or at least in a short space of time, the rest of the household were carried off, so much so that very often in one home ten or more ended their lives together, and in many houses the dogs and even cats died.

At the time when the epidemic prevailed in England[5] there was according to Knighton a great mortality of sheep, so much so that in one place there died in one pasture more than 5000 sheep, and they were so putrid that neither beast nor bird would touch them.

Similar accounts are given by Arab authors[6] as to its attacking animals and birds which ate the flesh of infected bodies that had not been buried.

Rats, moles, serpents, conies, foxes, badgers, martens, and adders are mentioned by later writers as having been observed to die before, or during plague epidemics, and the appearance of these in unusual numbers was usually considered to be the harbinger of plague.

Skeyne[7], in 1568, gives as a sign of impending plague the moles and serpents leaving their holes, "as quhan the moudeuart and serpent leauis the Eird beand molestit be the Vapore contenit within the bowells of the samin"; also he states, "quhan the domesticall foulis becummis pestilentiale, it is ane signe of maist dangerous pest to follow."

---

[1] *The Great Pestilence*, 1348–9, F. A. Pasquet, 1893.
[2] *Ibid.*   [3] *Ibid.*   [4] *Ibid.*   [5] *Ibid.*
[6] *Histoire des Huns*, Vol. v. p. 224. J. de Guignes.
[7] "Ane Breve Description of the Pest, p. 10, by Maister Gilbert Skeyne, Doctoure in Medicine, Edin. 1568." Edited by W. F. Skene and presented to the Bannatyne Club, 1860.

In treating of the plague in London, Lodge[1] mentions rats and moles and other creatures, accustomed to living underground, forsaking their holes and habitations, and attributes it to corruption of the soil.

Dr Hodges[2], in writing of the Great Plague of London of 1665, says " that subterranean animals, such as moles, mice, serpents, conies, foxes, &c. as conscious of approaching mischief, leave their burrows, and lie open in the air which is also a certain sign of a pestilence at hand."

It must be noted, however, that no mention is made of epizootics in accounts of many of the epidemics of plague in European cities, though it is curious that in most, rats, dogs and cats are ordered to be destroyed. Dr J. F. Payne informs me that in the plague on the Volga in 1878 and 1879, which he and Dr Colville investigated, a large mortality among rodents was observed, but its relationship to the epidemic of plague did not impress him at the time. Now he is inclined to think that the association was very intimate.

In the Káthiáwár epidemic in India of 1820 mortality and sickness in cattle is referred to, but was believed to be due to other causes.

On the other hand, Dr Forbes[3] mentions that in the Pali plague of 1836–38 the plague was preceded by a great mortality among the cattle, and that the most singular phenomenon was the death of all the rats in the village of Taiwali during the latter half of April, and just before the plague's first appearance. Mr White reports, " they lay dead in all places and directions in the streets, houses, and hiding places of the walls," and " this death of the animals attended or preceded the disease in every town that was attacked in Marwar, so that the inhabitants of every house instantly quitted it on seeing a dead rat."

The epidemic which prevailed in Kumaon, one of the endemic centres in India, in 1834–5 was, according to Mr Gowan, the Commissioner, preceded or accompanied by a great mortality of rats in the village. The same phenomenon was observed and commented on by Drs Planch, Francis, Pearson, Hutcheson and Thompson in several of the later outbreaks of plague, or Mahamari as it is called by the natives, in Kumaon and Gharwal.

In Yunnan in Western China, another endemic centre of plague, it is to be gathered from the reports of the French Missionaries who have resided there, and from M. Rocher who visited the province,

---

[1] *A Treatise of the Plague*, by Thomas Lodge, Doctor in Physics, 1603, cap. iii.

[2] *Loimologia*, or an Historical Account of the Plague in London in 1665, p. 42. By Nathaniel Hodges, M.D.

[3] *The Nature and History of Plague as observed in the North-Western Provinces of India.* By Frederick Forbes, A.M., M.D.

that a rat mortality preceded the several outbreaks of plague[1], and that other animals, great and small, such as buffaloes, oxen, sheep and deer, and sometimes also court-yard fowls, died of the disease.

Mr Davenport[2], who was in Yunnan a few years later, mentions cats, rats, mules, and other quadrupeds as being affected.

Mr Baber, of H.B.M.'s Consular Service, in his *Notes on the route of Mr Grosvenor's mission in Western China, Yunnan,* refers to the mortality among rats and poultry, pigs, goats, ponies and oxen.

Dr Lowry states[3] that in nearly every house in Pakhoi, where plague broke out, rats were observed to come out of their holes and die on the floor.

Coming to the present pandemic, a large mortality of rats was noticed in the first affected quarters of Canton before the plague appeared among human beings. Later on, the appearance of affected rats in portions of the city hitherto immune was the signal of the approaching disease, and residents who could afford to do so moved to the suburbs, or went to live in boats moored in the river. In Canton there is a very large boating community which remained for the most part free of plague. This comparative immunity of boating people was observed also in Hongkong, and has been noticed in the older epidemics of Europe. In the great epidemics of London many of the inhabitants took up their residence in boats, because of the freedom from plague which the boat population enjoyed. The great mortality among rats in Canton may be judged from the fact that 22,000 rats were taken out of one gate of the city and buried. In Hongkong there was a great mortality of rats during the plague epidemic of 1894, and the same occurred in the subsequent annual recrudescences.

The same seasonal influences have a corresponding effect on the plague epizootic and epidemic. From the chart for Hongkong in 1900 prepared by Dr Clark, Medical Officer of Health for Hongkong, and reproduced on the opposite page, it will be seen that the rise and fall in the epizootic is similar to the rise and fall of the epidemic. The very rapid rise in the rat mortality antedates the epidemic outbreak for several weeks; it reaches its maximum a week or so before plague and declines with the plague mortality.

In 1902 the examination of rats for plague was carried out in Hongkong on a most extensive scale by four bacteriologists engaged on no other duties. It resulted in demonstrating that the great majority

---

[1] *La Province Chinoise de Yunnan.* E. Rocher, Paris, 1879.

[2] *Commercial Reports from His Majesty's Consuls, China.* No. 2, 1877.

[3] Notes of an epidemic disease observed at Pakhoi in 1882. *Imperial Maritime Customs Medical Reports, China,* for the year ended Sept. 1882. June, 1883.

of plague cases in Hongkong in 1902 was preceded by rat plague. A
further enquiry on the same lines by Dr William Hunter[1] for 1903 confirmed this relationship.   The results for 1903 are shown in the chart

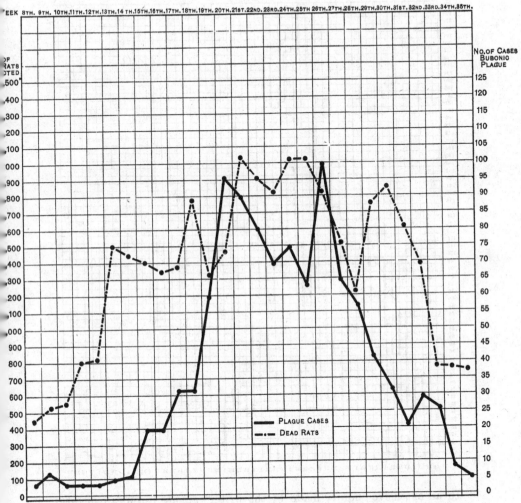

on the next page, which at the same time shows that the plague in rats
continues to exist at a low level throughout the non-epidemic period of
plague. The epizootic rises at the season when young rats are most
numerous.

Governed by the same seasonal conditions, the plague epizootics
differ in time only from the plague epidemics, preceding them slightly.

[1] *A Research into Epidemic and Epizootic Plague.*   By William Hunter, Government
Bacteriologist, Hongkong, 1904.

The precedence of the epizootic among rats which is exhibited in the charts has been observed also in the villages and towns of China.

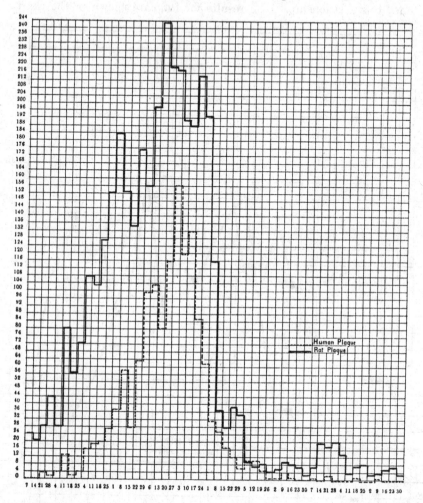

In an extensive enquiry made by the writer[1] among European medical men practising in Southern China and among others conversant with plague in the villages, into the occurrence of epizootics before or during times of plague, it was ascertained that the opinion was practically unanimous that the rat mortality is a precursor of plague. Not only is this opinion held by the medical men in Southern China experienced in

[1] *Report on the Causes and Continuance of Plague in Hongkong.* By W. J. Simpson, M.D., 1903.

plague, but it is also entertained by the Chinese whose villages or towns have been attacked with plague.

Dr A. Lyall[1] of Swatow, in referring to the order of occurrence in plague, states, " It is generally recognised by the Chinese that rats die first. During the year I have often been told that ' men are dying in such and such a street; rats have begun to die in another street, men not yet.'" In Taiwan, Formosa, Dr J. L. Maxwell's experience was that, shortly after hearing that rats were dying in such and such a house, he would be called to a case of plague in the same house.

In Uganda, recently discovered to be a separate focus of plague, Koch states that plague in man is preceded by plague in rats, and that the natives of Kisiba leave their huts on this sign.

Mice as well as rats are sometimes, but not often, observed to be affected during a plague epidemic. According to Yamagiva mice died of plague during the epidemic of plague in Formosa. The same phenomenon was observed at Yedda in 1898 when the plague was there.

Previous to the appearance of the epidemic of plague in Bombay, a heavy mortality occurred among cattle, sheep, and goats. What the exceptional mortality was due to was never ascertained. Pigeons and cats also sickened and died during the epidemic. The most conspicuous epizootic, however, was that which prevailed among rats, and which bacteriological examination proved to be plague. It broke out near the docks and gradually extended to other parts of the city. It preceded and ran concurrently with the epidemic of plague, and was accompanied by a great migration of rats from locality to locality, evidently induced by alarm on the part of these animals. In the town of Mandive[2] the inspector reported that in nearly 50 % of the houses he disinfected, he found dead cats and rats.

The epizootic among rats was observed in most of the towns and villages of India in which plague became epidemic. The same phenomenon presented itself in the Mauritius, Alexandria, Oporto, Naples, Cape Town, Port Elizabeth, East London, Durban, and in Sydney and Brisbane, precedent to and concurrently with plague prevalence.

Rats when they sicken with plague leave their holes and generally come out into the open. They look ill and are in a dazed condition; their eyes are watery, their coats are partially deprived of hair, and they hobble about with difficulty and stagger and fall. The nervous system is affected, showing itself most often in lethargy, sometimes in paralytic symptoms and sometimes in great excitement. They either make very little attempt

Plague-stricken rats, their appearance and behaviour.

[1] Simpson, *Ibid.*   [2] *The Plague in India*, 1896–98. Nathan, Vol. II. p. 222.

to escape when approached, or they may rush about madly or caper round the room, and their behaviour is so extraordinarily different from what is usual that the illness from which they are suffering may be at once suspected.

The glands of plague-infected rats, especially the submaxillary and praesternal, are enlarged, and these, together with the internal organs and blood, contain plague bacilli. The tissues are congested and of a dark colour, and as a rule have a sodden or macerated appearance. The lungs are congested, exude on section frothy blood, and at times contain pneumonic patches. The spleen is generally enlarged and engorged with blood; the liver is also enlarged and presents in portions of it a mottled appearance. There are petechial haemorrhages on all the internal organs and under the pleura and peritoneum. The plague bacilli on smear preparations often vary in appearance according to whether the rat is examined immediately after death or later, or has suffered from an acute or chronic illness. In the case of delay in death, or in examination, the bacilli are often found to have undergone involution changes.

Cats suffered from illness, accompanied with buboes and wasting, in Bombay, Karachi, Ahmednagar and Baroda. The Austrian Commission caused plague in three cats by feeding them with the bodies of animals dead of plague. One cat took the disease in an acute form, while the other two took it in a chronic form, having buboes on the neck and wasting.

Cats affected with plague.

In Cape Town there was also a great mortality among moles, but as these animals were not examined bacteriologically it cannot be definitely stated that the mortality was due to plague. Cats also contracted plague as proved by post-mortem examination and bacteriological examination, but not in great numbers. The type of plague was bubonic, affecting the glands of the neck and the submaxillary glands. There was sometimes extensive infiltration below the jaw, extending down to the neck.

The post-mortem appearances met with in the cats are as follows[1].

Cat I. Found dying in the street. Post-mortem showed glands in neck and throat much swollen and filled with well marked plague bacilli. Lungs congested and pneumonic, liver healthy, spleen healthy, mesenteric glands much enlarged but not congested, submaxillary glands much enlarged but not congested.

Cat II. Submaxillary glands enlarged, spleen enlarged, liver normal, glands along vertebrae enlarged, axillary and groin glands enlarged, blood dark in colour, bacilli in blood, enlarged glands and spleen.

[1] The post-mortems were made by Dr Robertson, Pathologist to the Cape Government, in the presence of the author.

Cat III. Submaxillary glands enlarged and congested. The praesternal lymphatic glands much enlarged and congested. Right lung presents patches of acute lobular pneumonia. Heart blood fluid and dark in appearance, liver much enlarged, clayish colour, spleen much enlarged, moderately firm in texture and congested, kidneys normal, intestines much inflamed in condition of enteritis. There is a general inflammatory condition of the respiratory and digestive organs. Inguinal glands congested, plague bacilli in the glands.

Cat IV. Cat found in a house, ran a little distance and then fell down dead. Submaxillary glands greatly swollen, great oedema of the subcutaneous cellular tissue of neck, mesenteric glands enlarged and congested, glands in the groin and praesternal swollen and congested, with oedema in the surrounding cellular tissues, spleen normal, digestive system normal, lungs with patches of pneumonia, plague bacilli in lungs and glands.

Cat V. Identical lesions to that of *Cat IV.* and typical plague bacilli, but not so numerous.

Cat VI. Cat which had died after having been noticed to be sick for four or five days. There was extensive necrosis of the tissues of the lower jaw. Post-mortem showed submaxillary glands very much enlarged, periglandular tissue oedematous, and veins over glands dilated. Praesternal glands on left side below pectoralis major were enlarged and pink ; lungs were congested, heart distended, liver dark, soft, and easily broken up, spleen not enlarged, kidneys very large and congested. Plague bacilli were found in glands and in lungs.

Cat VII. Found dead in a house. The submaxillary glands were much enlarged and there was an extensive infiltration of the colourless fluid into the subcutaneous tissue below the jaw and extending down to the neck, plague bacilli present in the glands, and infiltration.

Cat VIII. Found in a moribund condition in a house in which there was plague. The expression in the cat's face is almost typical, head being triangular in shape, owing to great swelling below jaw, lips thickened and eyes nearly closed.

On post-mortem the submaxillary gland on right side was yellow in colour and foci of pus were formed. The condition of the gland on the left side was not so advanced, but on section was soft. Surrounding the glands was much yellow fluid. The surface of the glands was of a deep red colour, and the vessels were dilated.

There was a very large soft congested gland on either side in praesternal region. The liver, spleen and abdominal organs were normal. The lungs were congested but not pneumonic. The heart contained some pericardial fluid, and petechia were on its inner surface, plague bacilli in buboes and tissues.

Cat IX. Killed because looking ill. Glands under jaw much enlarged, right submaxillary gland on right side suppurating. Plague bacilli present.

Cat X. Found ill in empty house. Submaxillary lymphatics much enlarged, contain plague bacilli.

Cat XI. Found ill in street. Submaxillary glands very large and haemorrhagic, contain plague bacilli.

Cat XII. Found dead in street. Submaxillary glands enlarged and haemorrhagic, praesternal gland enlarged, plague bacilli present.

Dr William Hunter[1] records a small outbreak of plague among cats in a warehouse in Kowloon, in which rats had been previously dying of plague. In the course of his investigations he found that rats fed on paddy soaked in the faeces or urine of plague-infected cats died of acute rat plague. The post-mortem appearances of cat plague were, in Hongkong, extreme congestion of all the tissues and organs, congestion of the lymphatic glands with the presence of cortical haemorrhages, and frequent bubonic swellings about the neck and the mesentery; but, as pointed out by Dr Hunter, the most interesting condition was found in the abdomen. The peritoneum was smooth and shiny. Very little fluid was found in the peritoneal cavity. The stomach was congested, particularly on its mucous surface which showed innumerable haemorrhages of varying size. No actual ante-mortem ulceration was found. The small intestine was in general reddened. The ileum was the seat of many small petechiae scattered through its entire length, the mucous surface of which was reddened and thickened. The thickening was chiefly due to oedema. The solitary follicles were visible, being pin-head in size and greyish-yellow in colour. Small areas of necrosis were present which appeared chiefly about the regions of haemorrhagic extravasation.

In one or two cases a distinct bubonic formation was found in the mesentery. Plague bacilli were found scattered throughout the body, and were specially abundant in the lymphatic apparatus and in all bubonic areas. The faeces and the urine also contained plague bacilli. Dr Hunter also observed cases of chronic cat plague, in which the cat became extremely emaciated, with the formation of buboes in various situations of the body, especially about the neck. The buboes are very chronic in growth, accompanied by extreme surrounding infiltration, and slowly break down with the production of thick creamy pus. The animals may live from two weeks to a month. It is a marasmus, and is well described by the term "Pest Marasmus."

Other animals such as pigs, goats, cattle, sheep, fowls and rabbits suffer from plague as well as man.

In Newchang[2], in the plague epidemic of 1899 two months after the

Other animals affected with plague.

first recognised cases of plague and at a time when many deaths were taking place, in the houses and shops in close

[1] *A Research into Epidemic and Epizootic Plague.* By William Hunter, Government Bacteriologist, Hongkong, 1904.

[2] *Imperial Maritime Customs Medical Report* for half-year ended 30th Sept. 1899, 58th issue, 1900. Dr C. C. Burgh Daly's *Report* on the health of Newchang.

proximity to foreign residences it was noticed that rats, chickens, ducks, geese, pigs, dogs, deer, and cattle were dying in unusually large numbers.

Dr Michoud, in describing the epidemic of 1893 at Mengtze in Yunnan, says, "We saw on some roads dogs and pigs feeding undisturbed on corpses which no one cared to bury. These animals fell victims to their voracity and succumbed to the scourge[1]."

Dr J. P. Maxwell, of Changpo in the province of Fokien, mentions the fact of dogs occasionally dying with glandular swellings during the plague epidemic; he had seen four. Surgeon-Major Lyons of the Indian Medical Service also reports that in the case of a dog which was examined in Bombay there was post-mortem evidence of it having been affected with plague.

In Cape Town a dog was found dying in a house. The post-mortem examination showed the lungs to be congested and full of froth and blood. There was lobar pneumonia. Heart was distended and full of tarry blood. Axillary and mesenteric glands were enlarged, with the surrounding areolar tissue congested. Liver was congested. Spleen healthy. Kidney enlarged and congested. Plague bacilli were present in the blood.

Additional evidence of the susceptibility of the lower animals to plague has been obtained experimentally. By feeding with cultures of plague bacilli, by inoculation with them, and by causing animals to breathe air containing plague bacilli, rodents, especially rats and guinea-pigs, have been found to be very susceptible. The disease produced in them may be acute or chronic. In the latter form it may exist for months. The significance of the disease in rats will become more apparent when treating of the continuance and spread of plague It will at present be sufficient to state that the rôle played by other rodents is small compared with that of the rat.

Result of experiments to produce plague in animals.

As regards susceptibility of other animals to artificially induced plague, experimenters have met with conflicting results, but in the main the positive are more important than the negative, and as such will be chiefly dealt with.

The following tabular statements give a summary of the experiments on different animals carried out by the German and Austrian Medical Commissions on their visit to Bombay.

---

[1] *Imperial Maritime Customs, China, Medical Reports* for the year ended 30th September. 1894, 47th and 48th issues, 1895

EXPERIMENTS BY GERMAN COMMISSION.

Arbeiten aus dem kaiserlichen Gesundheitsamte. Sechzehnter Band, 1899.

Animals	Manner of infection.	Material used.	Results.	Post-mortem appearances and bacteriology.
Rats	Simple inoculation.	Smallest quantity of plague cultures.	Death in a few days. Animals lose their appetite, sit huddled together in cage with hair and fall on side before death.	Site of inoculation infiltrated and glands in vicinity swollen, containing masses of B. pestis, spleen enlarged and containing B. pestis, lungs and liver hyperaemic.
Rats	Feeding.	Smallest quantity of plague cultures or rats dead of plague.	Death in 2 or 3 days.	*1st infection from the glands of the neck.* Glands at neck dark bluish red, swollen and containing numerous bacilli. The body presents picture of septicaemia, spleen enlarged, liver and lungs hyperaemic and containing bacilli; in some cases petechiae in stomach and intestine, but in the majority the mucous membrane was normal. *2nd type. Direct infection from alimentary canal.* Mucous membrane of stomach covered with numerous haemorrhages, and follicular swellings, villi and intestine filled with plague bacilli, mesenteric glands swollen, reddened and haemorrhagic, with plague bacilli. *3rd type. An aspiratory pneumonic plague.* The lungs exhibit fresh inflammatory centres in which there are numbers of bacilli; there is splenetic tumour and hyperaemia of liver.
Rats	Culture placed on (a) mucous membrane of nose, or (b) into conjunctivae. Subcutaneous injection.	Fresh cultures.	Death in 3 days.	(a) Bubo at neck, splenetic tumour containing masses of bacilli. (b) Bubo at neck and symptoms of septicaemic plague.
Mice	Subcutaneous injection.	Virulent plague cultures.	Death in from 3 to 4 days. Death in from 3 to 5 days In rare cases even after 2 days, and sometimes not until 6 or 7 days.	Enlargement of spleen, which was plethoric, dark red and containing great numbers of plague bacilli; sometimes buboes were visible; blood also contained bacilli.
Mice	Subcutaneous injection.	Very virulent, pure plague cultures.	No illness in quite rare cases. This result shows that mice must be used with caution for diagnosis of plague.	
Mice	Feeding.	Cadavers of mice dead of plague and swarming	No results.	

Animal	Mode of inoculation	Material	Result	Post-mortem appearances
...	into hind-foot.	rat.	—	...contained bacilli; the enlarged spleen contained bacilli; inguinal glands of infected leg enlarged and embedded in an infiltrated tissue.
Mongoose	Feeding.	Organs (containing bacilli) of a rat dead of plague.	Death in 5 days.	Glands at angle of jaw swollen and purulent, but no bacilli in same. Spleen large and indurated and containing bacilli. Mucous membrane of stomach and intestine pale and without petechiae; concluded infection through mouth and glands of neck leading to general septicaemia.
Squirrel	Subcutaneous injection.		Death in 4 days.	Inguinal glands dark red and embedded in viscid connective tissue, which, as well as the enlarged spleen, contained numerous plague bacilli.
Squirrel	Feeding.	Pure plague cultures.	Death in 6 days.	Spleen much enlarged and full of bacilli; mucous membrane of intestines and stomach pale, no petechiae; suprahyoid gland enlarged and containing plague bacilli; plague bacilli in urine.
Guinea-pigs	Subcutaneous injection at abdomen.	Plague cultures.	Death in 5 days.	Buboes present, embedded in caseous haemorrhagically infiltrated connective tissue; spleen much enlarged and permeated with innumerable minute yellow nodules; punctiform necrosis of liver; lungs pale and containing four yellow centres with hyperaemic zones, and buboes. Bacilli present in the organs.
Guinea-pigs	Feeding.	Virulent plague bacilli in broth.	No results.	
Guinea-pigs	Feeding.	Virulent plague bacilli in broth.	Death after a long time. (Chronic plague?)	Inguinal glands haemorrhagic, swollen and embedded in a viscid connective tissue, spleen enlarged and congested, with a few minute yellow nodules. Plague bacilli present in the spleen. Doubtful whether the infection arose from the alimentary canal.
Rabbits	Subcutaneous injection.	Virulent culture.	Death, as a rule.	Appearances of septicaemic plague.
Horses	Hind leg shaved and cut in various directions; then the material rubbed in.	Fresh plague cultures.	Temperature high soon after inoculation; sub-normal on the 6th day, then renewed rise of temp. and recovery on the 16th day. Animal showed very little indisposition, appetite was not good, eyes were red, seat of inoculation only slightly inflamed, glands not swollen nor painful.	

EXPERIMENTS (*continued*).

Animals.	Manner of infection.	Material used.	Results.	Post-mortem appearances and bacteriology.
Horse	Subcutaneous injection at neck.	Plague agar cultures.	Fever set in 4 hours after injection. Irregular fever on and off for 6 weeks. Oedematous swelling at spot of injection; submaxillary glands swollen; ultimately absorption and recovery. The horse showed signs of indisposition on 2nd day, appetite was lost, and eyes were red.	
Ox	Subcutaneous injection after inoculation with Koch's tuberculin.	Fresh plague agar culture, a few streptococci present in the broth.	Irregular fever and indisposition; swelling at point of injection, which terminated in absorption. Recovery in 15 days. No swelling of lymphatic glands.	
Ox	Scarification of skin and inoculation.	The same as above ox.	Irregular fever, scarified skin inflamed and painful, no glandular swelling. Recovery. General reaction unexpectedly severe. Eyes congested.	
Sheep	Subcutaneous injection.	Fresh plague culture.	Immediate rise of temperature followed by irregular fever, swelling at point of injection, which burst on the 8th day. Recovery. Animal was fairly ill and took very little food. Numerous plague bacilli found in pus of swelling.	
Sheep	Rubbing into scarified skin.	Plague culture.	High fever the day after injection. Irregular fever and swelling, in the centre of which an abscess appears which bursts. Recovery slow, as animal remains weak for a long time. Numerous plague bacilli found in pus of abscess.	
Goat	Rubbing into scarified skin.	Pure plague culture.	High fever and a large painful swelling on spot of injection, animal very ill; on the 7th day the swelling ulcerates, then slowly heals up. Recovery. Pus from ulcerations sterile.	
Goat	Subcutaneous injection.	Plague culture.	Course of disease and fever as previous goat, but there is a cough and accelerated respiration; purulent secretion from the nose; the animal finally became so ill that it had to be destroyed a month after it was injected.	
Cat	Rubbing into scarified skin.	Plague culture.	Fever for several days and swelling at place of infection; this, however, soon decreases. Rapid recovery.	Bacteria of various descriptions found in secretion from nose. No bacilli were found in the glands after death. The lymphatic glands of neck as large as pigeon eggs, pale, hard and like marrow on incision.

Dog	Subcutaneous injection.	Fresh plague culture.	formed an abscess. Pus from without sterile. Recovery.
Dog	Rubbing into scarified skin.		Local swelling, no affection of the glands. Recovery.
Dog	Feeding.	Fresh plague agar culture.	Slight inflammation at place of inoculation, and trifling rise of temperature, which set in on 5th day, the only symptoms of illness.
Dog	Feeding.	Plague cultures in meat.	No illness.
Pigs (2)	Subcutaneous injection.	Plague cultures.	Remained well for 9 days, then rapid emaciation and swelling of submaxillary glands, one of which was excised, was hard and size of a bean. The juice expressed from gland was found to be sterile. Recovery.
Pigs (2)	Feeding.	Rats dead of plague.	Slight rise of temperature. Recovery. No symptoms of disease. No reaction.
Pigeons (1), Hens (2) and Geese (2)	Subcutaneous injection into thoracic muscle.	Fresh plague cultures in broth.	Slight rise of temperature. Recovery.
Brown Monkey (*Macacus radiatus*)	Rubbing into scarified skin.	Fresh plague cultures.	Glandular swellings in axilla and in groins. Recovery.
Brown Monkey	Cutaneous injection.	Fresh virulent, fresh plague agar cultures.	On next day very ill, soft infiltration of cellular tissue in vicinity of seat of injection. Spleen enlarged and crammed with plague bacilli. Oedematous infiltration at spot of inoculation; many plague bacilli in all the viscera. Axillary glands on injected side larger than peas, dark red with punctiform haemorrhages. Intestines congested, mesenteric glands enlarged, with a few plague bacilli, groin glands also enlarged, spleen large, soft and hyperaemic; the liver and kidneys pale; serous fluid in the pleura; numerous plague bacilli were found in the viscera, plague bacilli in blood. Irregular fever, infiltration of cellular tissue. Death on the 4th day.
Brown Monkey	Subcutaneous injection.	Plague agar culture.	
	A series of cases of subcutaneous injection in monkeys produced the same results.		
Brown Monkey	Injection into the peritoneum.	Plague bacilli.	Death in 30 hours. Spleen enlarged, congested and containing many plague bacilli; small haemorrhages in the coat of stomach; the mucous membrane hyperaemic; lungs hyperaemic and oedematous; glands not swollen; numerous plague bacilli in spleen, lung, and peritoneal exudation.

EXPERIMENTS (*continued*).

Animals.	Manner of infection.	Material used.	Results.	Post-mortem appearances and bacteriology.
Brown Monkey (3)	Feeding.	(a) 4 c.cm. freshly prepared plague agar culture in broth.	(a) Death in 4 days.	(a) Septicaemic plague. Glands of neck, axilla and groin unchanged, lungs normal, spleen enlarged with many plague bacilli, mucous membrane of stomach covered with numerous small haemorrhages, entire mucous membrane of intestine hyperaemic with numerous minute haemorrhages, mesentery glands unchanged.
		(b) 1 c.cm. freshly prepared plague agar culture in broth.	(b) Death in 4 days.	(b) Lymphatic glands of neck unchanged, viscid oedema in region of the stomach, haemorrhagic infiltration in left inguinal region and a large swollen gland, the lungs hyperaemic, spleen typically enlarged, mucous membrane of stomach at the pylorus infiltrated with numerous punctiform haemorrhages, mucous membrane of small intestine haemorrhagically inflamed.
		(c) ·5 c.cm. freshly prepared plague agar culture in broth.	(c) Animal ill 3 days later, soft swelling of both submaxillary regions, nostrils covered with scabs. Death on 6th day.	(c) Glands of neck swollen, viscid oedema of the subcutaneous cellular tissue of the abdomen, swelling of the lymphatic glands in both inguinal regions, spleen typically enlarged, mucous membrane of stomach and intestines pale but unchanged. It is thought that this monkey derived its infection from injuries of the mucous membrane of the nose and mouth.
Large grey long-haired Monkeys (*Semnopithecus entellus*)	Cutaneous injection.	Plague culture in broth.	Vicinity of inoculation swollen as well as the glands. Death on the 3rd day.	Septicaemic plague.
Grey Monkey	Subcutaneous injection.	Plague agar culture, $\frac{1}{10}$ minim.	Death in 2 days.	Septicaemic plague.
Grey Monkey	Subcutaneous injection.	Plague agar culture, $\frac{1}{100}$ minim.	Death in 6 days.	Septicaemic plague.
Grey Monkey	Subcutaneous injection.	Plague agar culture, $\frac{1}{1000}$ minim.	Death in 6 days.	Septicaemic plague.

EXPERIMENTS ON ANIMALS.

(By Albrecht and Ghon, members of the Austrian Commission sent by the Imperial Academy of Sciences in Vienna.)

(Die Pest von Weil. Docent Dr H. F. Müller und Dr R. Pöch. Wien, 1900.)

Animals.	Manner of infection.	Material used.	Results.	Post-mortem appearances and bacteriology.
Guinea-pigs	Intraperitoneal.	Very virulent and less virulent cultures.	(a) Many plague bacilli in blood and all organs; viscid oedema at point of puncture often accompanied with haemorrhages; general condition is one of acute haemorrhagic septicaemia. When the material was less virulent the mesenteric glands exhibited the characters of primary buboes with splenic tumour. When the animal only died after 3 or 4 days, a purulent exudation was in the abdominal cavity, and yellowish white miliary nodules in the spleen and liver, and distinct parenchymatous degeneration. (b) Death in 24 hours in some, 3 or 4 days in others, and 5 or 6 days in others.	
Guinea-pigs	Subcutaneous.	Slightly virulent.	(a) Death in 2 or 3 days. (b) Death in 4 or 6 days. (c) Death from marasmus after a chronic course.	
Guinea-pigs	Cutaneous.	Plague bacilli and other bacteria.	Typical primary buboes. Acute infection can be caused by rubbing of plague material on an unshaven part. Pathological changes same as those in the intraperitoneal and subcutaneous injections.	P.M. (a) Round the site of injection haemorrhagic exudation with viscid oedema. (b) Oedema less, purulent necrotic state of seat of injection, and contiguous lymphatic glands exhibit primary buboes.

TABLE (*continued*).

Animals.	Manner of infection.	Material used.	Results.	Post-mortem appearances and bacteriology.
Guinea-pigs	Feeding.	Animals dead of plague.		(a) Mouth most frequently exclusive point of entrance. Glands of neck form the primary bubo. Alimentary canal only shows secondary changes. (b) The intestine alone is the point of entrance. In small intestines Peyer's patches are haemorrhagically infiltrated or necrotic in centre, the mesenteric glands resemble primary buboes. (c) When the virus is introduced simultaneously in mouth and intestines, the lymphatic glands of neck as well as the mesentery glands resemble primary buboes. If the intestines are the point of entrance the faeces contain masses of plague bacilli.
Guinea-pigs	Material introduced on mucous membrane of nose or eye.	Cultures.	Primary buboes in glands of neck. Catarrh of mucous membrane and plague bacilli in secretion.	
Rabbits	Intravenous.		Septicaemic forms can be induced and forms with localisation of plague virus in separate organs.	
Grey Rats	Feeding, intraperitoneal, subcutaneous, and puncture.	Rats dead of plague.	Death with or without convulsions, but in some cases no results.	Acute septicaemia with haemorrhages. Mouth infection the most frequent.
White Rats	Subcutaneous and intraperitoneal.		Catarrhal and haemorrhagic conjunctivitis frequent.	Same pathological changes.
White and grey field Mice	Feeding.		Rapid death with convulsions.	Degeneration of liver and hyperaemia of organs. No plague bacilli.
Jackal (*Canis Aureus*)	Intraperitoneal.	Plague bacilli in a solution.	Death in 48 hours of acute general infection, haemorrhagic type.	Large numbers of plague bacilli in the blood and organs.
Jackal	Feeding.	Large quantities of material with plague bacilli.	None.	
Dogs	Intraperitoneal injection.		Death in from 12 to 24 hours.	
Dogs	Subcutaneous injection.		Death after formation of typical buboes.	

Animal	Method	Material	Result	Remarks
Dogs	Feeding.	Large quantities of highly virulent material.	No reaction but B. pestis demonstrated in faeces.	After some time were killed, no signs of plague infection.
Hyena	Intraperitoneal.		Death.	Haemorrhagic septicaemia.
Hyena	Feeding.		None.	Haemorrhagic septicaemia.
Mongoose (*Herpestes Griseus*)	Intraperitoneal.		Death.	
Mongoose	Feeding,	Great masses of material containing plague bacilli.	None.	
Cats	Intraperitoneal.		Death in a few hours.	
Cats	Feeding.		Submaxil. bubo, infection local or death from general infection.	Plague atrophy in connection with cervical bubo.
Pigs	Intraperitoneal.	Material with B. pestis with splinters of glass and bone.	Rapid death.	Haemorrhagic septicaemia.
Pigs	Continuous feeding.		None.	
Monkeys	Intraperitoneal.	Very virulent.	Death.	Haemorrhagic septicaemia.
Monkeys	Intraperitoneal.	Slightly virulent.	Death.	Creamy peritoneal exudations.
Monkeys	Intraperitoneal.	Slightly virulent cultures.	Only slight reaction.	Typical appearance of spleen.
Monkeys	Subcutaneous.		Primary bubo of corresponding local lymphatic gland.	
Monkeys	Cutaneous.		Death.	General infection.
Monkeys	Pouring liquid with plague bacilli into mouth.		Death after 10 days.	Symptoms of primary pneumonic plague, the animal having coughed during process.
Pigeons	Intravenous and intraperitoneal.		Fatal general infection.	Acute splenetic tumour, degeneration and hyperaemia of liver, kidneys, plague bacilli in blood.
Pigeons	Intramuscular infiltration.		In addition to local infiltration paralysis of wings and feet.	
Pigeons	Feeding.		None.	
Vultures (2)	Intravenous, intrathoracic and intrapulmonal.		No infection but 1 bird showed symptoms of indisposition.	
Hens (5)	Intravenous, feeding and intraperitoneal.		No results.	
Snakes, Lizards and Frogs	Feeding, subcutaneous, and intrathoracic.		No results.	

In view of the intimate association of the inhabitants of a great many countries with their cattle, pigs, goats, and fowls, either in the farm or in their houses, it is important that the question should be decided as to whether these animals are susceptible to plague. The Chinese belief is that cattle, pigs, fowls, as well as rats suffer from plague, and it is in accord with the older views of Europeans when plague was epidemic. Both the German and Austrian Commissions failed to produce plague in oxen, pigs, and poultry. In the case of cats the German Commission failed to produce the disease, while the Austrian Commission succeeded by feeding. Dogs could not be successfully infected by feeding, but virulent plague bacilli were found in their **Haffkine's** faeces. Haffkine experimented on horses, cows, sheep, and **experiments.** goats by inoculation of plague cultures, but the goats alone, without developing any acute disease, lost condition gradually, wasted away, and after a considerable time many of them succumbed. Lowson experimented on pigeons, ducks, crossbills, yellow-hammers, linnets and canaries, and failed to infect them with plague. On the other hand, **Wilm's ex-** Wilm[1] in the Hongkong epidemic of plague in 1896 suc- **periments.** ceeded in infecting a pig fed with the spleen of a man who had died of plague; and a number of poultry fed by him with plague material and with pure cultures of the plague bacillus died in 3 or 4 days of plague. Piaxi and Posen[2] found, when pigeons and sparrows were starved, that they were susceptible to plague.

Further experiments on a large scale were carried out in Hongkong **Experiments** in 1902 by the writer[3], assisted by Dr Hunter, the Govern- **on a large** ment Bacteriologist, and Dr Matsuda, a Japanese medical **scale carried** **out in Hong-** man lent to the Government of Hongkong by Japan. **kong in 1902.** The result of these experiments was to establish the fact that calves, hens, turkeys, geese, pigeons, sheep and pigs were susceptible to plague both by inoculation and by feeding, and that pigs and poultry were susceptible in a high degree.

Plague material containing the plague bacillus and taken from a plague case was employed in preference to the use of cultures of the plague bacillus, which is more or less an artificial condition, and it is probably to the adoption of this method that the experiments were

[1] *Report on the Epidemic of Bubonic Plague in Hongkong in the year* 1896. By Staff-Surgeon Wilm.

[2] *Revista Interna d'Igene*, April, 1897.

[3] *Report on the Causes and Continuance of Plague in Hongkong and suggestions as to remedial measures.* By W. J. Simpson, M.D., Colonial Office, 1903.

attended with success. The material for experiment was always carefully examined before use in order to be certain of its nature. Each experiment was checked bacteriologically and by the effect produced by feeding rats on portions of the animal which had been experimented on. The bacilli were isolated, and cultures of them were made, and the effects of a few of the cultures were tested on guinea-pigs.

There were employed in the experiment 15 pigs, 7 calves, and 1 buffalo calf, 31 hens, 7 pigeons, 6 turkeys, 6 geese, 6 ducks, 3 redbeaks, 7 monkeys, 7 guinea-pigs, and 109 rats. The result is shown in the following statement which gives the number and percentage of the animals that died of plague :—

Of the 15 pigs experimented on 13 equal to 86 % died; of the 8 calves 7 equal to 87 % died; of the 31 hens 11 equal to 35 % died; of the 7 pigeons all died; of the 6 geese 3 equal to 50 % died; of the 6 turkeys 4 equal to 66 % died; of the 6 ducks all died; of the 3 redbeaks 2 died; of the 7 monkeys 5 equal to 70 % died; of the 7 guinea-pigs all died; of the 109 rats 72 % died.

In the case of the first 4 pigs experimented on, in which the infective material was derived from a human being, the time was so

Pigs.

long before the animals showed any signs of illness that, if it had not been that suspicion of illness arose from the daily temperatures recorded, they probably would have been disposed of at a date anterior to their illness and counted erroneously as failures. Of the 4 pigs first

CHART I.

Temperature of pig inoculated with emulsion from bubo of plague case on May 31st, and again with emulsion of plague pneumonic lung on June 2nd.

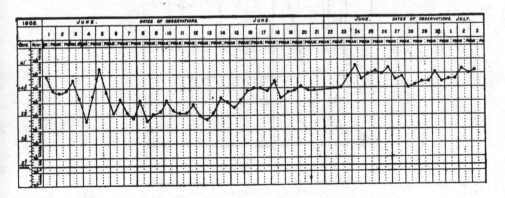

CHART II.

Temperature of pig fed with emulsion of bubo of plague case on May 31st,
and with emulsion of plague pneumonic lung on June 2nd.

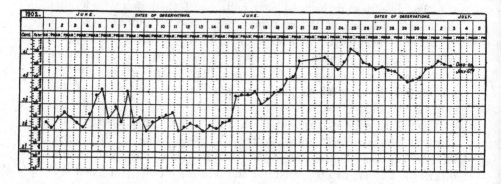

CHART III.

Temperature of a smaller pig inoculated with bouillon emulsion
of plague pneumonic lung.

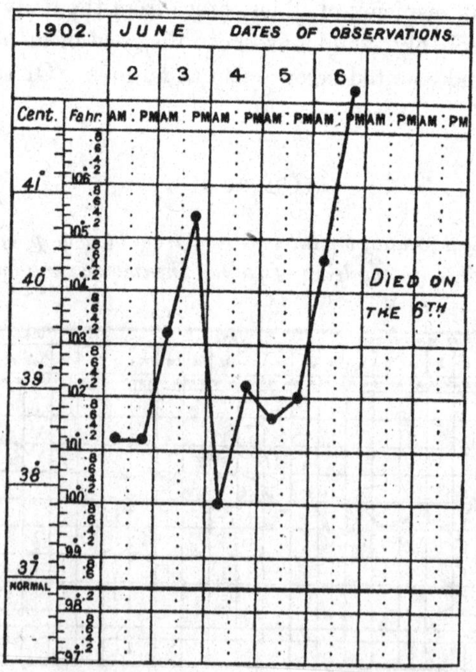

experimented on 3 were fed and 1 inoculated. The 3 that were fed
died in the 5th week, while the one that was inoculated was killed in
the 5th week, the seat of inoculation having become necrosed and the
inguinal glands enlarged. The temperatures were of much the same
type, rising on the 14th or 15th day and continuing from that time at a
higher range. Of this type Charts I. and II. are examples.

The type of disease varied in intensity, however, as is seen by Chart
III., which is that of a smaller pig which was inoculated at the same
time, with the same material and with the same dose as that used for
Pig 1, the only difference being that the larger pig had had a previous
inoculation two days before with emulsion from bubo of a plague case.

Feeding with the organs of pigs which had died of plague killed in
4, 8, and 17 days. Chart IV. represents the temperature of pig that
died on the 8th day.

CHART IV.

Temperature of pig fed with the organs and blood of a pig
that had died of plague.

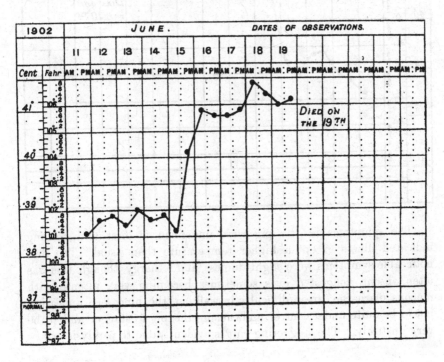

Scarification and vaccination on the abdomen of pigs with blood and spleen pulp of other pigs which died of plague killed with plague in 9 and 15 days; while the same process with the haemorrhagic glands of buffalo calf dead of plague killed in 9 and 19 days. A pig, fed with the organs of a hen which succumbed of plague, died on the 13th day.

Chart V. represents temperature of pig scarified and vaccinated with blood and spleen pulp, which died on the 9th day.

CHART V.

Temperature of pig scarified and vaccinated on abdomen with blood and pulp from spleen, heart, and gland of a pig which had died of plague.

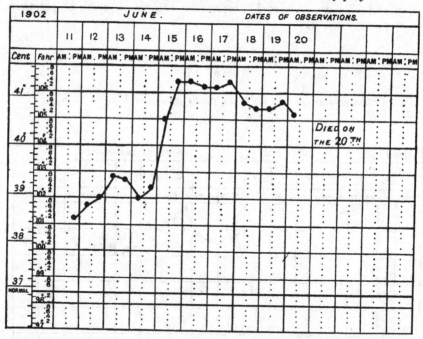

The symptoms in the pig were undefined at first and nothing indicated illness except a higher temperature than usual. The first noticeable symptoms were slight dulness, and lethargy, though this was often absent, congested eyes sometimes becoming very intense with mucous discharge, great difficulty in walking, the hind legs appearing not to be quite under control, and causing the pig to stagger and to be very unsteady. The staggering gait is evidently due to paralysis or loss of co-ordinating power in the nerve centres. The appetite was good up to the last. In some there was diarrhoea on the last day. Death as a rule was sudden, the symptoms of serious illness being of short duration in most of them.

The post-mortem appearances were great congestion and haemorrhagic condition of the glands; in two cases the neck glands were the worst affected. The large intestines were congested in those that had been fed, in the others they were healthy. The bladder was always congested. Plague bacilli were found in the blood, organs, and glands, and in scrapings from the bladder. They were also in the urine, and in the discharges from congested eyes.

In the calves experimented on the disease ran a more rapid course than in the pig when the infection was derived from a human case, and was considerably accelerated when the infection was conveyed from calf to calf. The symptoms were as ill-defined as in the pig. There was a certain amount of dulness, the glands felt swollen and were evidently tender, and the animal lost weight. Suddenly a comatose condition would set in. The post-mortem appearances were those of congestion and infiltration, especially in the region of the neck.

Calves.

Chart VI. represents the temperature of a calf fed on May 29th with emulsion of bubo from plague case and on June 2nd with emulsion of plague pneumonic lung.

Hens fed with plague material from human plague died on the 10th, 11th and 15th day; those inoculated died on the 15th day, while those inoculated or fed with material from a plague-infected hen, or from a calf, or from a pig, or a rat, died as rapidly as the 2nd or 3rd day.

Fowls.

Turkeys, geese and ducks suffered from an acute or chronic form of plague; one type being fatal in a few days, the other in a month to 7 or 8 weeks.

An interesting experiment was the feeding of a monkey with a banana, the inside of which was smeared with the blood of a rat which had died of plague. The symptoms were in all respects similar to those induced by inoculating a monkey with the same material. Both showed a rise of temperature on the 3rd day, with dulness, weakness and death on the sixth day. The post-mortem appearances were general congestion of the organs of the body, congested glands without any marked symptoms of enlargement and bacilli in blood and organs.

Monkeys.

CHART VI.

*Temperature of a calf fed with emulsion of bubo from plague case,
and 4 days later with emulsion of plague pneumonic lung.*

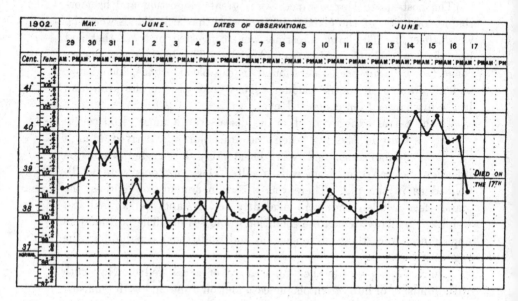

Another monkey fed in a similar fashion on another occasion remained well. The positive experiment demonstrates, however, that rat plague is communicable to the higher animals. A similar experiment in 1896 by Wilm, in which a monkey was given a piece of sugar-cane infected with a pure culture of the plague bacillus, and died in 5 days, showed in the post-mortem examination a very slight swelling of the inguinal glands, great congestion of the intestines, and swelling of the mesenteric glands and of the spleen.

In another experiment a rat dead of plague, with no visible fleas about it, but which had been opened for post-mortem examination, was placed in a cage with a monkey. The temperature of the monkey rose on the third day; great dulness set in at the same time, which continued for three days, after which it lessened, and the monkey appeared to be getting better. There was later a relapse, and death occurred on the 10th day. There were the same post-mortem appearances as in the monkey inoculated or fed with plague material, and there were plague bacilli in the spleen and glands, but only a few in the blood.

The exact manner in which the monkey with the plague-infected rat in its cage became infected it is difficult to decide. It may have been by inoculation caused by scratching, or by infection of the mouth, the fingers of the monkey becoming infected by touching the rat; or it may have been possibly though unlikely due to fleas from the rat passing to the monkey, or it may have been caused by the fleas of the monkey passing to the rat, and then again settling on the monkey.

With the object of endeavouring to settle this point, two monkeys were placed in specially constructed cages along with rats dead of plague but so separated as to prevent any possibility of contact. The cages each consisted of three compartments, the middle compartment being separated from those at each end by rails. which, while permitting small objects to pass between them, effectually prevented the monkey in the compartment at one end putting his hand through to reach or touch the rats in the compartment at the other end. The walls of the

CHART VII.

Temperature of monkey inoculated with blood from a rat dead of plague, which had died from feeding on the organs of a plague-infected buffalo calf.

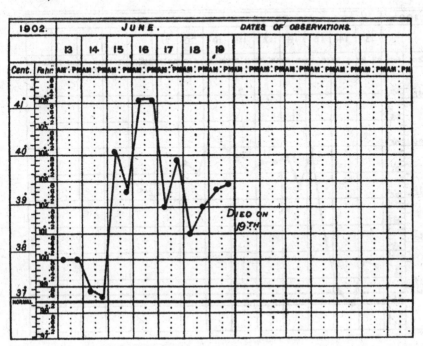

cages were constructed of mosquito wire netting, which prevented fleas
in the cage getting outside, though they might readily pass from one
compartment of the cage to the other.

In one cage a monkey was placed in one compartment, and a rat
sick of plague in the compartment at the opposite end. This rat was
covered with fleas. Taken out three days after, there were no fleas on
it. The monkey on the 4th day had a temperature of 104·6 deg. It
became dull, did not eat, and was evidently sick, remained in a drowsy
state with its head down on its breast, and with its hand to its head;
but after this illness had continued for nearly a week it recovered. In
the other case a monkey was placed in one compartment and four dead
rats in the compartment at the other end. The monkey on the 3rd day
had a temperature of 103·8 deg. It also became dull and drowsy and
was evidently sick, but in a few days it also recovered.

CHART VIII.

Temperature of a monkey placed in the same cage as a rat dead of plague and
which had been opened and examined. Rat was quite free of fleas.

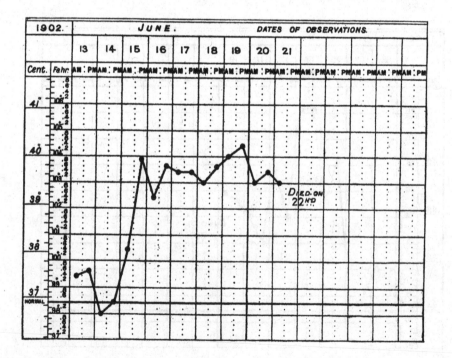

The temperature and course of the disease induced by the several methods employed are seen in Charts VII., VIII., IX. and X. The type and duration of the disease are much the same, irrespective of the channels of infection.

CHART IX.

Temperature of monkey placed in cage, having a rat dead of plague in adjoining cage, but with impossibility of contact. Rat was covered with fleas.

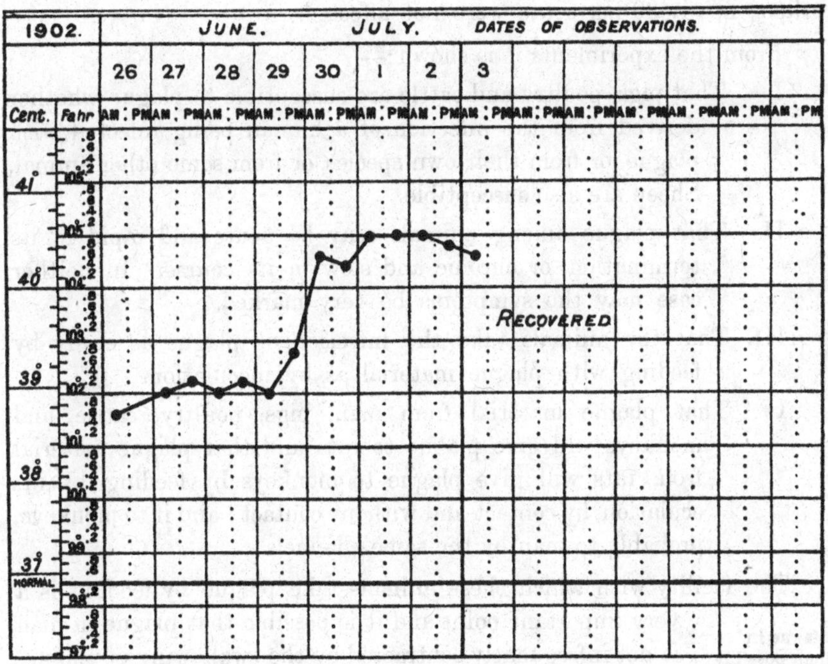

1902.		JUNE.							JULY.						DATES OF OBSERVATIONS.						
		26	27	28	29	30	1	2	3											
Cent.	Fahr	AM PM	AM PM	AM PM	AM PM	AM PM	AM PM	AM PM	AM PM	AM PM	AM PM	AM PM	AM PM	AM PM	AM PM	AM PM

A sheep fed with a bouillon emulsion of spleen from a septicaemic case died of plague in 34 days, while another sheep fed on blood from a calf which died of plague was affected, and died of plague on the 10th day. The chief symptoms were difficulty of breathing and great weakness. Post-mortem showed the spleen and internal organs congested, glands haemorrhagic, lungs much congested, with black patches, bladder healthy, large intestines haemorrhagic, small intestine and stomach healthy. Plague bacilli were found in blood, spleen, kidneys, bladder and glands.

Sheep.

Dogs. Three dogs fed with material from a bubo remained well, apart from a rise in temperature. The German Commission and Ogata likewise failed to produce plague experimentally in dogs. The Austrian Commission, though unable to cause illness in dogs fed with plague-infected material, recovered highly virulent plague bacilli from the excreta of the dogs.

Variation in susceptibility was observed in rats fed with the organs of animals which had died of plague. Some rats took the disease rapidly and were dead of plague by the second day; others did not die for a week, a fortnight, or even 3 weeks after they were fed, while others, nearly 30 per cent., were not affected.

From the experiments it is shown :—

I.　That pigs, poultry and cattle are susceptible to plague whether derived from the infection of a human being infected with plague, or from their own species, or from some other animal. Sheep are also susceptible.

II.　That plague among animals may be acute and rapid in its termination, or chronic and slow in its course. In neither case may the symptoms be very marked.

III.　That the animals take the infection of plague as easily by feeding with plague material as by inoculation.

IV.　That plague material from man, pigs, poultry, cattle, and monkeys will give plague to rats, and that plague material from rats will give plague to monkeys by feeding, by inoculation, by contact and without contact; and if to monkeys, probably to man by the same channels.

Plague in man possibly not infrequently caused by food contaminated with plague infection. The facility with which these animals take plague by feeding is a very important point and it is possible that plague in man is not infrequently contracted by the swallowing of plague-infected food contaminated by an infected rat, or by the uncleanliness of those preparing the food; the frequently congested condition of the stomach and intestines of plague patients, as well as the occurrence of tonsillar plague, serve to give countenance to this view. Emphasis has recently been given to this opinion by Dr Hunter of Hongkong, who has observed diarrhoea, vomiting or colic to precede the fever in a number of cases of plague. Since these experiments were made, and more attention directed to the markets in Hongkong on account of the knowledge as to the susceptibility of poultry, some of the poultry exposed for sale there have been discovered to be affected with plague during the plague season.

The chronic and ill-defined character of plague among some of the animals perhaps also explains the endemicity of the disease in those localities in which pigs and poultry share the living-rooms of the inhabitants, and by their close association become, under favourable circumstances, subjected to the risk of contracting each other's diseases. The same character probably also explains the apparent absence of plague in a locality during the non-epidemic season.

While these enquiries were proceeding, opportunity arose of examining into a fatal epizootic among cattle which has occurred every year since plague began in Hongkong. Investigation showed that it was not plague, nor was it that rinderpest which visited South Africa, but that it was a systemic disease manifesting itself mainly in the intestinal tract and causing at times a haemorrhagic condition of the lymphatic glands. The causal agent was apparently a diplococcus or diplobacillus present in the organs of the body, in the urine and in the excreta, and probably infecting the fodder.

Further investigations of this disease by Dr W. Hunter, Government Bacteriologist, and Mr A. Gibson, Colonial Veterinary Surgeon, confirm the results obtained in the preliminary research and prove that the micro-organism is constantly present. They conclude that the disease is a form of haemorrhagic septicaemia and is allied to Pasteuralosis. Apart from the importance of the identification of this haemorrhagic septicaemia and the differentiation from other diseases of cattle, the prevalence of such a disease when plague is epidemic shows that epizootics other than plague may be readily and erroneously taken for plague; and that nothing but a careful bacteriological examination of the animals affected can decide the question.

Similar experiments to those carried out in Hongkong were repeated in Natal[1] by the medical authorities, but these experiments failed to produce the disease in pigs, fowls, or cattle. There may be several explanations of this. In the first place the experiments were not carried out during the epidemic season, which is always an important factor, and secondly the plague microbe in the epidemic of Natal may not have had that virulence which belongs to the bacillus in China. The great difference in severity of symptoms and fatality of the plague in China and that in South Africa has already been referred to. There may also be a more or less comparative racial immunity among animals

[1] *Report on the Plague in Natal*, 1902–3, by Ernest Hill, Health Officer for the Colony.

in one country as compared with another, similar to that prevailing among human beings.

The susceptibility, which the animals referred to exhibit in regard **Plague in ani-** to experimental plague, is not confined to the laboratory **mals under** any more than it is to the rat, but occurs at times **conditions of** **natural** under natural conditions in the form of epizootics. How **infection.** frequently and under what conditions has still to be ascertained.

Epizootics of plague other than among rats and cats, and under natural conditions, have been positively demonstrated in a few instances. In China pigs and poultry have been discovered to have been attacked by plague under natural conditions. In Hongkong[1] it was demonstrated in 1896 by bacteriological evidence that a ship-load of pigs, imported from a locality infected with plague, died of the disease.

In 1903[2] poultry in the markets of Hongkong were proved to have died of plague. In Kunkhal[3] near Hurdwar in the north-west provinces, and in Jawalapur in 1897, and in Gadag near Dharwar in 1898, monkeys were observed to fall from the trees and die in the streets, and on examination were found to be plague-stricken. Some had buboes on them, and the plague bacillus was isolated from their tissues. Monkeys were also observed to be attacked by plague in other localities in India.

In Gadag a squirrel[4] was proved on bacteriological examination to have died of plague, and squirrels died in Hubli, in Poona, in Bangalore, in Baroda, and other places during the occurrence of plague in those localities.

In Sydney in 1902[5], during the second outbreak of plague in that city, eleven animals in the Zoological Gardens were positively ascertained to be infected with plague. These consisted of four wallabies, one wallaroo, one pandemelon, one tree-kangaroo, one Indian antelope, and three guinea-pigs.

There is considerable evidence[6] to support the view that a fatal

[1] *Report of the Epidemic of Bubonic Plague in Hongkong in the year* 1896. By Staff-Surgeon Wilm.

[2] *Report to the Sanitary Board of Hongkong*, June, 1903.

[3] *Thirtieth Annual Report of the Sanitary Commissioner of the North-West Provinces and Oudh* for the year ending 31st December, 1897.

[4] "Plague in Monkeys and Squirrels," by Alice Corthorn, M.B., *Indian Medical Gazette*, 1899.

[5] *Report of the Board of Health on a second outbreak of Plague at Sydney*, 1902, by J. A. Thompson, M.D., D.P.H.

[6] "Plague in Siberia and Mongolia and the Tarbagan (Arctomys bobac)," by Frank Clemow, M.D., *Journal of Tropical Medicine*, Feb. 1900.

sickness, which sometimes prevails in a epizootic form among a species of marmot known as the Tarbagan (Arctomys bobac), is plague, but hitherto there has been no direct bacteriological proof of this. This disease has been observed to affect the tarbagans in Aksha, in the Siberian province of Transbaikal, and also in the valley of Solenko in Eastern Mongolia to the north-east of Pekin.

In the different epidemic manifestations of the existing pandemic no important epizootic other than that prevailing among rats has been observed, such as is recorded in some of the older plague epidemics. But the examples cited indicate that there is always a possibility of plague becoming prevalent among many of the lower animals on the occasion of a severe epidemic, and that the disease among these animals may be an important agency in the maintenance and dissemination of plague in an infected locality. In this connection the chronicity of plague in some of the animals experimented on in Hongkong, the chronic form of plague as observed in guinea-pigs by Albrecht and Ghon in their experiments, and the chronic plague existing in rats for months as shown by Kolle and Martini are important as explaining the prolonged continuation of plague in endemic centres.

CHAPTER VI.

DIFFERENT VIEWS AS REGARDS THE ETIOLOGY OF
PANDEMICS AND EPIDEMICS OF PLAGUE.

THE discovery of the plague bacillus has as already stated put an end to the theory of the cause of plague being a gaseous emanation from the soil, and to the possibility of spontaneous generation independent of the plague bacillus. The power of growth and rapid reproduction which the bacillus displays when sown on a favourable medium supports the view that the infective agent of plague, notwithstanding its feeble resistance to many hostile influences, is able to maintain its existence, in at least some quarters of the globe, and there to flourish in man, in animals, or in the soil. The continuity of plague as thus understood, and its connection with homes of plague, temporary or permanent, are in direct opposition to the doctrine of the spontaneous origin of plague from particular or local conditions. This latter hypothesis arose in great measure from failure in the past to be able to trace a connection between great epidemics in different places. But as plague became rarer in Western Europe during the 18th and 19th centuries, and nearly every plague epidemic was traceable to a fresh importation from the East, the doctrine of the spontaneity of plague in a non-infected locality was considerably weakened, to be still further weakened by the facts ascertained in the present pandemic, when the facilities for tracing of cases and for chronicling them have been better than at any previous period. The specific nature of the infection, its differentiation from those infections causing other diseases, such as typhus, relapsing fever, malaria, and typhoid fever, which were formerly confused with plague, and the facilities for tracing the course of plague from one locality to another, are factors which have assisted in establishing the non-spontaneity of the origin of plague.

The present pandemic has exhibited an insidious, slow, steady, and widely distributed dispersal of the infection from infected centres to healthy localities, and it can be definitely stated that as far as modern plague is concerned there is no such thing as spontaneous origin in a non-infected locality, and that an outbreak, except in an endemic centre, is invariably due to importation of the bacillus. On the other hand in endemic regions the possible long vitality of the plague bacillus, the facilities which the microbe obtains of passing through the lower animals, without attracting any special attention either on account of the slightness of the symptoms or the chronicity of the disease produced, together with the variability of the bacillus in losing and acquiring virulence in some unknown way, certainly clothe the origin of plague in man with an apparent spontaneity.

A knowledge of the nature of the infection may be decisive enough in negativing the spontaneous origin of plague, but it does not settle questions closely allied to that of spontaneity, viz. how does the bacillus retain or acquire its specificity and virulence, and what are the determining factors in the diffusive qualities of plague? Virulence of the microbe is an inconstant factor, and may be so weakened as to lose the power of producing a recognisable specific disease. In what way can that virulence be retained or exalted? It is from this aspect that the older views of the origin of plague may be considered.

Some questions related to spontaneity.

For centuries the origin of the virus or infection of plague has been suspected to be due to putrefaction of dead bodies brought about by improper disposal, or by great physical disturbances in the phenomena of nature. The disturbances themselves, or their effects, have also been held to be not only the originators of plague, but also the cause of pandemics and epidemics.

Origin of plague long attributed to putrefaction of dead bodies, or to great physical disturbances.

Pariset[1], who was one of the Commissioners from France to study the plague in Syria and Egypt in 1829, first gave scientific shape to this old hypothesis that putrefaction of the bodies of the unburied or imperfectly buried is, under certain conditions, the origin of the plague virus.

Observing on the occasion of his investigations into plague in Egypt the condition of corpses buried in a soil subjected to inundations, Pariset came to the conclusion that these putrefying corpses and the putrid emanations from them were the source and origin of the plague virus, and the cause of the endemicity

Pariset's theory.

---

[1] *Mémoire sur les Causes de la Peste et sur les moyens de la détruire.* Par M. Étienne Pariset. Paris, 1837.

of plague in that country, which he took to be the birth-place of the disease. In the elaboration of his views he enters into the history of Egypt in regard to the disposal of the dead, showing that the ancient Egyptians down to the Christian era were most careful of their dead, embalming them and thus preserving them from the putridity which burial in a water-logged soil brings about. With the advance of Christianity these precautions gradually passed into desuetude. Pariset says: "The admirable police arrangements for sepulture were abolished. What a false zeal accomplished at Constantinople, at Rome, at Milan, in all the towns of the two empires, was done also in Egypt. The bodies of the martyrs and of the faithful filled the houses, the churches and the cemeteries as at the present day, and after a century, or a century and a half, the new method of honouring the dead caused one of the most terrible plagues in history to break out at Pelusium."

Following this up he shows that under the Arabian, and particularly the Turkish rule, Egypt gradually lost its high estate, sank from a fertile country with a healthy and highly civilised population into one in which the inhabitants were more or less slaves, ill fed, badly housed, and uncleanly; dwelling in huts and houses, damp and over-crowded, and so built as to be without fresh air or sufficient light. It was under these conditions the Copts had their family vaults in their houses, and every time one of the family died the slab of the vault was raised and a new corpse deposited on the older. Sometimes these vaults contained 80 to 90 bodies, and the family was only separated by a plank. There were at the time of the enquiry 300 Coptic houses in Cairo, nearly all occupying the centre of the city. To these insanitary conditions, more particularly the poisonous emanations from putrefying bodies in a wet soil, and in the vicinity of dwellings, Pariset ascribes the endemicity of plague in Egypt.

Creighton, 50 years afterwards, adopts a similar view as to the origin **Creighton supports Pariset's views.** of the plague virus, which he believes to be derived from the crude products of cadaveric decomposition polluting the soil and sub-soil. Earth-born in this wise, the plague virus could be carried by merchandise and by persons to localities in similar conditions as regards putrefaction to those in which the virus was generated, and finding them favourable for development infect the soil and the emanations from it, causing thereby an outbreak. With this special affinity for the products of cadaveric decomposition the virus of plague in the great epidemic of 1348 found in England a congenial soil in the monasteries and in the homes of the clergy. It may be remarked, however, that the monasteries were the centres of record, and accordingly it would be of them that the most details of the ravages of the epidemic would be given.

"Within the walls of the monastery, under the floor of the chapel or cloisters, were buried not only generations of monks, but often the bodies of princes, of notables of the surrounding country, and of great ecclesiastics. In every parish the house of the priest would have stood close to the church and the churchyard. One has to figure the virus of the Black Death, not so much as carried by individuals from place to place in their persons, or in their clothes and effects, but rather as a leaven which has passed into the ground, spreading hither and thither therein as if polarising the adjacent particles of the soil, and that not instantaneously like a physical force, but so gradually as to occupy a whole 12 months between Dorset and Yorkshire. Sooner or later it reached to every corner of the land, manifesting its presence wherever there were people resident. Such universality in the soil of England we have reason to think it had. But it appears to have put forth its greatest power in the walled town, in the monastery, and in the neighbourhood of the village churchyard[1]."

The mortality of rats and other animals in endemic centres of plague

Mortality of rats from plague not against Pariset's theory. antecedent to, or during an outbreak of plague, has always lent support to the theory that the soil is the probable manufactory of the plague virus. It was not, however, until 1894, that the two diseases were proved to be identical. The discovery of the plague bacillus disproves the emanation hypothesis, though it does not affect the question as to the soil being the seminary and seed-plot of the microbe. It rather strengthens it than otherwise. The fact that the rat suffers from a septicaemic variety of plague, occasioned sometimes at least by cannibalistic propensities, puts a new aspect on the subject of the relationship of plague to the soil. It not only shows that the older observers were partly right in their observations as to there being a connection between plague and the soil, but it also explains what that connection is, and how the plague can reach the dwellings of the inhabitants. Plague is carried slowly hither and thither by rats containing the plague bacillus in their bodies and in their excretions. Burial of plague corpses in endemic centres is always imperfect, as is the case with the burial of the dead generally, and it is within the range of probability that some rats at least acquire their infection from dead bodies of—men

[1] *History of Epidemics in Great Britain*, Creighton, p. 175, 1891.

and animals. In Cairo the Coptic vaults were not likely to have been quite safe against the attacks of these vermin.

It would appear that plague is a disease that under certain circumstances attacks animals other than rats as well as man. It may then be that the bacillus regains or acquires its virulence from an animal or series of animals through which it passes, and that some animal strains are more capable than others of infecting the general animal kingdom. In the pandemic of 1348, more than any other, except, perhaps, the Justinian or Byzantine plague, animals of all kinds seem to have been as susceptible as man. These questions are unhappily at present in the domain of speculation and they must remain there until money is expended in scientific research for their elucidation.

Great calamities of a cosmic or telluric nature have been assigned as the cause, not only of the generation of the plague virus, but also of the virulence and diffusiveness necessary to render the disease epidemic or pandemic. Plague may manifest itself in one city or district by a few cases; in another by a great epidemic; or it may overrun a province or country or one or two hemispheres. It is obvious that other factors besides the mere presence of the causal agents of plague must come into play in determining such very different results. Volcanic eruptions, earthquakes, the unusual conjunction of certain planets, irregular seasons, floods, droughts, famines, and the putrefaction of dead bodies, have, one and all, been brought into requisition as special causes, but to an age which is, more or less, unfamiliar with any continuous succession of extraordinary physical disturbances, the causes appear to be somewhat remote in their action and fantastical in their conception. The list includes influences which are likely only to have a subsidiary effect. The two great consequences of these catastrophes are the ensuing putrefaction of the dead, and the miserable condition of the living, whose homes and food have been destroyed. These depressing conditions are generally favourable to the revivification and to the rapid and wide extension of any endemic disease. India furnishes a number of instances in which cholera has broken out in epidemic form after a destructive inundation, as for example in the severe epidemic which affected the survivors of the great tidal wave which swept over the Sunderbunds in Bengal in 1879. The natural resistance of those who escaped the flood was probably reduced by the shock which they had suffered and by the depressing influence of inadequate shelter and insufficient food.

Origin of plague attributed to great calamities cosmic and telluric.

The antecedents in Asia of the great pandemic of 1348, given in Deguignes' *Histoire Générale des Huns*, and made use

The Black Death preceded by great disturbances in the balance of nature. of by Hecker in his *Epidemics of the Middle Ages*, are a succession of extraordinary and exceptional events denoting some great deviation from the ordinary sequence characteristic of the phenomena of nature and its seasons.

Deguignes follows the Arab historian Mahassin, who records the commencement of the plague in Tartary and its connection with the smell of corpses arising from the perishing of men, beasts, and even birds in the disastrous floods. The infection thus produced obtained a ready means of transport westwards by the northern caravan route, whose European marts were on the Caspian and the Black Sea, and by which gateway it entered Europe.

Hecker places the commencement of the Black Death in China, and attributes the virulence of the disease and its pandemicity to the mighty revolutions of the earth which are recorded to have preceded it.

"[1]From China to the Atlantic, the foundations of the earth were shaken. Throughout Asia and Europe the atmosphere was in commotion and endangered by its baneful influence both vegetable and animal life." He writes of a succession of inundations, earthquakes and famines, which, commencing in China, spread over the greater part of the known world, and it is in China the great pandemic is held to have originated.

Creighton, while accepting the origin of the plague virus from the decomposition of corpses, is perplexed, like many others

Creighton places the origin of the Black Death on the borders of the Euxine or Black Sea. who have given the subject their attention, to find that though in China from 1333 to 1352 there are records of great physical disasters with great mortality ensuing, there are no entries in the chronicles of a great plague until the latter year. For this reason, and because there were special conditions at the European entrepots on the Black Sea favourable to the development of epidemic disease, he shifts the place of commencement to the marts on the Black Sea. What were then the conditions of the emporia or European termini of the trade from the Far East to cause them to be suspected as the principal factors in the generation and birth of the Black Death?

Creighton[2] describes these conditions on the authority of the

---

[1] *The Epidemics of the Middle Ages*, p. 11. By J. F. C. Hecker, M.D.

[2] *History of the Epidemics of Great Britain*, Vol. I. p. 144. By Charles Creighton, M.A., M.D., 1891.

manuscript of Gabriel de Mussis, a jurist of Piacenza, who had been practising as a notary or advocate among the Genoese and Venetians trading around the shores of the Euxine and Caspian.

It was at a time when these shores and the country north of them were harassed by the Tartar hordes. Among other incidents, the Italian merchants were besieged, first at Tana, then at Caffa. The siege of the latter town was maintained for three years, and caused those invested to be put to great straits. Plague broke out in the Tartar army and the dead bodies were thrown by the besiegers from their war engines into the town, so that the infection took hold of those within the fort. The mortality, however, became so great among the Tartars that, panic-stricken, they fled from the siege and spread the plague wherever they went. It was then that some Italian traders, and Gabriel de Mussis with them, escaped from Caffa in a ship and arrived in due course at Genoa, where plague broke out in a most deadly form a few days after, *although none of those on board were suffering from the disease.*

In making a choice between the origin of the plague virus among the Tartar hordes besieging the merchants within the walls of Caffa and the pre-existence of that virus for a long time latent among the goods or effects of the besieged, Creighton gives the preference to the latter hypothesis on the ground of advantage in probability; why the latter should be chosen rather than the former is not very clear. Three or more years is a long time for the virus to be latent in towns with the conditions prevailing in Tana, Caffa, and Sarai, whereas it is not an uncommon event for plague to be associated with armies in the field in that part of the world. The explanation is a reasonable one if the facts and conditions set forth by de Mussis were correct, but unfortunately there is a doubt as to the accuracy of the account given by him, who is looked upon rather as another Daniel de Foe than a recorder of facts of which he himself was an eye-witness. The lower region of the Volga was the scene of an intense exaltation of the plague virus as recently as 1879, when a mild manifestation of plague in Astrakhan suddenly assumed a most virulent form, but this was in the depth of winter and without any attendant decomposition of a special character and without the acquisition of diffusive powers. As a matter of fact it was a self-limiting plague, though the virulence was extremely violent.

The account given by Creighton cannot be said to literally agree with that given by de Mussis in his manuscript, for instead of no one on board suffering from the plague it states that on departure there were a few sailors on board infected with the pestilential disease, and out of a thousand passengers and crew in the several ships scarce ten survived when the ships arrived at Genoa. Literally translated by Dr J. F. Payne from the Latin manuscript, a copy of which is given by Haeser, the account is as follows:

"[1]In the year 1346 innumerable tribes of Tartars and Saracens perished in these regions by an inexplicable disease. Whole tracts of country, innumerable provinces, splendid kingdoms, cities, camps, and towns abounding in population were attacked by a horrible death, and in a short time denuded of their inhabitants. Now a town called Thanna, in the eastern region towards the north, a place trading with Constantinople, was besieged and conquered by a great army of Tartars; and it happened that the Christian merchants, driven out by force, took refuge within the walls of Caffa, which the Genoese had formerly built in that region. Suddenly the infidel tribes of Tartars, collecting from all sides, surrounded the city and besieged the Christians, who were shut up there for nearly three years; when lo! a disease attacked the Tartars, and the whole of the besieging army fell into a state of weakness and disorder so that many thousands of them died daily. It seemed to the besieged Christians as if arrows were shot out of the sky to strike and humble the pride of the infidels, who rapidly died with marks on their bodies and lumps in their joints and several parts, followed by putrid fever; all advice and help of the doctors being of no avail. Whereupon the Tartars, worn out by this pestilential disease, and falling on all sides as if thunderstruck, and seeing that they were perishing hopelessly, ordered the corpses to be placed upon their engines and thrown into the city of Caffa. Accordingly were the bodies of the dead hurled over the walls, so that the Christians were not able to hide or protect themselves from this danger, although they carried away as many dead as possible and threw them into the sea. But soon the whole air became infected, and the water poisoned, and such a pestilence grew up that scarcely one out of a thousand was able to escape.

"Thus were the Orientals in all parts, both those who lived on the southern shore and those on the north, struck down by this pestilential disease, and almost all of them died. So great was the mortality that Kathayans, Indians, Persians, Medes, Armenians, Georgians, Turcomans, Arabs, Saracens, and Greeks throughout the whole of the East, gave themselves up to clamour, weeping, and sighs, and remained in this

[1] *Plagues Ancient and Modern.* St Thomas' Hospital Reports. Vol. XVII.

distress from the above-mentioned year to 1348, expecting that the Day of Judgment was at hand.

"Now it so happened that a ship left the aforesaid land of Caffa, having on board a few sailors (who were also infected with the pestilential disease), and made for Genoa, some other ships going also to Venice and others to other parts of Christendom. Marvellous to relate. whenever the navigators arrived at any land, as if some malignant spirits accompanied them, wherever they mingled with other men the latter perished. Every city, every town, every country, and their inhabitants of both sexes, poisoned by the pestiferous contagion of the diseased, fell a prey to sudden death, and when one began to be sick, soon falling and dying, he poisoned the whole of the family. Those who came in to bury the bodies perished by the same disease. Thus whole cities and castles were made desolate, and only the waste places themselves were left to mourn for their dead inhabitants.

"Alas! when our ships arrived at any city, and we entered our houses, our relatives, our connections and neighbours flocked in to see us from all sides, because we were still in bad health, and out of a thousand who sailed with us scarce ten survived; but alas! we carried with us the arrows of death. And while they were embracing and kissing us we could not help pouring out poison from the lips with which we spoke. So they, returning to their houses, soon poisoned their own families, and within three days the whole household, struck down, succumbed to the dart of death, and the number of the dead increased so much that the ground was not sufficient for their graves. Priests and doctors, whom their great care for the sick compelled to be present at the death-bed, alas! returned home sick themselves and quickly followed the deceased."

The account by de Mussis as literally transcribed consorts more or less with other contemporary authors who mention the prevalence of the pandemic in Central Asia and India before its entrance into Europe. The disease being accredited as having begun in Tartary may mean any part of Asia, for the vast empire of Kublai Khan still remained, though broken up into many sections and ruled over by his descendants and lieutenants. There were Tartars everywhere in power from Hungary in Europe to the eastern coast of China. The westward wave of that great invasion of Mongols begun by Gengiz Khan had not yet ebbed, and Tartar and Turkish kingdoms were established on the coasts of the Persian

Considerations showing the difficulty and even the impossibility of now locating the origin of the 14th century pandemic.

Gulf and the Black Sea as they were around the Caspian. It is difficult enough at the present day in times of peace, and with the facilities which steam and electricity afford, to locate the origin of any pandemic. We have examples of this in the pandemics of cholera and influenza of the 19th century. They were never traced to any particular source, or to any special set of conditions. The source of the recent pandemic of influenza became a very movable affair if the localities from which it is believed to have originated are taken into account. It was ultimately supposed to come from Russia or some part of the Russian dominions which extend over the greater part of Northern Asia, and it has even been pushed back further to some remote and unknown part of China. The tendency at all times is to locate the origin of rare diseases in some distant and unknown country. Plague in recent years has been given a theoretical endemic area in Thibet, a country into which no one, until the British Expedition of 1904 forced its way in, has been permitted to enter, and about which nothing is known. Once creating an imaginary home in this unknown country plague is supposed to have travelled down to Yunnan in China on one side, and Kumaon and Garhwal in India on the other. These are all matters of assumption which it is impossible to affirm or deny. Until the world is circled with the telegraph, and that which has happened even in remote places is immediately known, it will not be easy to locate the exact place where a pandemic takes its origin. All that is known of the origin of the plague of 1348 is, that having prevailed in a malignant form for several years in the East, it entered Europe by the Black Sea, and probably also by the caravan routes of Mesopotamia and Asia Minor, and that it occurred at a time when the division of the Mogul or Tartar empire on the death of Kublai Khan caused large portions of Asia to be a constant seat of warfare.

Volcanic eruptions have on occasion apparently given rise to disease in a limited degree. Humboldt relates that in an eruption of Cotopaxi so many fish of the order Pimelodus were ejected that they poisoned the air all round, and it is recorded by Pouchet that near the end of the 18th century the town of Bourra was ravaged by a malignant fever, which was attributable to the miasmata arising from the decomposition of an enormous number of these fish vomited by a neighbouring volcano. Humboldt again relates in his travels that at the end of violent earthquakes the herbs that covered the Savannahs of Tucuman acquired noxious properties, and that an epidemic disorder broke out

Volcanic eruptions are recorded to have rendered plants and herbage poisonous.

among the cattle, and a great number of them appeared stupefied or
suffocated by the deleterious vapours exhaled by the ground. If herbs
can be rendered poisonous in this way, it may be possible that low
vegetable organisms such as bacilli can acquire virulent properties under
similar conditions, or disturbances of Nature.

Atmospheric causes of a far-reaching character, which are followed
by lean and fat years of famine and plenty, are not without
their influence on germ life in the lower plant orders.
Droughts, floods and other cosmic disturbances which are
destructive to the grain and food of man and animals, and
which are productive of famines and general misery, do
not appear to be injurious to the germs of disease. On the contrary,
while the higher orders of plants wither and die, the lower orders, among
which may be included the plague bacillus, appear to find in the
exceptional circumstances conditions highly favourable to a rapid and
luxuriant growth.

Great multiplication of disease germs associated with lean or famine years.

Exceptional circumstances of weather and other adverse events
were not wanting in Hongkong, in India, in Bombay or
in the Cape to favour the development of plague, once the
infection was introduced. Some time previous to the
outbreak of plague in 1894 several extraordinary phenomena were noticed in Hongkong. The year before extreme
cold prevailed during the winter, and for three days the
Peak was covered with ice to within about 400 feet of
the sea level, and the hills on the mainland opposite Hongkong were
covered with snow. In the autumn of 1891, 1892, 1893, and 1894, an
epidemic of caterpillars[1], *Thialleta signifera* and *Pharazia bicarsisatis*,
attacked the trees and grass in Hongkong in such multitudes that the
Government employed men to gather them, for which they were paid
at a certain rate. Then the flowering of the male bamboo was noticed,
and this, combined with an eclipse of the sun and the other phenomena,
presaged, according to the Chinese, an epidemic of some kind.

Exceptional meteorological conditions preceded the epidemic of plague in Hongkong.

If the signs of the times could have been read aright, they would
have indicated that India was under conditions specially
favourable to the maintenance and spread of some epidemic
disease. In 1896 there was failure of the crops over a considerable part of the country, creating scarcity and a rise in the price
of food. Large numbers of famine-stricken or destitute people flocked

Scarcity preceded plague in India.

---

[1] *Reports of the Botanical and Afforestation Department for Hongkong*, 1892, 1893, and
1894.

from the famine districts into Bombay. In 1897 the famine area became more extensive and there were severe earthquakes in the eastern parts of India. The inference is not that either of these was the cause of the plague, but that their occurrence showed an abnormal atmospheric and terrestrial condition which was likely to favour the epidemicity of plague once introduced into the country.

Cases of plague occurred in Bombay as early as May 1896, but it was not until the following October that the disease attracted any special attention and began to spread. The local phenomena which preceded the epidemic are described by Dr Weir, the

Abnormal season preceded epidemic of plague in Bombay. Health Officer[1]. The mean temperature of the year was 80·70, which was the second highest on record during the previous 51 years. The total fall of rain amounted to 87·6 inches, which was 15 inches above the average. It was not only above the average, but it was abnormal also in distribution and in duration. The heavy rainfall, owing to an obstruction in the sewage outfall, flooded with sewage the low-lying portions of the city, through which the polluted streams rushed in swirling currents, leaving banks of mud and sludge behind to ferment or dry slowly, and although the monsoon practically ceased in August, the shady sides of the streets in crowded portions of the city remained damp long afterwards. In September only 1·6 inches of rain fell, being as much below the average as the earlier months had been above. Even in the famine years of 1876–77 the September rainfall was not less than 4 inches. An abnormal September was followed by an abnormal October, dry and warm. In September the godowns in Mandvie, the district in which plague first broke out epidemically, were still damp.

The city appears to have been in an exceptional plight due to an abnormal season of rainfall, that lasted only about half the normal period, and which produced an abnormally high level of sewage in the arterial sewers, and soakage of the grain in dark and damp godowns or granaries underneath human dwellings. All traffic to the island was interrupted for five days. The grain lay in the wet. The low-lying portions of Bombay were under water. At the most distant points on the esplanade, near the head of the drainage system, water welled up through the man-holes. The subsoil water welled up where it had never been seen before, and wells overflowed that had never previously been full. Dr Weir lays stress on the fact that during this period wet

[1] *Report of the Health Officer for Bombay for* 1896, p. 610.

grain was stored in wet granaries with no means of ventilation. These, he remarks, are the conditions most favourable to the generation of disease, and had it been necessary to cultivate the microbe, it would not have been possible to have created artificially more favourable conditions, *i.e.* organic matter, moisture, warmth, and darkness. These were the conditions which existed in the granaries, in the floors above which the disease first became epidemic.

A similar abnormal season preceded the epidemic outbreak of plague in Cape Town in 1901, which occurred at a time of war and scarcity. The season at the beginning of the year was altogether exceptional. It was cold when it should have been hot, wet when it should have been dry, and in every way it was abnormal. The rainfall in January was abnormal, and was the heaviest recorded since 1842 when observations began to be made. In this respect the conditions of Cape Town corresponded with those of Bombay in 1896, when the outbreak of plague in September was preceded by an exceptional season and abnormal rainfall in July and August. In Cape Town a rare comet was visible for several nights.

Unusual season preceded epidemic of plague in Cape Town.

It will be seen that the explanations of the causes of the origin and development of pandemics and epidemics, as distinguished from the conditions which have been generally observed to favour their continuance and spread, are all within the region of speculation. To-day we are no nearer their explanation than our predecessors, who ascribed them to the anger of the gods, to astronomical conjunctions, to putridity, to epidemic influences, and to numerous other causes. All that is definitely known is that pandemics and epidemics are generally associated with unusual seasons which bring distress and misery, with war and famine and their attendant ills, with political, social or economical conditions which are the reverse of prosperous, and which produce general depression in the community, and also with a laxity or absence of sanitary administration which prevents or hinders prompt dealing with the earlier cases. They also acquire their ascendancy owing to incomplete knowledge as to the different modes by which they spread, and as to the laws governing these. Some of the modes are known, but others being unknown there is always the risk, even when administrative action is prompt, of the preventive measures employed being only partially successful in checking and controlling the disease.

Conclusion.

CHAPTER VII.

VARIATION IN POWERS OF DIFFUSION OF EPIDEMICS AND THE EFFECT OF SEASONAL INFLUENCES ON THEM.

VARIATION in powers of diffusion is indicated by the terms sporadic, epidemic, and pandemic, which are applied to plague.

Variation in diffusive powers. When the disease is imported into a country it is impossible to foretell which quality it will assume, or how long it will continue to retain the quality it first displays. There are

Self-limiting plagues. self-limiting plagues and there are plagues which possess great powers of diffusion, but the exact conditions under which each obtains, or which determine the one or the other, or by which the one is distinguished from the other before its results are known, are, as will be surmised, still a matter for research. The factors controlling the diffusion of plague are really unknown. The Cyrenaic, Mesopotamian, and Persian outbreaks during the fifties, sixties, and seventies of the 19th century were shown by Tholozan to be self-limited. They spread to a certain extent and then stopped, not because of the preventive measures taken, for they were usually applied either too late or not at all, but because of some general law which is not yet understood. The plague at Vetlianka was a self-limiting plague. When alarm was aroused most energetic measures were applied, but not until the disease had spent itself. Like the local outbreak at Benghazi in Northern Africa and in the Assyr district in Western Arabia, the outbreak at Vetlianka began and ended within a comparatively circumscribed area.

The existing pandemic, though it may seem paradoxical to say so, possesses comparatively small diffusive qualities, notwith-

The existing pandemic possesses comparatively small diffusive powers. standing its success in reaching a large number of countries. Its tendency in most places where it has acquired a footing is not to spread to any great extent. This may be only a temporary characteristic, for India is an exception. But even in India, with the rapid means of intercommunication which the country possesses, the extension of the disease is comparatively limited, and does not compare with the progress of the 14th century or the 6th century epidemic, or with the pandemics of influenza and cholera of the 19th century. On the whole the manifestation of plague in different places has been, with the exception of India and China, more sporadic than epidemic. Nowhere as yet have the great ravages common to the towns and villages of India and Southern China been repeated elsewhere.

A great sowing of seed has been effected, but apparently for the most part on ground which is barren or only slightly favourable to growth. Telegraphic and postal communications have brought civilised countries into such intimate relationship with one another that outbreaks of plague of any considerable size are immediately heard of, and their progress followed in a manner that was never possible before. Never before has there been such an opportunity of watching so closely the gradual scattering of the seed over an area of the globe which has for centuries been free of plague. The European powers at the Venice Convention of 1897 agreed to notify to each other any case of plague in their respective dominions coming to their official notice. The result has been the possibility for the first time of tracing the different movements and gradual progress of the plague, and with it certain features in the epidemiology of plague have become conspicuous. These are the slowness of the progressive advance, the evident difficulty with which new centres are formed, and the absence at present of any special tendency to severe epidemics. They are features probably not new to plague, for they are likely to have been overlooked at earlier periods when the facilities for obtaining information were less than they are now. If it be true that plague has generally such a vanguard of sporadic cases when spreading in pandemic form, these sporadic cases may be the missing links which are so frequently wanting in tracing the connection between concurrent epidemics in widely separated places.

There is one noticeable feature belonging to the existing pandemic and which presages danger in the future. It is that notwithstanding its apparent inability to cause in any one place a great epidemic, it exhibits in some places marvellous powers of recrudescence and resistance to all known measures of prevention, and this, even when the cases are few. This tenacious capacity combined with its transportability makes it formidable because its slow progress, few cases, and possibly slight mortality, accustom the people to its presence, and lull the authorities into a frame of mind of looking upon it as a very manageable disease. In the meantime it gradually dots itself over different parts of the country, securing a firm hold in some localities which again form fresh centres for its activity, until, in the course of a few years, it is fairly established in the country at many centres, and only awaits the conditions necessary for its development into an alarming epidemic. In this respect its behaviour, when established in a country, is likely to be similar to small-pox in an unvaccinated country in which there are a series of years with a few cases followed by one or two epidemic years. In Africa and South America the dotting stage appears to be in progress.

The danger of the existing pandemic lies not so much in its present aspects with its slight diffusive powers, but in the oppor-tunities which it may meet with of acquiring both virulence and diffusive qualities. Such opportunities would arise in the case of distress on a large scale from economical or political causes, from atmospheric conditions giving rise to scarcity, or from war. None of these will themselves give rise to plague, but with plague spreading as at present, any one of them would serve to render it formidable.

The danger of the existing pandemic.

It is because of these dangers that the plague in India with its extensive area of infection may at any time become a menace to Europe, for it possesses all the potentialities which once developed would give it those diffusive qualities that have characterised former pandemics. It has at present reached Cashmere and is not far from the borders of Afghanistan. Should it attack and pass through the latter country, it then reaches the high road through which so many epidemics have entered Russia and Europe. There is always the possibility of the plague in India assuming the influenza type, and should this ever occur then there is nothing to prevent a repetition of the ravages that plague committed in the sixth and fourteenth centuries.

From an epidemiological point of view there are two varieties of plague. Between them are plagues which approximate more to the one or to the other variety. The first and the most common is that which frequents the more or less endemic areas and their neighbourhood, with small tendency to spread. It may possess considerable powers of ex-tension once it has passed beyond the bounds of the endemic area, but it seldom displays any great contagious qualities, most frequently re-taining the characters of its origin. The second is on the other hand a plague of an expansive and diffusive character, manifestly contagious both to man and to many kinds of the lower animals, and is capable of causing wide-spread destruction to both.

PLAGUE EPIDEMICS AND SEASONAL INFLUENCES.

The season of the year has a very powerful influence on the prevalence of plague and the duration of the epidemic. There
may be in any locality a few cases of plague all the year
round, for instance in Bombay and in Hongkong there is
not a month without a case, but it is only at certain
seasons that the disease becomes epidemic. This season may vary
somewhat in different localities, but it is nearly always the same in
the same locality, and has a tendency to become earlier the further
south it occurs. Plague may occur in endemic centres such as in the
mountainous regions of Assyr or Kurdistan under conditions of intense
cold; but intense cold or intense heat are generally inimical to the rise
of an epidemic, though they do not prevent the occurrence of sporadic
cases even outside the endemic areas, when these sporadic cases are the
remnants of a preceding epidemic or the harbingers of one that is
impending. An occasional outbreak of pneumonic plague such as the
Vetlianka outbreak may take place in the depth of a severe winter, but
it is seldom of any great dimensions. Similarly small epidemics have
occurred in Sindh with a temperature of between 110° F. and 120° F.,
but they are exceptions.

Plague epi-
demics occur
at particular
seasons of the
year.

The development and decline of the epidemic of plague in Bombay in
1896 are shown in Diagram A on the next page, taken from the report of
the Health Officer on the outbreak, and is an excellent type of the usual
characters of most great epidemics of plague. First of all there is a
period of hesitancy more or less prolonged; then there is a sudden but
fluctuating rise which reaches its highest point in the course of three
months or in a shorter time; and then there is a decline possessing
much the same character as the ascent but often less prolonged; and
finally the disease lingers in a sporadic form for some months.

The duration of any of these stages may vary somewhat, being
either lengthened or shortened, so that within the plague season there
may be epidemics lasting from 4 to 8 months. If the epidemics themselves were analysed, they would be found to be more or less a series
of epidemics invading at different times different districts of the same
city. The months of epidemic prevalence in several towns, the month
in which the epidemic reached its maximum and the duration of the
epidemic, are shown in Diagram B on page 148.

DIAGRAM A.

Weekly Total and Average Mortality.

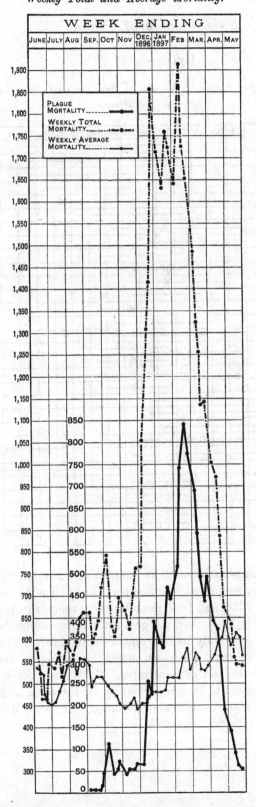

Diagram B.

*Duration of Epidemics and Months of their greatest Intensity in
different Localities.*

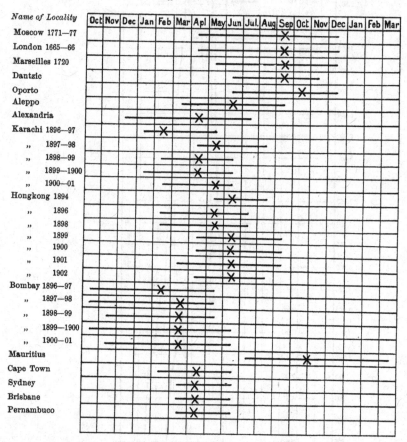

Name of Locality	Oct	Nov	Dec	Jan	Feb	Mar	Apl	May	Jun	Jul.	Aug	Sep	Oct	Nov	Dec	Jan	Feb	Mar
Moscow 1771—77												✕						
London 1665—66												✕						
Marseilles 1720												✕						
Dantzic												✕						
Oporto													✕					
Aleppo								✕										
Alexandria						✕												
Karachi 1896—97					✕													
„ 1897—98							✕											
„ 1898—99						✕												
„ 1899—1900						✕												
„ 1900—01							✕											
Hongkong 1894								✕										
„ 1896							✕											
„ 1898							✕											
„ 1899								✕										
„ 1900								✕										
„ 1901								✕										
„ 1902								✕										
Bombay 1896—97					✕													
„ 1897—98						✕												
„ 1898—99						✕												
„ 1899—1900						✕												
„ 1900—01						✕												
Mauritius														✕				
Cape Town						✕												
Sydney						✕												
Brisbane						✕												
Pernambuco						✕												

In Europe great epidemics occur in summer and autumn, the worst
months being usually August and September. In London the epidemics
of 1603, 1605, 1625, 1636, and 1665 resembled one another in beginning
in June and ending in December, the greatest number of deaths being
between the latter part of July and the end of September. In Marseilles
the epidemic of 1720 took a similar course, beginning in June and
declining rapidly at the end of September. In Moscow the epidemic
of 1770 raged from April to December, but by far the worst month was
September, when 21,000 deaths were recorded. In Asia Minor the

epidemic season is generally spring and summer. The Syrian epidemics
usually began in March or April and ended in August, the worst month
being June. The Egyptian epidemics generally commenced in December
or January and terminated in June or July, the highest mortality occurring in March or April. At other periods of the year the disease
was more or less quiescent, the last half of the year having comparatively
few cases. Recent epidemics in Egypt have shown similar seasonal
characteristics. In Hongkong plague prevails epidemically in the late
spring and summer and reaches its height in May or June.

DIAGRAM C.

Chart showing the mortality from the Plague for the year 1903
compared with the average of the previous 5 *years.*

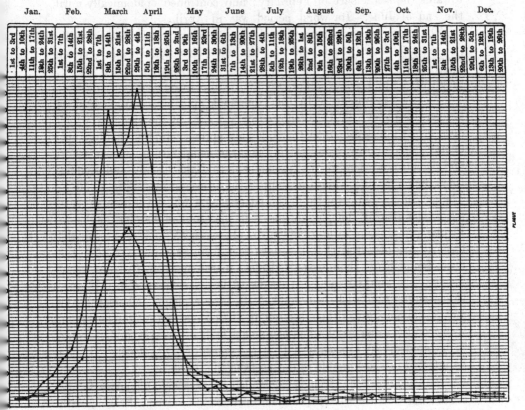

In India there may be two epidemic seasons: one in January,
February and March, and another in August, September, October and

November. In Bombay plague prevails from October or November to May or June and reaches its height in February or March. In Calcutta it prevails a little later than in Bombay and reaches its height in March or April. The seasonal occurrence of plague in Calcutta is shown in the Diagram C taken from the report of the Health Officer for Calcutta for the year 1903.

On the other hand the epidemics at Poona have been later in the year.

In the Mauritius it is epidemic from July to March, arriving at its climax usually in October or November. In the southern hemisphere epidemics manifest themselves during the first half of the year. In Cape Town plague was epidemic from February to June, being worst between the end of March and the first weeks of April. It was much the same in Brisbane and in Sydney, where the plague was first detected towards the latter part of February; and continued epidemically until the end of June. Its worst period was in April.

The range of temperature favourable to plague varies considerably in different localities, the most favourable being between **Temperature affects the endemicity of plague.** 56° F. and 75° F.; mean temperatures above 85° F. and below 50° F. are as a rule unsuitable for epidemic prevalence. In the Hongkong epidemics any continuous temperature above 83° F. is followed by a decline of the epidemic which does not begin again until the following spring. In the Bombay epidemic there is always a fall when the mean temperature is above 82° F. and sometimes when it reaches 80° F. In Cape Colony and Sydney there was a decline when the temperature lowered to a mean of 50° F. The maximum temperature in the latter places was never so high as to check the rise of the plague once the disease had become epidemic. Plague prevailed most at temperatures between 55° and 70° F. In the Cape it was observed that ten days to a fortnight after a rise in the mean temperature there was an increase in the number of plague cases.

No very marked influence seems to be exerted by rain. If anything, slight rain with heat appears to favour plague, whereas heavy and continuous rain, although often an antecedent of a plague outbreak, seems, on the other hand, when plague has broken out, to be unfavourable to its epidemicity especially if it is the cause of large floods. It may be infected rats are unable to escape from the floods.

Why plague is so strongly controlled by seasonal influences is one **Season a composite force.** of the many problems still to be solved. Season, with its meteorological factors, is a composite force, and as such operates in more than one way on the agents and media connected with

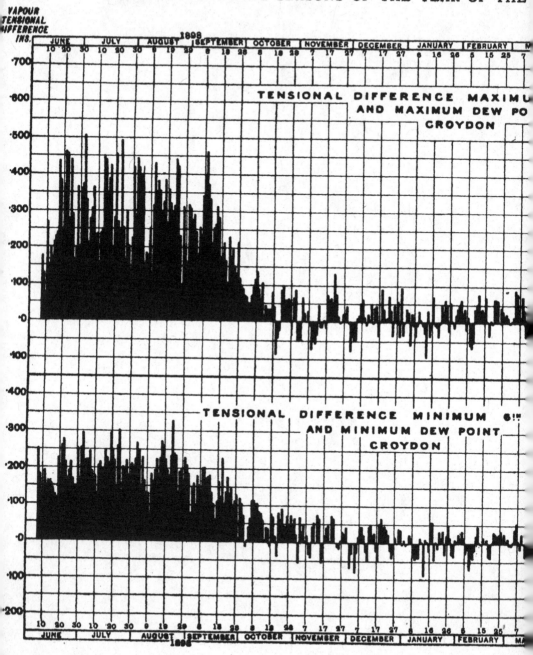

TENSIONAL DIFFERENCE MAXIMU
AND MAXIMUM DEW PO
CROYDON

TENSIONAL DIFFERENCE MINIMUM 6ᴵᴺ
AND MINIMUM DEW POINT
CROYDON

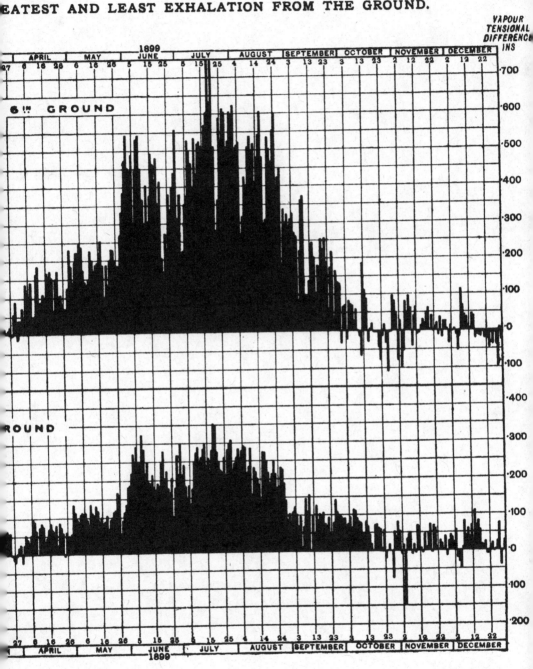

plague. For instance it affects a man's constitution and powers of resistance against infective diseases in various ways through its influence on the air, soil and food which react on man; it affects the plague bacillus in regard to reproduction and virulence, and it affects animal and insect life as well. The difficulty lies in differentiating the main factors of which season is composed, and in determining the exact influence of each on man, the plague germ, and on animals and insects concerned in the spread of plague.

The older writers observing seasonal variations in plague were content in attributing it to an "epidemic constitution," and did not attempt to analyse what that constitution was. We are no further advanced to-day in this respect. The only serious investigation into the influence of different climatic factors on plague is that carried out by Mr Baldwin Latham[1]. He found no particular tem-

Mr Baldwin Latham's analysis of the influence of climatic factors on plague.

perature of the air nor temperature of the ground to have any marked connection with the incidence of plague, but that plague prevailed at a period of the year when exhalations from the ground were greatest, and ceased at a time when the ground exhalations were slightest. Diagram D shows the season of the year when the vaporous exhalations are highest and lowest in Croydon. Comparing these with the weekly number of deaths from plague in London in the years 1564, 1592, 1603, 1607, 1636, 1642, and 1665, and also with the vaporous exhalations in London during a period of 15 years, he finds, as is shown on the diagram on page 152, that there is a strong marked parallelism between the tensional differences which are the cause of vapours rising from the ground and the plague epidemics which formerly occurred in this country.

An interesting point is that a similar investigation into the tensional differences in Bombay and the prevalence of plague there brought out a similar result, although the period of the year in which plague occurred in London was not the same as in Bombay. It was demonstrated that the forces that gave rise to earthy exhalations only came into operation in Bombay as in London at the particular times that the plague was rife.

Experimenting with cylinders filled with earth freely suspended in a perforated tube within the earth, at depths of 1 foot and 2 feet below the surface, it was ascertained that the hygrometric

[1] "The Climatic Conditions necessary for the Propagation of Plague." By Baldwin Latham. *Quarterly Journal of the Royal Meteorological Society*, Vol. xxxvi. No. 118, Jan. 1900.

condition of the ground varied according to the temperature of the air and the temperature of the ground. The earth cylinders increased in weight when the air was warmer than the ground, and lost weight when the temperature of the air fell below that of the ground, or in other words when the air was warmer than the earth condensation took place, but when the earth was warmer than the air evaporation took place.

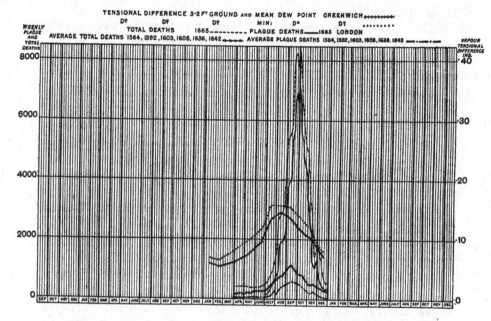

The periods of the year when exhalations escape from the ground and the quantity that then arises were then determined. Numerous observations were made by which the temperatures of the ground at different depths were compared with the temperatures of the dew point, and the factors thus obtained were employed for calculating the tensional difference between the ground air and the temperature of the dew point. At all times the exhalations take place in proportion to the tensional differences. The results, as stated, compared with the period of the year of plague epidemics in Bombay and London, showed that the rise and fall of the tensional differences between the ground temperature and the minimum dew point agreed in a remarkable manner with the rise and fall of plague. Mr Baldwin Latham deduces from his observations that a high temperature of the air, by raising the temperature of the dew point, and causing condensation to take place, stops plague; while a fall in temperature means a fall in temperature of the dew point, and the tensional difference between a low dew point and a high ground temperature, which would at once lead to exhalations which Mr Baldwin Latham thinks would cause liberation of plague bacilli from the ground. There is no evidence at present as to the possibility of plague bacilli being lifted from the soil by these forces. The facts are against it, but the question needs to be scientifically settled by experiment. It sounds like the old hypothetical cause of malaria which the investigations of Laveran, Ross, Manson and others have completely destroyed. If the vapours have any influence, it is probably in the direction of favouring a condition productive of susceptibility of the organism in man or the lower animals or in both.

The phenomena observed recently of strong electrical currents in the earth disorganising the telegraph service indicate that the conditions of the soil are influenced considerably by meteorological changes, and that the conditions of the soil at different times may possess powerful properties.

The varying hygrometric condition of the soil and its fluctuating temperature are just the conditions likely to affect the multiplication and possible virulence of the plague bacillus. At the same time they may exercise a great influence on the life of insects which may carry infection to and between animals susceptible to plague such as rats. An instance of certain seasonal conditions, bringing into activity swarms of insects, is to be seen in the annual but sudden appearance of green flies in Calcutta near the end of the rains. So great is their number that for several nights it is impossible to read with comfort except under a mosquito curtain. They get into the food and drink, swarm around the lamps, and it is impossible to be comfortable for the few nights of their ephemeral existence. The flies disappear almost as suddenly as they come. They are the harbingers of the cold weather. It is possible that insect life of a different order, useful in assisting the spread of plague by acting as carriers, may be brought into activity by certain conditions of the soil. In relation to this it is interesting to note that Dr Tidswell[1], when collecting different species of fleas infesting rats, had no difficulty during the epidemic of plague of finding many fleas on rats, but as soon as the epidemic was over the rats appeared to be exceptionally free of fleas. The egg, larva and

The varying condition of the soil and its fluctuating temperature, likely to have an effect on microbic and insect life.

[1] "Ecto-parasites of the Rat." By Frank Tidswell, M.B. *Report of the Board of Health on a second outbreak of Plague at Sydney*, 1902. By J. Ashburton Thompson, M.D., President.

pupa of fleas on rats are probably affected in their development by the seasonal temperature and moisture of the soil, which vary in time in different places but recur about the same time yearly in the same locality.

That a mean temperature of 83° F. should exert so marked a control over an epidemic of plague, while the bacillus flourishes in man at

The temperature of the air itself not directly influential. 98° F. and in birds at 107° F., leads one to suppose that the influence is not a direct one on the plague bacillus itself, which appears to be able to develop at considerably higher temperatures than 83° F. Especially is this view emphasised when it is considered how much the infection is a house infection, where direct sunshine plays a very unimportant part, the microbe being never exposed to any very high aerial temperature, or to any exceptionally low temperature which might destroy it.

Connected with seasonal influences is also the peculiar fact that, on

At the end of the plague season infected articles lose their infectivity, but may regain it the following season. the decline of an epidemic, infected articles and houses in the infected locality lose their power of infection for the time being, until the favourable season comes round again. The best examples of this are from epidemics belonging to an earlier period than those of the existing pandemic, because the latter are not dissociated from active measures for the suppression of the disease. The fact is, however, discernible in all, whether old or recent. In the plagues of London, Marseilles, Naples and Egypt the inhabitants who fled when the epidemic was increasing have flocked back to the infected houses towards the end of the epidemic, have slept in infected beds, and have worn the clothes of those who have died of plague, yet beyond a number of accidents here and there that general infection which was to have been feared has not taken place; and yet when a recrudescence takes place in the season of the following or a subsequent year, the infection is frequently, as in Hongkong it was largely, connected with plague in the same house in the previous year or in the year previous to that.

That healthy persons run great risk of contracting the disease during the epidemic season by sleeping in beds previously occupied by plague patients was shown in Cairo in 1835, when on the 15th of April two criminals, Ibrahim Assan and Ben Ali, condemned to death, were taken from the citadel in Cairo and given beds to sleep in which had been vacated by two patients suffering from well-marked plague. On the 19th of April, Ibrahim was attacked by plague with bubo and carbuncle. He died on the 23rd. Ben Ali was also attacked at the end of the 3rd day with the ordinary symptoms indicating the invasion of plague, but the illness aborted and convalescence commenced on the 4th day.

The rapid loss of infection at a time when the plague bacillus is
most widely distributed in a town is shown by the following
Instances.   passage in Hodges' *Loimologia*: "[1]About the close of the
year, that is in the beginning of November, people grew more healthful
and such a different face was put upon the public that, although
the funerals were yet frequent, yet many who had made most haste
in retiring, made the most to return and came into the city without fear; insomuch that in December they crowded back as thick as
they had fled: the houses which were before full of the dead were now
again inhabited by the living; and the shops which had been most
part of the year shut up were again opened, and the people again cheer-
fully went about their wonted affairs of trade and employ, and even,
what is almost beyond belief, those citizens who were before afraid,
even of their friends and relations, would without fear venture into the
houses and rooms where infected persons had a little before breathed
their last; nay, such comforts did inspire the languishing people and
such confidence, that many went into the beds where persons had died,
even before they were cold or cleansed from the stench of the disease."

It is not that some of the people so exposed to infection were not
attacked but the vast majority escaped, a contrast to that which
happens when the epidemic is raging: Then the infected house is
dangerous.

The arrival in Bombay of between 250,000 and 300,000 immigrants[2]
during the months of April, May and June, when the first epidemic was
declining exercised, as will be seen from the chart showing the fluctuating rise and decline of plague and the general mortality of Bombay, no
check on the decrease of the plague, once that disease had commenced to
decline. Although the majority of these immigrants were people who
had fled from the city when plague was becoming epidemic, yet a large
proportion consisted of destitute country labourers, who had flocked into
the city from the famine districts of the Presidency in search of work.
Labour was scarce and the price of grain was high. Notwithstanding
the opening of relief works and the payment of those put on to them
of subsistence allowance, the city contained a large number of feeble,
half-starved and ill-fed persons who crowded into houses many of which
had been declared unfit for habitation. In spite of these circumstances
peculiarly favourable to plague, it was not until the next season in

---

[1] *Loimologia, or an Historical Account of the Plague in London in* 1665. By Nath.
Hodges, M.D., p. 27.

[2] *Report of the Bombay Plague Committee on the Plague in Bombay* for the period
extending from the 1st July, 1897, to the 30th April, 1898.

November that the plague once more began to show signs of becoming epidemic. The disease had lost the infectivity it possessed in November, December, January and February. This is a very striking feature of plague, not explainable by lessened opportunity of exposure to infection from the plague bacillus in the houses or in the sick persons. The microbe is able, as before, to develop and multiply in the human body if once introduced, as is to be seen by the residual number of persons who continue to be affected with plague, but there is some important factor or factors wanting which it possessed just before, and endowed it with its active qualities of infectivity and extension.

The variation in power of infectivity was well known among the inhabitants of the Levant and Egypt, and the Franks or merchants, taking advantage of this knowledge, shut themselves up in their houses, whenever the disease began to show signs of progress, and continued to do so until there was a marked decline in the disease. Little dread was felt for the disease when it arrived at the more or less sporadic stage.

In Cairo the plague used to rapidly decline in the month of June, and Russell, in some criticisms which he passes on the observation of Prosper Alpinus that the disease then suddenly ceases, remarks: "[1]It is agreed by all that about the 24th of June, at Cairo, there is a remarkable sudden alteration in the contagious property of the plague, as well as in the malignity of the disease itself to whatever cause it is to be ascribed"; and "the second part of Alpinus' observation that at the same time the pestilence ceases, the furniture in infected houses suddenly loses all powers of communicating the disease to the inhabitants, so that health and tranquillity are at once restored to the city, agrees in some measure with the general experience of other places in Turkey, where it is well known houses or goods undergo little or no purification; but this is to be understood with some restriction."

The restriction is that there are a fair number of exceptions. For instance, it was ascertained that those taken ill at the close of the epidemic of 1720 at Marseilles were mostly persons of the lower class who had rashly exposed themselves in handling infected goods or in communication with the sick. The fact, however, still remains that the infective qualities of plague rapidly disappear at a time when the bacillus is most widely distributed over the locality attacked. The loss of infectivity is independent in a large degree of the measures taken to destroy the bacillus. The behaviour of plague in this respect is the

---

[1] *A Treatise of the Plague.* By Patrick Russell, M.D., F.R.S., pp. 268, 269.

same in Canton, where no special purification of houses and household effects is carried out, as in Hongkong, where particular attention is paid to the disinfection of the premises.

Referring to the practice of the Turks and Moors in Egypt, Mr Bruce in his travels says: "[1]The Turks and Moors are known to be pre-dictionists....Secure in this principle they expose in the market-place, immediately after St John's day, the clothes of the many thousands that had died during the late continuance of the plague, all of which imbibe the moist air of the evening and morning, are handled, bought, put on and worn without any apprehension of danger, and though these consist of cotton, silk and woollen cloths which are stuffs the most re-tentive of the infection, no accident happens to those who wear them from their happy confidence."

A very different picture from this presents itself at an earlier period when blind faith in inevitable destiny led to practices during epi-demics, not only in their stages of decline but also in their stage of rise and crisis, which were most disastrous. It was not uncommon for Turks to use immediately, while even damp with the death sweat, the clothes and linen of persons dead of plague. "If it be God's will I should die of plague it is unavoidable, if it be not his will it cannot hurt me," represented their feelings on the subject, and from such a standpoint the practical effect was that whole families were exterminated. The same superstition spread to Cairo, and took such firm hold there that a traveller remarked that: "Through this Turkish belief plague occasion-ally rages so severely at Al Cairo, and such a large number of people fall victims to it that, on different occasions, over 500,000 persons have died of this fatal disease within 6 months[2]."

A similar loss of infectivity as that observed with plague on the decline of an epidemic was noticed in Calcutta at certain

The same ob-servation has been made in regard to small-pox and vaccine. seasons of the year in regard to small-pox. There were cycles of four or five years in which there was a rise and fall of small-pox, and it was noticeable that if small-pox was introduced by returning pilgrims from the Hedjaz, as it often was, while the disease was on the descent no precautions were necessary to prevent the spread of the disease. A case of small-pox might be in a building with a hundred others, and yet at the most there might only be one or two infected, but more frequently none at all, notwithstanding intimate exposure. While, if small-pox was on the

[1] *A Treatise of the Plague.* By Patrick Russell, M.D., F.R.S.
[2] *The Great Epidemics of the East from Arabian Sources*, p. 30. Kremer.

upward grade, the danger to the inhabitants was very great if the case was not immediately isolated. The same observations were made with reference to the infectivity of vaccine. During the spring children and calves showed beautiful vesicles on the vaccinated parts, while in the rainy season there was the utmost difficulty in maintaining the vaccine of either children or calves, the vesicles showing signs of degeneration from the normal, and the lymph not taking when transferred.

The regularity in the seasonal periodicity of plague in an infected locality has been attempted to be explained by the seasonal breeding period of the rat. Gotschlich, in discussing this subject as regards Egypt, points out that there are two types of plague prevalence in that country, the winter or pneumonic type, due to infection from individual to individual, and the summer or bubonic type, due to rat infection. The bubonic form according to this observer is always the initial disease in man, the primary pneumonic arising in the course of an epidemic from secondary plague pneumonia in a bubonic case. In examining 6500 rats in the course of a year, Gotschlich found from November to February, *i.e.* during the plague-free winter months, that only 2 % of the rats were pregnant; in March and the first half of April there was a gradual rise, reaching in the second part of April 6 %, and to 12 % by the middle of May, after which there was a rapid fall, the percentage being at the end of September 5 % and in October 2 %. It was also observed that in the plague-free months, many of the older rats suffered from a latent or chronic form of plague, while when the younger rats came into existence these young rats were susceptible to the acute disease[1].

Seasonal periodicity of plague, and seasonal breeding period of the rat.

---

[1] Neue epidemiologische Erfahrungen über die Pest in Aegypten von Prof. Dr Emil Gotschlich. Festschrift zum sechzigsten Geburtstage von Robert Koch, 1903.

CHAPTER VIII.

VARIATION IN VIRULENCE OF PLAGUE EPIDEMICS.

A GREAT mortality in a country may not be synonymous with virulence; for example, the epidemic of Egypt of 1834–35, though it caused some 50,000 deaths from plague in the country, had an average case mortality of about 33 per cent., contrasting in this respect with some of the earlier epidemics, when it was nearer 70 per cent. A comparison of epidemics of plague with each other shows that no standard can be equally applied

Variation in virulence.

to all, for they differ very considerably in their respective severity, some epidemics being remarkably benign, others extremely malignant, and between these extremes there is every variety approximating more or less to one quality or the other. Nor is the difference in type peculiar only to different epidemics, for the same epidemic may be at one stage malignant and at another mild.

The attention which malignant plague epidemics attract almost excludes the consideration of mild epidemics, and yet the latter are equally important from an epidemiological point of view, for, as will be seen later, the mild may develop gradually or suddenly into the severe, and the severe attenuate into the mild. Great epidemics and high mortality are so written into the history of plague, that it is difficult to realise they are the history only of great epidemics, and that the disease may be associated with neither of them. The most con-

Mild epidemic of plague at Astrakhan and Vetli-anka.

spicuous outbreak of plague of a mild nature on record is that which occurred in the Delta of the Volga in the city of Astrakhan and its environs in the summer of 1877[1]. Some 200 persons were attacked and only one died. The symptoms were malaise, fever, sometimes acute, running in a few cases to as high as 104° F., and swellings of the lymphatic glands in the neck,

[1] *Ninth Report of the Local Government Board*, 1879–80. *Supplement by the Medical Officer*, p. 49.

groin or arm-pit. The swellings ended either in resolution or suppuration. When the glands began to swell the indisposition usually disappeared, the appetite and general functions of the body became normal, and the patient, except for the swelling impeding motion, was rarely disabled and prevented from going about. The cases ran a course of from 10 to 20 days, sometimes longer. The disease seems to have recurred in the summers of 1878 and 1879, but there are no details given.

This epidemic would never have attracted special attention, had it not been followed in the autumn of 1878 by a severe outbreak of plague at Vetlianka, a Cossack settlement higher up the Volga in the province of Astrakhan. The outbreak is notable for its malignity, and for the alarm which it caused in Europe. Malignity did not, however, characterise its commencement. From October to the middle of November, the malady presented similar symptoms to the non-fatal outbreak in the city of Astrakhan, viz. fever, slight but debilitating, and glandular swellings. Dr Döppner, who saw the cases at the beginning of November, states that they were marked by two or three paroxysms of shivering, and succeeded by a hot stage, and by swellings of the inguinal and axillary glands, often ending in suppuration. The sick persons were afoot with good appetites, the organic functions undisturbed, and sleeping well. They had abscesses of the lymphatic glands, either of the groin or the arm-pit, which were suppurating freely. The duration of the sickness was from 10 to 20 days, and all the cases recovered. In the middle of November a second phase in the disease

The Vetlianka outbreak suddenly acquires great virulence. manifested itself, and the symptoms became so violent that they proved fatal in from 12 hours to three days. From November 27th to December 9th of 100 persons attacked 43 died and 14 recovered[1]. From the 9th of December the malady became more acute. New patients, whose general state appeared good, were seized with violent palpitation of the heart, a pulse that could not be counted, vertigo, praecordial anxiety, haemoptysis, and vomiting of liquid uncoagulated blood. The face was pale, expression apathetic, and eyes heavy and sunk, with dilated pupils. In the course of a few hours extreme prostration supervened, violent feverishness set in with somnolence, slight delirium, constipation and suppression of urine. From the 10th of December were added to these symptoms, in

---

[1] Report of Dr Döppner, the Principal Medical Officer of the Cossack troops in the Province of Astrakhan on the outbreak of Plague in Vetlianka in November and December 1878. *Ninth Annual Report of the Local Government Board*, 1879–80. *Supplement by Medical Officer*, p. 52.

some cases, spots upon the skin varying in size from a millet seed to a ten copec piece; the patients exhaled a peculiar odour like honey, became collapsed and died during a state of lethargy. There was no *rigor mortis*, and decomposition set in at the end of two or three hours. From the 9th of December the rate of mortality increased from day to day, and on the 14th of December every person attacked died.

In the Vetlianka outbreak it is evident that a transformation had taken place from a mild bubonic form of plague to the septicaemic and pneumonic varieties, the symptoms being those that are to be recognised in patients suffering from these types of the disease in the existing China epidemic. There was in the Vetlianka outbreak a gradual ascent from the non-fatal cases of Astrakhan to the bubonic form of plague, more or less malignant, which in turn reached the septicaemic and pneumonic type. It is possible that the pneumonic cases first showed themselves as secondary pneumonias in bubonic cases and that these secondary pneumonias gave rise by their infective sputum to the contagious primary pneumonic type. Plague of this malignant type is rarely accompanied by buboes, and accordingly it is not surprising that some of the medical men were inclined to think that the latter manifestations were not plague, but *typhoid pneumonia* or *typhus complicated with pneumonia*. It was only in 1897, during the first epidemic of plague in Bombay, that the *pneumonic* form of plague, the most fatal of all forms, was clearly differentiated by Dr Childe of the Indian Medical Service. In addition to a description of its symptoms and of its pathological appearances he showed the sputum of the patient suffering from it to be filled with plague bacilli, and the disease to be extremely contagious. It was not the first time the pneumonic form of plague had been recognised. Guy de Chauliac of Avignon[1] in 1348 described the epidemic of plague which ravaged Avignon as consisting of two types. The first, the most malignant and contagious, prevailed during the first two months. The symptoms were constant fever, cough, and spitting of blood, the illness ending fatally in three days. The second caused no symptoms of spitting of blood, but buboes appeared in the groin, under the arm, or in the neck, and the patient gradually succumbed on the fifth day. The second type seems only to have been observed two months later than the pneumonic type, and appears to have lasted five months. In this instance it was an attenuation or decrease of the virulence and not a development or augmentation as in the preceding.

Early malignity of the Avignon epidemic of 1348, with its pneumonic symptoms followed by a less malignant type.

---

[1] *La Grande Chirurgie de Maistre Guy de Chauliac.* Par M. S. Mingelon Saule, Traité II. cap. v.

Different types with varying degrees of virulence may be seen running concurrently or following one another in the same epidemic. At Káthiáwár in 1820 pneumonic plague and ambulant plague, which is generally the mildest form of plague, were observed in the same

Different types with varying degrees of virulence may be seen running concurrently or following one another in the same epidemic.
epidemic. Dr Whyte [1], in writing of the varieties of plague which he and Dr Gilder met with in the outbreak of plague in Káthiáwár in 1820, describes the pneumonic form as follows: "The characteristic symptoms of this variety are slight cough, pain of the chest, and haemorrhage from the mouth attended with fever, but with no buboes." He also mentions a mild bubonic variety; he saw a great number who had buboes without any fever, and was told that upwards of a hundred and twenty had suffered in this way. "These people walked about without either alarm or inconvenience, for none had died and not many of the buboes suppurated."

Dr Forbes [2] in his account of the Indian epidemic of 1836 in which

Four different types of plague in the Pali epidemic of 1836.
plague broke out in Pali, a town in Marwar, divides the types of plague seen by him into four forms: first, an ordinary bubonic; secondly, a more virulent and malignant; thirdly, a most fatal pneumonic in which there was scarcely any febrile excitement, slight cough and bloody expectoration, with oppression at the praecordia being the chief symptoms; and fourthly, an extremely mild form in which the glandular swellings made their appearance with little constitutional disturbance, and were attended only by languor, debility, and a great feeling of indisposition. In the latter buboes went on slowly to suppurate and health was only gradually restored. Dr Forbes' description of this mild form is similar to that given by Foderé, as applying to the benign plague observed in the Levant and in Marseilles in 1720, and concerning which Foderé declares that it is no less plague than the other forms, and equally demands the attention of the physician and of the magistrates. This plague of Marseilles was divided into five classes by the physicians

Five degrees of severity noted in the Marseilles epidemic of 1720.
who reported on it. The first class included the most malignant cases ending in speedy death, and was observed specially at the commencement of the epidemic, but towards the end there was observed the fifth class characterised by few signs of illness and ending always in recovery. "This fifth and last class contains all such infected persons, as

---

[1] Report by Dr Whyte to the Secretary to the Medical Board, Bombay, 1820.

[2] *Nature and History of Plague as observed in the North-West Provinces*, by Frederick Forbes. A.M., M.D.

without perceiving any emotion, or there appearing any trouble or lesion of their natural functions, have buboes and carbuncles which rise by little and little and easily turn to suppuration, becoming sometimes scirrhous, or, which is more rare, dissipate insensibly, without leaving any bad effect behind them; so that without any loss of strength and without changing their manner of living, these infected persons went about the streets and public places, only urging themselves a simple plaster, or asking of the physicians and surgeons such remedies as are necessary to these sorts of suppurating or scirrhous tumours[1]."

Samoilowitz[2], in his account of the plague in Russia in 1771, says

Three degrees of severity observed in the Russian epidemic of 1771. the disease varied according to the stage of the epidemic, which he divides into three periods: that of invasion, that of the middle, and that of the end or decline. The milder degree of the disease corresponded with the period of invasion, in which the patients suffered from headache, vomiting, and buboes which suppurated. Samoilowitz saw several persons at this stage who recovered without medical assistance. Towards the middle of the epidemic the disease assumed its most terrible and fatal form. Then the patients had carbuncles, petechiae, headache, delirium followed by prostration, constant vomiting, diarrhoea and incontinence of urine. Sometimes it was impossible to stop these two last excretions. At other times it happened to women that the menstrual flow could not be stopped, and when pregnant they miscarried, the orifice of the womb relaxing and opening with ease. On the decline of the epidemic milder cases again occurred, similar to those of the period of invasion.

In the epidemic of Cairo in 1834 and 1835 investigated by Clot Bey[3],

An Aura Pestilentiae noticed in the Egyptian epidemic of 1834-35. Gaetani Bey, Lachese, and Bulard, different degrees of severity of the disease were observed at different stages of the epidemic, and it is stated that the great majority of the population felt the influence of the epidemic, though not actually attacked with plague. Thus, among those suffering from the Aura Pestilentiae, as it was called, painful glands were felt in the groins, or arm-pits, the pain being usually slight, but increased by pressure, muscular contraction or movement of the limbs,

---

[1] *An Account of the Plague at Marseilles, its symptoms, and the methods and medicines used for curing it.* By MM. Chicoyneau, Verney, and Souillier. Translated from the French by a Physician. London, 1721.

[2] *Mémoire sur la Peste qui, en 1771, ravaga l'empire de Russie.* Paris, 1783.

[3] *De la Peste observée en Égypte.* Par A. B. Clot Bey.

and appearing or disappearing, to reappear again with malaise, want of appetite, white tongue, nausea and giddiness. The expression of the face was altered. Those who were thus affected, without ceasing from their business, were not infrequently in danger of being attacked with the disease.

In the first variety of the disease which was encountered in the middle, and especially in the decline, of the epidemic, in **Three degrees of severity in the Egyptian epidemic of 1834–35.** addition to the phenomena belonging to the Aura Pestilentiae, there were observed slight feverishness, frontal headache, altered expression of the face, nausea, which was sometimes followed by vomiting, and buboes and superficial carbuncles, which appeared together or one after the other in different glandular regions. The buboes terminated by resolution, suppuration, or induration. The patients seldom took to bed, the perspiration was easily established, and the termination was never fatal.

The second variety was characterised by shivering vertigo, headache, depression more or less profound, general lassitude, staggering gait, as if intoxicated, lumbar pains, dazed condition, dull gaze, injected eyes, embarrassed speech, frequent respirations, nausea, vomiting of mucous and bilious matter, which sometimes and at a more advanced stage was blackish, with or without heat of skin, frequent pulse, sometimes delirium, tranquil or agitated, restless and tiresome dreams, slight pain in epigastrium, moist tongue with white fur and red at tip and edges, becoming after the second or third day dry and red, or black in centre, and cracked, fuliginous teeth, diarrhoea sometimes declaring itself after the first vomiting, and the urine red, sometimes with blood, and diminishing towards the end, even becoming suppressed. On the second or fourth day this variety was distinguished by appearance of buboes in the arm-pits, groin, or neck, very rarely in the popliteal space, and of carbuncles and of petechiae, continuous delirium, coma and death on the fourth or fifth day.

On the other hand if the patient improved the symptoms lost their intensity, the tongue became moist, the skin soft, the pulse stronger, the buboes went on to resolution, suppuration, or induration, the carbuncles, if any, stayed their necrotic action, the petechiae resolved themselves in the manner of enchymoses, and the patient entered into a state of convalescence on the sixth or eighth day. Sometimes the illness was prolonged, the tongue remained dry, red or swollen, its centre was covered with a blackish coating, the teeth became more fuliginous, the abdomen swollen up, diarrhoea persisted, the motions were foetid, sweating and dryness of the skin alternated, the pulse was frequent and irregular, sleep was disturbed, sometimes delirious, the buboes went on slowly towards suppuration, and when it occurred it was serous and foetid. The patient became convalescent about the fourteenth or twentieth day, or the symptoms became aggravated and the issue was fatal. This variety predominated towards the middle and decline of the epidemic.

In the third variety there was an exaggeration of all the preceding symptoms. It was characterised by an air of hébétude, extreme mental and physical prostration, restlessness, trembling, pains in the loins, almost normal heat of skin, short and rapid respiration, quick, small and full pulse, moist, large and bluish tongue, bilious vomiting, sometimes black, no pain in epigastrium, often petechiae of dark colour, stammering speech, wandering delirium, affected intelligence, extreme anxiety, with coma, death in 24 or 48 hours, rarely longer, with a cyanosed aspect and without pain. If the patient lived beyond this period there was a reaction. The pulse became stronger, the tongue red and dry, the skin hot, the face flushed, the eyes injected, and towards the third day there was an eruption of buboes, rarely of carbuncles. Then were established some chances of recovery, and the patient might present similar symptoms to those at the termination of the second variety, but this termination was rare. Buboes, petechiae and carbuncles may be absent in this variety. This form was found during the first months of the epidemic almost exclusively, although it was also seen at every stage.

In the Marseilles epidemic of 1720, and the Cairo epidemic of 1834-35, the most malignant cases occurred at the commencement of the epidemic, and the disease became milder in the later stages. This is usually the most common behaviour of an epidemic, but is by no means a general law, for exactly the opposite sometimes occurs, the epidemic beginning with mild cases, as happened in the Russian epidemic.

Sporadic cases of mild plague may precede severe epidemics of plague, or they may bridge over the intervals of epidemics.

Mild cases are described by Dr Dutheuil as occurring sporadically in Mesopotamia during the years 1856–1867, and were generally set down as typhus or malarial fever with glandular swellings. One physician proposed to give them the name of bubonic fever, or Febris intermittens bubonica, a term which was applied also to the earlier cases of plague in Bombay because of their comparative mildness.

That the cases in Mesopotamia were not typhus nor malarial fever with buboes, but mild cases of plague, was shown afterwards by the investigations of Tholozan and Cabiadis. The mild type of plague was carefully studied by Tholozan in regard to the Persian, Mesopotamian, and Benghazi outbreaks, and he formed the opinion that they, by their sporadic occurrence, bridged over the intervals between different epidemics. In writing of the plague in Hiudieh Tholozan remarks, "It was a question here of a severe bubonic plague which destroyed in several months about the third of the population of the encampment attacked. I do not speak of light sporadic cases of bubo without fever which manifested themselves in 1856, 1858, 1859, 1860, 1861, 1864, and 1865. One of our distinguished colleagues, Dr Batailly, saw at Bagdad, in the spring of 1867, a great number of buboes, especially inguinal and almost always without fever, which lingered on till autumn. Other observers, especially Dr Colville, have recognised the same fact. At Hillah two military doctors declared that at this time the buboes prevailed in the regiments, and that they had never given rise to any case of death. Dr Dickson says that buboes or swellings of the glands of the groin, axilla, or neck prevailed in the whole province of Bagdad in the spring of 1867, and that according to native tradition this frequency of buboes indicated the appearance of plague. At this time also Dr Palladin observed at Divanié spontaneous buboes in the groin of two soldiers, a gendarme and a custom-house officer. The four patients recovered, but they all had a burning fever, a vivid thirst, a slight delirium at night, and diarrhoea. Dr Palladin, who communicated these facts to me in 1870, considered them then as cases of plague. It may be contended it is not the complete plague, but the larval or embryonic plague, and the facts demonstrate the slow or gradual preparation of the illness and the wide primary diffusion of the germs[1]."

The Mesopotamian epidemic of plague in 1876–77[2] was also preceded by *glandular swellings free of fever.* The swellings showed themselves in the groin, arm-pit, or neck, and were not accompanied by other symptoms. They began to appear among the inhabitants at the end of autumn, and continued through the winter. On the cessation of fatal plague *apyretic glandular swellings* reappeared, precisely similar to those which had preceded the outbreak, and they continued to manifest themselves for about two months longer. These glandular swellings

The import of glandular swellings before and after plague prevalence.

---

[1] *La Peste en Turquie*, Tholozan, p. 86.

[2] "On the character of epidemic plague in Mesopotamia in 1876–77." By E. D. Dickson, M.D. *Transactions Epidem. Society*, Vol. IV., 1879.

were frequently met with, and were distinct from the chronic adenitic swellings met with in subjects of a scrofulous tendency, and evidently unconnected with any special diathesis.

It is curious how often these glandular swellings have been set down as malarial fever or typhus fever with buboes. In this connection it has been held that plague was an aggravation of either of these diseases, and that the one could pass into the other. The pathological confusion which gave rise to these doctrines has now passed away, and it is known that each disease has its own specific causal agent, and that nothing will change a malarial fever or a typhus fever into plague unless the specific plague bacillus has been superadded. In India and in South Africa during the epidemics of plague prevailing there the plague bacillus has been found in the affected glands of the ambulant type, *i.e.* in those cases in which the symptoms were so mild that the patient did not require to take to bed. There are other cases in which it has not been found, and in which it may be taken that, though the bacillus was in sufficient numbers to irritate and enlarge the gland, it was overcome by the *vis medicatrix naturae*.

Dr Tinno[1], in describing the small outbreak of plague at Naples, points out that in June and July of 1899 and 1900 a considerable mortality occurred among the rats in the port together with a strange illness among some of the workmen of the port. This illness was characterised by the presence of buboes, which were taken as venereal manifestations and treated as such, and it was not until October, 1901, that the real nature of the disease was recognised in a mild case, which had also been mistaken at first as venereal.

Dr Tinno recalls the fact that, in the plague at Noia in 1815, Dr Morca relates that in the preceding year there were many benign cases, whose nature escaped completely the attention of the profession and the laity. It was only after the terrible explosion of the disease, when the symptoms were rendered familiar to all, that it was recognised that in the preceding year plague was in the city and the province.

Cantlie has pointed out that previous to the outbreak of plague in Hongkong and Southern China there was an unusual prevalence of glandular enlargements which attracted some discussion at the time as to their nature and cause. In Bombay, as has already been mentioned, the epidemic of plague in its early stages was called bubonic fever rather than plague, because of the glandular enlargements and comparative mildness of the symptoms. In Calcutta some of the first cases

---

[1] *Archives de Médecine expérimentale et d'Anatomie pathologique*, Jan. 1904.

in 1896 were of so mild a nature that a controversy arose on the subject. There can be no doubt, however, that they were cases of plague, and that the mortality of rats in the native mercantile quarters of Calcutta, where the produce from Bombay was stored, was due to plague.

Not only may the type and virulence of plague vary in different epidemics, but symptoms may be present in one epidemic which are absent in another; for example carbuncles, which appear to have been an important feature in many of the older epidemics and an indication of severity, have not been conspicuous for their presence in the epidemic of to-day. When occasionally carbuncles have been present in the existing pandemic, they have, as in the plague of Egypt in 1834–35, rather indicated mildness than severity. The tokens, also, that were so constant in fatal cases in the Great Plague of London in 1665 have not been observed in recent epidemics. Clot Bey, alluding to the presence in some epidemics and absence in others of particular symptoms, points out that in the epidemic of the sixth century, to the buboes, carbuncles and black boils or pustules there were added affections of the throat and withering of the limbs; that in the fourteenth century lung affections were common, and that in the sixteenth and seventeenth centuries sweats were a distinguishing feature. In the Plague of London of 1665 there were profuse and extraordinary sweatings in addition to the ordinary symptoms, such as shivering, vomiting, delirium, dizziness, headache, stupefaction, fever, sleeplessness, palpitation of the heart, bleeding of the nose, great heat about the praecordia, blains, buboes, carbuncles, which according to Boghurst did not appear until July, spots and tokens.

Presence and absence of certain symptoms in different epidemics.

Hodges, referring to this particular symptom, says: "[1] These sweats also of the infected are not only profuse but also variously coloured; in some of a citron hue, in others purple, in some green or black, and in others like blood, which I take to be from the various dispositions of the mortified venom to give different tinctures to the humours; and by this means some experienced nurses could prognosticate the event of the distemper from the colour of the cloaths or linen tinged with the sweat. The sweat of some would be so foetid and intolerable from a kind of empyreumatick disposition, possibly of the juices, that no one could endure his nose within the stench; some-

Extraordinary and coloured sweats in the plague of London.

---

[1] *Loimologia, or an Historical Account of the Plague in London in 1665.* By Nath. Hodges, M.D.

times it was sharp and in a manner caustick, and hence it was easy to judge from what origin the pestilence derived its qualities, viz. from a sharp and burning ichor that would even excoriate the parts, and sometimes vesicate them as if scalding water had been poured upon them, sometimes cold sweats would break out while the heat raged inwardly and excited unquenchable thirst." The variation of symptoms in individuals and seasons is remarked on by Creighton, who quotes Woodall's experience of London plague in 1603, 1625, and 1636. A letter is also quoted by Creighton on this variability: "[1]The practitioners in physic stand amazed to meet with so many various symptoms which they find among their patients; one week the general distempers are blotches and boils, the next week as clear skinned as may be, but death spares neither; one week full of spots and tokens and perhaps the succeeding bill none at all."

In the Moscow and Jassy epidemics it is recorded that the sweat had a sour odour and so much viscosity as to leave on the skin a thick and mealy coating. In the plague observed in Egypt at the end of the 18th century, during the French expedition there, the skin was observed by the French medical men to be covered with a gummy or sticky coating, and there were frequent haemorrhages. In the pandemic of to-day, although occasionally gangrene, pustules, petechiae, haemorrhages, pneumonia, and slight perspirations are seen, yet none of them are so frequent or so predominant as to give any special character to the different epidemics; on the contrary their absence may be considered to be the distinguishing feature, and their presence as exceptional. In this respect the present pandemic may be viewed as wanting in some of the more terrible features of plague; whether this is a sign of attenuation or degeneration, or one in which further time and opportunity are needed for more mature development, it is impossible to say.

The epidemic at Bombay in 1896–97 is an example of plague beginning in a comparatively mild form, and in the course of the outbreak exhibiting a progressive rise and fall in virulence.

Plague may increase in virulence if it appears in the same locality in successive years.

Thus at the municipal hospital the average percentage of case mortality which was 61·5 was for the different months:

Sept.	Oct.	Nov.	Dec.	Jan	Feb.	March	April	May
52·23	52·23	66·67	74·12	69·00	81·64	67·35	56·66	38·46.

[1] *History of Epidemics in Britain*, p. 677. By Charles Creighton, M.A., M.D., 1891

The type of the disease in the recrudescence of the following year was however of a more fatal character, and there has been a gradual increase in virulence with successive epidemics.

In the second epidemic of 1897–98 the case mortality was from 78·55 % at the Arthur Road Hospital to 79·26 % at the Grant Road Hospital. The third epidemic of 1898–99 was still higher, in its case mortality being from 78·97 % at Arthur Road to 81·40 % at the Modikhana Hospital. The average mortality in 5836 cases treated at the Modikhana, Maratha, and Arthur Road Hospitals during 1898–99 was 80·39 %. During the fourth epidemic of 1899–1900 the non-serum cases at Arthur Road Hospital gave a mortality of 79·54, while at the Maratha Hospital the mortality on 2599 cases was 80·95. The normal plague mortality at the public hospitals is, as observed by Dr Choksy[1], now about 80 %.

The virulence of plague became more severe in Bombay in the epidemic of 1900–1901, and manifested itself in a much larger proportion of cases with multiple buboes, and in a greater number of septicaemic cases. In previous epidemics multiple buboes were only to be seen in 13·95 % of the cases treated in hospital, whereas in 1900–1901 they reached 63 %, forming as the epidemic advanced the bulk of the admissions; 45 % of the cases were proved by examination of the blood and culture of the bacillus to be already septicaemic at the time of admission. Dr Alfons Mayr[2] in Bombay examined the blood by culture of 1014 patients on admission at the Maratha Hospital during 1902, and found that 437, equal to 43·09 %, were septicaemic cases. None of the septicaemic cases recovered. The pneumonic cases only formed 2·44 % against 4·10 % in previous epidemics. In contrast to this was the very exceptional occurrence of septicaemic cases in the Cape Town epidemic, their existence to the extent of only 5 % in Sydney, and their absence in the Brisbane epidemics. In Cape Town the pneumonic types formed 7 % of the admissions and furnished a mortality rate of 70 %.

Variation in the virulence of the disease dependent on conditions to which the microbe and those attacked are subjected.

Variation of virulence of the disease is probably not wholly dependent on the degree of virulence of the microbe which changes with the physical conditions it meets in nature, and the opportunity it has of passing through susceptible animals, but also on the differences in the

---

[1] *The Treatment of Plague with Professor Lustig's Serum.* By N. H. Choksy, M.D. Bombay, 1903.

[2] *Ibid.*

predisposition or susceptibility of those attacked. The facilities for the plague microbe to become attenuated or exalted in the great laboratory of Nature are not fewer than are to be observed under artificial conditions in the laboratory. In the latter a race of microbes so virulent as to cause the death of a monkey or other animal if introduced into the body by a mere puncture under the skin, can in a short time become so weakened as to be unable to cause death or any marked symptom even when given in larger doses. This weakened race of microbes can in their turn be exalted to virulence.

Different degrees of susceptibility to plague are observed when experimenting with the same microbe on different animals at the same time, and even when these animals are of the same species; one will take the disease almost at once, another will only take it after a long period has elapsed, while others will not be affected. This varying predisposition has an important influence on the type of plague and in the extent to which it spreads in man. The variation is seen in different races, in different communities, in different families, and in members of the same family. It is also, as stated, seen in animals that are the subject of experiment, some of which exhibit a strong resisting power to the plague microbe, while others succumb readily to its power of attack. This resisting power or natural immunity which belongs to the majority unless the microbe has acquired an exceptional virulence, or has been received in overwhelming quantities, is seen in every outbreak, but there are no infallible means of recognising it in the individual before the ordeal has been passed. Even then the same individual, who has successfully resisted the plague at one time, may not do so on another occasion, so that the resisting power, natural immunity, or non-susceptibility varies in the same person at different times.

Natural immunity has been the subject of many researches made to Natural immunity. ascertain in what it consists, but these researches have not yet attained the object in view, except in the discovery of the presence of protective substances in the blood which are recognisable mainly by their physiological effects. The production of artificial immunity by injection of bacteria and their toxines, and the subsequent discovery of bactericides and antitoxines thus formed in the blood, have materially assisted these enquiries. The views generally held, founded in large part on Ehrlich's experimental work, are that the specific bacteria or toxines thus injected merely furnish a stimulus to the functional activity of the cells of the body, causing them to form immune bodies in larger quantities than usual; that the property of forming specific protective bodies is not, as it seems, a newly acquired quality caused by the specific bacteria or their products which can produce nothing in the body which is not already preformed in the constitution of the specific cell protoplasm, in other words that immunisation is only the augmentation of faculties already existing in the cells, that these inherited faculties or specific properties of the cells, strengthened or weakened by adaptation and selection, are brought into every-day action by normal forces, and that the protective substances in the blood are formed by the assimilation of food, and will according to Hueppe vary within certain limits with nutrition, environment and personal hygiene.

According to this view predisposition, natural immunity, and acquired immunity are different manifestations of the same faculties of the specific cells of the body. This elaboration of protective substance in the blood, which produces natural immunity, like all other inherited properties varies in different individuals, and is exalted or weakened by natural forces, to which the individual is subjected. Foods, habits, environment, climate, physical labour, and mental effort, when suited to the organism, are evidently stimulants which increase the natural elaboration of these protective substances, while when unsuited to the organism and accompanied by misery, starvation, depression and anxiety, they tend to weaken or diminish the production. It is on this hypothesis that the varying degrees of susceptibility of communities is explained, that the influence of race, age, sex, comes into play, and that social and political forces, so far as they affect the food, welfare and condition of the people, are important factors in the spread of plague. Plague has nearly always committed its greatest ravages on people whose vitality has been depressed by war, internecine conflicts, scarcity and famine.

Plague commits its greatest ravages on people subjected to depressing influences.

The ravages committed by the two great pandemics of plague in 543 and 1348, and the great prevalence of plague during the Mahommedan supremacy in the East and in Eastern Europe, have been attributed to social, economical, and political conditions, which at the time caused a decline in the general prosperity of the people affected, and rendered them more susceptible to the disease.

In the present pandemic variation in virulence is observable in different countries. Thus in Hongkong the mortality of the epidemic ranges from 89 to 96 % of those attacked; in India from 70 to 85 %;

in the Mauritius from 68 to 78 %; in South America at Ascension it was from 50 to 66 %; in Kashmir it was 53 %; in South Africa it was only 48 %, though for the coloured population it was 56 %; in Australia it was 34 %; and in Chili it was 33 %.

Notwithstanding this variation in virulence of the epidemics in
White people have a fairly uniform mortality from plague wherever they may be attacked. different countries the case mortality among Europeans in different countries is extraordinarily similar, and would indicate that predisposition and all it implies is a very powerful factor in combating plague.

	Total plague mortality among Europeans	Plague mortality of Europeans treated in hospital
Hongkong	34·6 %	
Bombay	30 to 40 %	
Cape Town	33·3 %	24·3 %
Sydney	32·4 %	
Brisbane	31·6 %	
Oporto	34·5 %	
Glasgow	44 %	28·5 %

It is possible that this greater resistance of the white is only of comparatively modern development, and it is a question how long it will continue once the microbe adapts itself to European conditions. In Bombay there was evidently, even in the case of natives, a greater resistance to the first epidemic than to subsequent epidemics.

The clinical features of plague in China, in India, and in South Africa, though presenting in common glandular affections and nervous incoordination, exhibited great differences in intensity as a whole. The difference in severity and in type was conspicuous, and it is possible that this difference in severity accounts for the somewhat conflicting accounts as regards mode of conveyance, channels of infection, and the extent to which animals are affected in the different countries. The disease in Hongkong is more virulent among the Chinese, and in Bombay among the Indians, than it is among the coloured population of South Africa, being about 90 %, 80 %, and 60 % respectively.

Locality and environment seem to have some influence, for if these
Susceptible races may become less susceptible out of their own country. susceptible races are attacked elsewhere the mortality is often much less. If one may judge of the account of the plague in Iquique in Chili, given by Dr J. M. Clarke in 1903 after personal observation, the plague there is even more modified than in South Africa or Australia. The disease seems to have had very much its own way, little effort being

made to combat it; 500 or 600 cases out of a population of 30,000 would indicate that it was a self-limiting plague. Whether the mildness was due to Iquique being in the rainless zone of South America and only 20° from the equator remains to be seen. The nationalities at Iquique are very mixed, consisting of Chilians, Peruvians, Bolivians, Indians and Chinese, but the disease was confined mainly to the yellow and dark-skinned races and to the half-breeds.

Personal cleanliness is at a discount among the lower orders, many of whom never wash the whole of their bodies. In the case of the women and children a garment or dress is put on when new and allowed to remain on until it falls into rags; in some cases when a new dress is bought it is fitted over the top of the old one. Dr Clarke states that the single men scarcely ever own a room or portion of a room alone. The climate being good they live in the daytime out of doors; at night a half-dozen or even more will occupy one room in which there is no window, and sleep on pieces of sacking spread on an earthen floor, and this sacking is never swept, turned over, or brushed. Closets and urinals being unknown among the lowest orders the natural functions are performed outside and in proximity to the house. Still, even under these conditions, the disease was of a mild character, the young were most frequently attacked, females formed 66 % of the cases. For the most part the fatal cases occurred between the ages of 16 and 22, and often death did not take place until the lapse of 20 to 25 days. There was great confusion between plague and venereal cases, the former being put down to the latter.

Even in India with its usual mortality ranging between 70 and 85 %, **Susceptibility may vary in the same race in different localities.** there are instances in which the mortality was exceedingly small, not at the beginning but throughout the epidemic. The outbreak among the Souttars of Kosumba village is a case in point. Here, according to Dr Dyson[1], the Sanitary Commissioner of Gujarat, the disease was of a mild type characterised by slight fever of two or three days' duration, and the formation of buboes, chiefly in the groin. "Fully three-fourths of the thirty-one cases which occurred were of this type, and during one visit to the village I found two boys about 12 years of age with buboes in the groin whose fever had been so slight as to escape observation, and they had not been recognised as 'plague.'" Race was here not a factor in the attenuation, for in neighbouring villages the disease was virulent.

---

[1] *Account of Plague administration in the Bombay Presidency* from September 1896 till May 1897, p. 243. By M. E. Couchman, 1897.

Some local conditions connected either with environment or food or both appear to have affected the constitution of the inhabitants and rendered them more resistant or to have modified the virulence of the attacking microbe.

Variety of type is seen in all infectious diseases. Cholera at one time will become epidemic, causing between 70 and 80 % of a mortality, while at another time the mortality only reaches from 18 to 20 %. The same is seen with small-pox. In one epidemic it is of a malignant character and very fatal, while at another it is mild and with a small death-rate. Scarlet fever has changed within the last 20 years from a comparatively malignant and serious disease to one that is so mild at times as to be scarcely recognisable. Mildness is no more permanent than severity, and with the ever-changing conditions of nature variation in type becomes a general law. It is impossible to say when a mild form of plague will become virulent, or this in turn become mild. The transformation is, nevertheless, a real one though the conditions which bring it about are unknown. Another cause of increased virulence may be the association of the plague microbe with other microbes. There can be little doubt that the early decomposition to which plague bodies are liable in some epidemics, and the offensive smell that is stated to arise from the patients, are due, not to the disease of plague alone, but to mixed infection. Plague may begin in a mild form in a new locality, then pass to a virulent variety which on reaching epidemic proportions gradually declines, and in the stage of decline loses its malignity and returns to the mild form; or it may commence in a severe form and continue to be severe throughout the epidemic or gradually become milder; or it may begin in a mild form and remain so to the end.

(marginal note) Variety of type is seen in all infectious diseases.

CHAPTER IX.

FOSTERING CONDITIONS OF ENDEMICITY AND EPIDEMICITY.

WHILE the duration of individual epidemics varies, so also does the duration of the existence of plague in a country which it has invaded. A city may be visited by a short and sharp epidemic lasting only one season as in Cape Town, or it may continue year after year as in Bombay. It is often difficult to determine when the recurrences of

Discrimination between recrudescence and endemicity. plague in a locality merge into endemicity, or in other words into the acclimatisation and the development of the disease in a new centre. There are few epidemics that are not followed by one or more recrudescences of smaller or larger dimensions during the subsequent year, and some of these recrudescences may occur for several successive years. Certain localities may even suffer from periodical and frequent epidemics, and yet the disease may not be endemic though it may have all the appearances of such, because the locality by its situation may be exposed to fresh importation and may have scarcely recovered from the effects of one epidemic with its recrudescences before it is subjected to the onset of another. These though often viewed as endemic areas do not come under the category of those localities in which the disease manifests itself sometimes sporadically, sometimes epidemically, for a long series of years.

It is possible that this was the case with Egypt, which for centuries was viewed as one of the birth-places of plague. It is remarkable, however, that when Egypt was politically cut off from Mesopotamia and stood in its relations to the region of the Euphrates valley in an isolated and independent position, it remained free of plague for nearly 300 years. It is, moreover, curious that when quarantine was introduced into the Ottoman Empire plague soon died out in Egypt and in Turkey. Before quarantine the epidemics of Turkey infected Egypt and *vice versa* the epidemics of Egypt infected Turkey. Quarantine was introduced into the Turkish dominions in 1838, and in Alexandria an International Sanitary Council for maritime and quarantine purposes was established in 1831. Plague disappeared from both countries by 1845, assisted no doubt by the decay into which the trade and commerce of Bagdad with the West had fallen. A similar relationship exists between Canton and Hongkong, by which new infections are introduced and epidemics maintained. When plague becomes dangerous in Canton, large numbers leave for Hongkong and bring to the colony fresh and virulent infection, and when plague increases in Hongkong, people leave for Canton and take with them virulent plague.

There are certain localities, however, in which the disease has
Endemic   prevailed for many years. Such are Kumaon and Garhwal
centres.   in India, and Yunnan in China, Assyr in Western Arabia, and Irak Arabi in the valley of the Euphrates. There are other localities where it reappears without trace of importation, such as in the Benghazi district in Northern Africa and in the highlands of Turkish Kurdistan. New foci have also recently been discovered in the Trans-baikal province in the neighbourhood of Lake Baikal, and also in the vicinity of the great lakes of Uganda.

Perhaps when more is known of these endemic centres it will be found that endemicity even in relation to them is only a relative term and that there are no endemic areas in the sense of plague never being absent from them. At all events this and other kindred questions of epidemiology and etiology will only be decided by lengthened investigation in some of these so-called endemic centres.

The old endemic areas in the region of the Tigris and Euphrates valleys are still centres in which plague is endemic, but since the
                discovery of plague in the highlands of Kurdistan, it has
Kurdistan.   been suggested by Tholozan that Bagdad and the surrounding towns and villages receive their plague from Kurdistan, which is the actual endemic centre of this region. Babylon and Bagdad under these circumstances from their important commercial relations are likely to have been the distributing centres to Syria, Egypt and Persia, just as Canton and Hongkong are to-day the distributing centres of the plague from the endemic centre of Yunnan. The endemic areas, as now known, are chiefly distinguished for their high altitudes, for the poverty and filth of the inhabitants, and for the promiscuous manner in which the cattle, fowls, and domestic animals are permitted to live in close association with human beings, the former often occupying the same room as

the latter. It is found also that the plague lingers longest in low-lying countries in which the habits of the people are similar to those of the highlands.

Apart from epidemics in India, there has existed in the North-west Provinces since 1823, probably longer, an endemic plague centre in the **Kumaon and Garhwal.** districts of Kumaon and Garhwal situated on the southern slopes of the Himalayas. These districts, the snow-clad peaks of which rise to an elevation of 23,000 to 26,000 feet, are bounded on the north by the Himalayan range and by the Thibetan frontier, and on the south by the plains of India. They lie between latitude 28° 14′ 15″ and 31° 5′ 30″ and east longitude 76° 6′ 30″ and 80° 58′ 15″ and embrace an area of over 11,000 square miles, in only half of which are found localities adapted for cultivation; of this half, three-fifths are always covered with snow, one-fifth is cultivated, and the remainder is not[1]. The average altitude of the mountain ridges is about 7000 feet above the level of the sea. The greater part of the population lives at from 3000 to 6000 feet above sea level and consists mainly of Hindús. The villages are scattered over the mountain side, exposed to the pure air of the hills and supplied with water from mountain streams. Villages thus situated are about the last places which one would expect to find to be the seat of an infectious disease such as plague, yet it is here that the disease is known to have prevailed in 1823, 1834, 1835, 1846, 1847, 1849, 1850, 1851, 1852, 1853, 1854, 1859, 1860, 1870, 1876, 1877, 1884, 1886, 1887, 1888, 1891, 1893, 1894, 1896 and 1897[2]. The local names by which it is known in the Himalayas are Mahamari,.and Gola or Phulkiya Rog. The symptoms and post-mortem appearances of Mahamari are identical with those of plague and are thus described by Dr Pearson: "Chilliness, giddiness, unusually severe headache, pain and throbbing of the temples, trembling of the limbs, inability to **Characteristics of the outbreaks.** remain in the erect posture, great prostration of strength, fever continued, thirst, tongue foul, chalky white, eyes heavy, watery and injected, breathing hurried, pulse small, frequent and unequal, nausea, vomiting and purging of bilious matters, urine high-coloured, clammy perspiration and heat and burning of praecordia, occasionally yellowness of the skin and eyes, wandering delirium, buboes in the groins, glandular swellings in the axilla, or neck, carbuncles, petechiae, expectoration of blood, convulsions,

[1] "Endemic Plague in India." By Surgeon-General C. R. Francis, M.B. *Transactions of the Epidemiological Society of London*, Vol. IV. 1879–80.
[2] *The Plague in India* 1896 *and* 1897. By R. Nathan.

coma terminating in death on the third or fourth day." The earlier cases are often without buboes, being evidently of the septicaemic and pneumonic varieties, and the later with buboes but evidently of a virulent type. In a recent outbreak of plague in Garhwal in which the disease was not imported from the plains, film specimens and cultures made by Dr Chayton White were identified by Haffkine and Hankin as plague bacilli. The view that Mahamari and the Black Death are different diseases from bubonic plague can no longer be entertained.

The disease varies in its diffusive power, sometimes being more or less sporadic and confined to a few houses or to a village, at other times extending to many villages or even down to the plains, as occurred in 1853–54. In the 1853–54 epidemic there were about 8000 deaths. It is for the most part very virulent, ending in death in the third or fourth day. In Dr Renny's report[1] of 1850 it is stated that "the mortality from Mahamari is very great, not so much in actual numbers as relatively to the small amount of the population. The recent mortality has been estimated by the civil authorities to be probably 25 % of the total population. Recent enquiries show it to have been even greater, but the statistical details are most defective. In certain places the destruction has been very great, of which an example has been given of 14 deaths out of 16 people in one place. In the village of Sarkoto in 1846–47, if the reports of the inhabitants can be trusted, out of a population of 65 in all, 43 died, two only recovered and 20 remained without infection."

Probably during the intervals of the virulent type there are mild cases. When Mahamari descended into the plains in 1853 so mild were the few cases at Kasheepore that Dr Stiven was of opinion that the swellings in the groin and arm-pit were not in the least suggestive that the cases were analogous to Mahamari. On further experience he formed an opposite opinion and he believed that they were cases of Mahamari modified by the diluted nature of the infection. Whenever the disease breaks out in a village the inhabitants leave their houses and encamp at some distance on the hill side until they think the infection is over. But as the first cases are frequently without buboes the village may not be vacated until a fair number is attacked and glandular swellings appear as one of the symptoms. A precursory sign which almost invariably appears is the death of

[1] *Medical Report on the Mahamurree in Garhwal in* 1849–50, and Appendices, p. 18. By Dr C. Renny, Superintending Surgeon, Meerut Division, Agra, 1851.

rats in a village before plague breaks out. It is seldom that the inhabitants avail themselves of the sign. Dr Hutcheson[1] mentions the case of a village where the inhabitants vacated their houses on account of a great mortality among rats and mice, and thus an outbreak of Mahamari was in all probability averted.

That plague should prevail endemically in high altitudes and in sparsely populated districts with a salubrious climate, and with the natural surroundings of the villages exceptionally healthy, would be

Poverty of the inhabitants, exceptionally insanitary houses and close association of animals and men.

perplexing were it not that the effects of these hygienic conditions are completely defeated by the singularly bad conditions under which the people live in their houses and which are highly favourable to the maintenance and dissemination of disease. It has already been stated that the people in endemic areas are usually poor and ill-nourished. To these may now be added exceptionally insanitary surroundings. For Garhwal and Kumaon there is the testimony of Drs Renny, Pearson, Francis and Planch who have at different times investigated some of the outbreaks. Each of them agrees in emphasising the extraordinary filthiness of the dwellings and the uncleanliness of the inhabitants owing to the houses accommodating men and animals together.

In 1850 Dr Renny[2] reported that "the filth is everywhere in their villages, their houses and their persons. It destroys the otherwise pure quality of the air and maintains ever round the inhabitants that contaminated atmosphere so favourable to the condensation of infectious emanations. Their dwellings are generally low and ill-ventilated except through their bad construction; and the advantage to the natives in other parts of India of living in the open air is lost to the villagers of Garhwal from the necessity of their crowding together for mutual warmth and shelter against the inclemency of the weather. The food of the majority is bad and insufficient." Dr C. R. Francis[3], who investigated the disease in 1853 along with Dr Pearson, in discussing the cause of Mahamari and how it is propagated, says, "I am afraid that we have no better answer to the first question than we had thirty years ago. We now know indeed, as we presumed then, that insanitation

[1] "Mahamari, or the Plague in British Garhwal and Kumaon." By J. Hutcheson, M.D. *Transactions of the First Indian Medical Congress*, 1894.

[2] *Medical Report on the Mahamurree in Garhwal in* 1849–50, and Appendices, p. 11. By Dr C. Renny, Superintending Surgeon, Meerut Division, Agra, 1851.

[3] "Endemic Plague in India." By Surgeon-General C. R. Francis. *Transactions of the Epidemiological Society*, Vol. IV. 1879–80.

fosters the disease and doubtless invites outbreaks; for a relaxation of hygienic regulations (partly as a result of the mutiny of 1857 and partly, it must be added, in consequence of the chief civil authorities in Kumaon not believing in and therefore not rigidly enforcing them) always has been followed by the reappearance of the disease in as violent a form as ever. From 1854 to 1857, during which period owing to the energy of Mr (now Sir John) Strachey in Garhwal sanitary progress was there most vigorous and effective, the plague was comparatively quiescent; but in 1859 and again in 1860 it visited the Northern Pergunnahs in Kumaon with great severity; and in these years 1000 persons died from the disease. Again in 1876–77 there occurred 291 cases of which 277 were fatal—a death-rate of about 95 per cent.! (The official returns show that 3600 deaths from Mahamari have occurred since its first appearance in 1823.) Until hygienic measures were adopted, the general uncleanliness of the people in their persons and *entourage* was incredible. A small stone dwelling (built upon a surface 13 feet square) consisting of two rooms each about 5 feet high, one above another—the upper chimneyless and practically windowless—tenanted by the entire family of often more than half-a-dozen in number and by huge baskets containing the family grain; the lower compartment (a wooden floor, full of cracks serving as media for the effluvium from below, dividing the two) being occupied by the family herds consisting of cows, goats and pigs; a row of such dwellings (sometimes they are single or double) spread over an irregular surface similarly tenanted and flanked at either extremity by the ancestral heap of manure from which streamlets of liquid filth were flowing in different directions; the cottages covered with cucurbitaceous creepers, as cucumbers, pumpkins, melons and the like; a small forest of hemp, some 8 or 10 feet high, luxuriating in the immediate neighbourhood of the village; a growth of underwood including nettles, &c., between the two, and more or less surrounding the latter; and unwashed Pater-familias, seated in front of his fig-tree, having submitted his head to be divested of the light infantry skirmishing in his unkempt hair! Conceive such a village situated towards the base of a mountainous slope, well within the range of whatever noxious influences may emanate from the valley below; located where there would be the veriest minimum of ventilation; and we cannot be surprised then when sickness does come, it should run rampant."

Dr Francis' description of the houses.

In 1876 Dr Planch[1] says of the infected village of Kumaon: "The

[1] *Report of the Sanitary Commissioner for the North-West Provinces for* 1876.

houses were double-storied, one room below and one above, close,
Dr Planch's description of the houses. ill-ventilated tenements. The lower room was used as a cow-house, the upper room for family occupation.
In the lower room, about 5 feet high, it had been customary to lodge from 4 to 8 head of cattle or goats at night, and indeed in some instances as many as the room had standing room for; the only opening being the small doorway of entrance, tight closed and barred at night. These rooms were seen to be littered for about a foot in depth with decaying straw and much manure, moistened by the fluid excrement of cattle, and the entrance way on each side and the stone platform facing the lower story were piled with heaps of manure which had been drawn out of the lower room as necessity required and there left for eventual removal to the land in the ploughing season. The upper room was noticed to be roughly divided by wooden slabs into a front and back portion; the former used as the family sleeping place, the latter as a granary. The doorway, and in some instances a round hole in the front, and a small round hole for the exit of smoke through the roof of the house, all commonly closed at night, were the only openings. The floor was made of thin wood, with pretty numerous cracks so that the warmth generated by the cattle below could reach to the sleeping people above, afterwards locally described as beneficial."

Dr Francis in his description adds pigs to the number of domestic animals occupying the lower floor of the house.

The similarity of the description of one endemic centre to another is very striking, whether it is in India, China, Persia, Mesopotamia, Arabia, or North Africa.

Yunnan, the endemic centre in China, has already been described.
Conditions in Yunnan. Like Kumaon and Garhwal it is some 5000 to 6000 feet above the level of the sea, the inhabitants live crowded in their dwelling-houses, and are much associated in their domestic life with their cattle, pigs, and poultry. The same phenomenon of mortality among rats precedes an outbreak of plague as in Kumaon and Garhwal. The rats leave their holes, lose their timidity, stagger about and then fall down dead. Large numbers die under the floor, where, putrefying, they give rise to most offensive smells. The inhabitants, knowing the signs, immediately begin to take precautions by burning charcoal in their rooms, and in certain places they abstain from eating pork. In connection with the abstention from eating pork at these times attention may here be drawn to the custom of eating raw meat. Such a custom may assist in maintaining the endemicity of plague.

Marco Polo says: "[1]Let me tell you also that the people of that country (Yunnan) eat their meat raw, whether it be of mutton, beef, buffalo, poultry or any other kind. Thus the poor people will go to the shambles, and take the raw liver as it comes from the carcase and so eat it; and other meat in like manner raw, just as we eat meat that is dressed." Besides rats, other animals such as buffaloes, oxen, sheep, and deer, and sometimes court-yard fowls have been observed to take the disease. The disposal of the dead, both of man and animals who die of this disease, is defective.

The endemic centre in the plateau of Assyr, Western Arabia, is **Conditions in Assyr.** also situated upon a range of high mountains, the affected villages being some 5000 to 6000 feet above the level of the sea. Dr Dickson, quoting the report of Dr Nouri, who proceeded on a mission of enquiry in 1879, referring to Namasse, the seat of government of this district, says: "The climate of this region is cold and damp, but the soil is fertile and well watered with pure limpid springs. It has no commercial transactions of any consequence with other places, and the inhabitants merely cultivate what is needed for their own immediate wants. The houses are built of stone and adjoin one another. They consist of two stories and contain one or two rooms with or without one or two apertures to let in the light. The ground-floor is used as a stable, and as the winter is very cold, the inhabitants live in it together with their animals in a disgusting state of filth."

In the six villages of the district Dr Nouri found that, in 1874, out of a population of 8000 persons 184 had been attacked, 155 had died, and only 29 had recovered. All these patients were said to have suffered from general "malaise" and fever, or from shivering followed by fever, more or less from headache, in some cases from great thirst and want of appetite, diarrhoea, vomiting, pain in the groins, and in other parts of the body, with or without buboes, with or without red or black specks, broken dreams, delirium, and insensibility lasting for several days. There is no mention of a rat mortality.

It is noticeable that the inhabitants of the so-called endemic centres live usually on the borderland of privation, any severe drought or inundation placing them at once in a state of misery. In the Benghazi outbreaks of 1858 and 1874 those first attacked were nomadic tribes of Bedouin Arabs living in encampments with their cows, sheep, and goats, but owing to preceding droughts and failure of crops brought to the verge of famine, and later by the inclemency of the weather

[1] *The Book of Marco Polo.* Book II. p. 53. By Colonel Henry Yule, C.B., 1875.

reduced to a state of great misery. In the Assyr outbreak of 1874 the localities had previously been visited by famine. In Mesopotamia in 1867 it was after an excessive flood of the Euphrates and inundation of the marshes that plague reappeared. Poverty and lack of nourishing food seem to play an important rôle in the susceptibility of a community to plague, and the conditions which favour the prevalence of relapsing fever and typhus fever also favour the endemicity of plague.

The fostering conditions of plague once the disease has been intro-
Fostering con- duced into a locality are similar to those already described
ditions of as being found in the endemic centres. The conditions
plague preva- may not everywhere present precisely the same aspects,
lence similar custom and race modifying them, but they are nevertheless
in exotic associated with poverty, overcrowding, bad ventilation of
localities to houses, and filth, and the concomitants of these. Though
those in en-
demic centres. perhaps not exactly the agents which disseminate plague they are the auxiliaries which facilitate its progress. To-day they are found in their greatest intensity in Eastern countries which are in the same condition of sanitation as Europe was in the 16th and 17th centuries.

Thus London with its great plague epidemics of the years 1603,
London in the 1625, 1636, and 1665, with their respective mortalities of
17th century. 36,000, 35,000, 10,000, and 68,000, was then ill-constructed,
with narrow and crooked streets, many of them being unpaved. The houses were built of wood and lofty; they were dark, irregular and ill-contrived, with each story hanging over the one below, so as almost to meet at top, and thereby preclude as much as possible all access to a purer air; they were, besides, furnished with enormous signs which by hanging in the middle of the street contributed not a little to prevent ventilation below. The sewers at the same time were in a very neglected state and the drains all ran above ground. The metropolis, which now enjoys such a plentiful supply of water laid on into every house, had till many years subsequent to the bringing in of the New River in 1613 been but scantily furnished with this first of luxuries. The condition of the town is stated to have been offensively dirty[1].

There were plague epidemics in Paris in 1619, 1631, 1638, 1662, and
Paris in the 1668; about the latter period Paris was paved, the streets
17th century. were widened and the city began to be kept cleaner[2].
Oporto in the These fostering conditions are far from being absent even
19th century. now from the great centres of population in the West.

---

[1] Maitland's *History of London.*

[2] *Observations on the increase and decrease of different Diseases and particularly of the Plague.* By Wm. Heberden, Jun., M.D., F.R.S.

When Oporto was attacked with plague in 1899 it prevailed in those portions of the town which were densely populated, overcrowded, and with inadequate means for the disposal of excrement and refuse. "[1]In the low class quarter of the town the houses are irregularly built and closely packed together so as to obstruct the free circulation of fresh air and prevent the entrance of sunlight into the dwellings. Some of the houses are built back to back, the ground-floors being damp Rotten garbage and other offensive matter are thrown out upon the street and are trodden into the soil and add to the unpleasant odours of the streets. Some houses are sub-let in tenements, a family occupying each room; often the ground-floor is used for the stabling of animals, such as pigs and goats."

Canton in the 19th and 20th centuries.

Hongkong in the 19th and 20th centuries.

However bad this may be from an European point of view it is not to be compared with the narrow and crooked streets of Canton, the ill-ventilation and darkness of the houses and the filth of the streets; nor with the overcrowding in Hongkong. The conditions in Hongkong which favour the prevalence of plague, apart from its proximity to an infected part of China, consist in its being a great emporium with immense warehouses filled with stores and infested with rats susceptible to the disease, and its containing a very high proportion of poor people essentially of the labouring and migratory class, and who like all people of this class in Eastern towns live under very insanitary conditions. Hongkong is peculiar in possessing a greater proportion of these insanitary classes and in housing them on a smaller space than even Bombay. Narrow streets and high houses abound in which light and air are obstructed. So closely packed are the buildings in the older portions of the town and so overcrowded are the houses that in one district the density of the population reaches 840 persons per acre, which is more than three times the most crowded area of Calcutta. Apart, however, from too many houses erected on too small a space, the evils attendant on the overcrowding of a dirty class of people are accentuated by the kind of buildings erected. Narrow streets and high houses are not peculiar to Hongkong. They are the means by which many towns manage to house a large population. But in Hongkong in the Chinese quarters defects in the construction of the houses intensify the obstruction of light produced by crowding together of buildings, while subdivision of the rooms serves to increase the over-crowding. The rooms are long and narrow with a window at each end, the front window looking into a wide and covered verandah and the

[1] "Reports and Papers on Bubonic Plague." By Dr R. Low, Local Govt. Board, 1902.

back window into a small open space at the back which forms a sort of well between two houses. Sometimes these small spaces do not exist, so that the buildings are back to back. The lower floors of many of the houses are remarkable for their darkness as well as being frequently damp. Many of the lower floors of the worst kind have been changed into store-rooms to contain the goods and merchandise for which Hong-kong is an entrepot. These store-rooms as a rule are infested with rats, which at times find their way up to the rooms on the higher floors. The basements are generally rat-ridden, both floors and walls, and from the walls being often hollow it is easy for rats to reach the upper floors.

The admission of light into the dwelling-rooms of Chinese tenement houses is still further obstructed by the subdivisions into several cabins or compartments, sometimes numbering up to six, which every room is subjected to. Each cabin is let out to a separate tenant and not infre-quently accommodates a separate family. The compartments or cubicles are windowless rooms and are often so dark that it is impossible for any-one coming directly from the light outside and drawing the curtain or opening the door of the cubicle to see from the passage if the cabin is occupied. Fresh air and sunlight never get into the cubicles except perhaps the compartment at each end of the room opposite the window. The cubicle system as described leads to overcrowding in its worst form and under the worst conditions, for wherever more than two cubicles are in a room the compartments become so dark as to render it impossible to be kept clean.

Many of the conditions which exist in Hongkong are also to be **Bombay in 1896.** found in Bombay, but on the whole the latter city contains proportionately fewer houses with windowless rooms and with so much overcrowding. There are, however, many buildings as bad, and many worse than in Hongkong, but they may in relation to the size of the city be considered as few in proportion.

Bombay, like Hongkong, is a port with large warehouses and stores, and it was in that quarter where grain and rice are stored in godowns and which are infested with rats that plague showed itself first in epidemic form. The Hindú low castes were the greatest sufferers from the plague in Bombay. They are so poor that they may often be seen searching among refuse for food; their dwellings are situated in the most crowded localities and several families not infrequently live in one room. They usually sleep on the floor on a thin sheet, and the ground on which they sleep is damp and mouldy and nearly as damp as the street outside. In one district of Bombay it is stated by the Health Officer, Dr Weir, that 75 % of the buildings were more or less unfit for human habitation by reason of imperfect ventilation, darkness, and dampness. Most of the buildings consist of double rooms separated by a narrow and dark passage which ends in a small open space in which is located the privy on one side and the water-tap on the other. All the clothes of the house are washed in this yard and the dripping of the water and the washing of the clothes render the outside walls damp. The rooms on each side of the passage may be further subdivided, so that the centre rooms are in darkness, while the front and back receive but little light.

The chawls of Bombay enjoy an unenviable reputation for being
The chawls of Bombay. huge warrens in which human beings are packed under conditions which, though not resembling the unhealthy dwellings of the inhabitants of Kumaon and Garhwal, are in no respect better as regards light and air and overcrowding. They frequently consist of high buildings of five or six stories, sometimes more than 100 feet in depth, and not more than three or four feet from adjoining buildings of a similar type. The entrance door leads to a long passage or corridor which runs from end to end of the building. On each side of this passage are rooms with windows occupied by one or more families. A staircase leads to the higher stories, which are also arranged on the same plan of a long passage and rooms on either side. The passages receiving light from the door and windows at the end are dark and badly ventilated, and the rooms abutting on these passages are also dark and badly ventilated, owing to the narrowness of the intervening gully between the buildings adjoining. In some inspections in which the writer joined, having for their object the discovery of plague cases, lamps had to be used to light the way in these houses, although it was day outside, and notwithstanding the light on one occasion he stumbled over a sick person crouched in the darkness. Each room has one or more occupants, and sometimes the inmates in the building amount to some hundreds.

Some of these buildings are described by the Health Officer[1].

"In the crowded buildings in Mandvi, in which the disease first appeared, we had over 100 people in many buildings, and as many as 600 people in one building, one family living their life in one room, opening on to a common passage in which the grain was ground, and
The crowded buildings in Mandvi. at one end of which was the water-pipe under which the clothes were washed, splashing the walls and the floor around. We take for explanation one building in Clive

---

[1] "Report on the plague of 1896–97 in Bombay." By Brigade-Surgeon Lieut.-Col. T. S. Weir, Municipal Health Officer, p. 735.

Road. There are 116 rooms, and say there are four persons to each room; it gives nearly 500 people to the house, and underneath this mass of people densely pressed in one building, with the foulness that must come from human beings, are three godowns and shops, and yet this is not by any means the most crowded and densely populated dwelling in the city. No-one can look at the size of the buildings, and the number of rooms in each building in this locality, as shown in this statement, without having a feeling of astonishment that the mortality has been so low. They are most thrifty people, the Jains and other classes who come here for business from Gujarat or Káthiáwár and live in these buildings; they suffer as much from thrift as other classes from want of thrift; they seldom eat fruit, and they use very little vegetables, unlike most Hindús. They are so thrifty that they collect rags and rubbish in the passages of the dwellings, and so careful of animal life that they fear to sweep near the rags they have with

The Jains and their indifference to death.

much pains bound in bundles. I have never seen any people so indifferent to the sight of the dying and the dead. This is what the Committee appointed by Government saw one evening during the inspection of a building. In one

A scene in a building.

room of a large building with double rooms on each floor was a patient ill from bubonic plague. In the next room was a man singing. In the room after that there was a dead body. And in a room almost after this a group of women were laughing at us. It was often pathetic to see the anxiety of some people to save an insect from disinfecting fluid."

The number of cases in buildings in Mandvi Bunder is seen in the annexed return, and the incidence of the disease by dwellings can be studied from it. " It shows

(*a*) the fatality by dwellings,

(*b*) the effect of the measures taken in the beginning.

" The mortality has been so small in proportion to the numbers and

Mortality from bubonic plague small owing to measures adopted.

the pressure of the population and the density of the houses that it has been suggested by some authorities that there may be another severe epidemic. All who have seen the charts of mortality have ascribed the repressions in the mortality to the influence of the sanitary measures adopted. There can be no doubt that the measures adopted have reduced and lightened the mortality. There is no reason except the influence of the measures carried out why in this city, more densely crowded than any city in the British Empire, the mortality has not been much greater.

" STATEMENT SHOWING THE NUMBER OF CASES OF BUBONIC PLAGUE AND THE DATE OF ATTACK AND DEATH IN BUILDINGS ON MANDVI BUNDER.

	Street	House No.	KEY Roman figures indicate date of attack and italics indicate date of death
1	Broach Street	58 A	25.8—*31.8*; 11.9—*16.9*; 12.9; 18.9; 22.9; 28.9—*1.10*; 8.10—*12.10*; 23.12—*30.12*; 31.3; 25 4—*28.4*
2	Argyle Road	172–176	16.9—*18.9*; 20.9—*21.9*; 22.9—*26.9*
3	Cullian Street	33	17.9—*20.9*; 18.9—*24.9*; 18.9; 21.9—*25.9*
4	Bhandup Street ...	9–13	18.9—*24.9*; 19.9; 20.9—*25.9*; 22.9; 28.9; 4.4
5	Akbar Street	Shed	18.9—*25.9*
6	Musjid Siding Road ...	50–54	20.9—*23.9*; 25.9—*27.9*; 16.10; 16.10; 17.10; 21.10; 21.10; 22.10—*26.10*; 30.10—*2.11*; 2.11
7	Do. ...	22	20.9—*24.9*; 22.9—*24.9*; 23.9—*28.9*; 25.9—*30.9*; 25.9—*27.9*; 26.9—*30.9*; 27.9—*29.9*; 27.9—*4.10*; 28.9; 30.9—*3.10*; 30.9—*3.10*
...	Do. ...	22	1.10—*3.10*; 1.10—*3.10*; 2.10; 2.10—*3.10*; 2.10; 2.10
8	Argyle Road	22	20.9—*25.9*; 20.9—*27.9*; 27.9—*29.9*; 28.9—*30.9*; 30.9—*30.10*
9	Musjid Station Road...	25	20.9—*23.9*; 27.9—*30.9*; 2.10; 25.10—*26.10*
10	Argyle Road ...	47	20.9—*24.9*
11	Musjid Station Road ..	24	21.9; 28.9; 28.9—*3.10*; 1.10; 1.10; 7.10; 20.10; 27.3; 11.5
12	Clive Road	45	21.9—*29.9*; 21.9—*26.9*; 22.9—*25.9*; 23.9—*25.9*; 26.9—*5.10*; 26.9; 27 9—*1.10*; 27.9—*30.9*; 28.9—*30.9*; 28.9—*4.10*; 29.9; 30.9—*5.10*; 6.10—*15.10*; 7.10; 29.9; 16.3—*22.3*; 24.3—*27.3*; 15.4—*17.4*; 29.4; 18.5—*23.5*
13	Sholapur Street ...	Shed	21.9—*25.9*
14	Broach Street	70	22.9; 27.9; 27.9—*28.9*; 28.9; 10.4—*11.4*; 11.4
15	Bhandup Street ...	17	22.9
16	Broach Street	80	25.9—*27.9*; 2.4—*10.4*; 12.4—*14.4*; 24.4
17	Cullian Street	45	26.9—*27.9*; 2.10—*4.10*; 3.4—*6.4*; 2.5; 25.5—*27.5*; 12.6—*13.6*; 18.6—*21.6*
18	Broach Street	60	26.9—*27.9*; 27.9—*30.9*; 17.10
19	Musjid Station Road .	8–9	26.9—*1.10*; 26.9
20	Argyle Road	56	26.9—*29.9*; 27.9—*30.9*; 7.10; 8.10—*10.10*; 8.4
21	Baroda Street	80	26.9; 27.9; 27.9—*29.9*; 29.9—*2.10*; 30.9—*1.10*; 2.10; 24.10—*27.10*
22	Bhandup Street ...	1–7	27.9—*28.9*; 27.9—*30.9*; 28.9; 16.10—*25.10*; 16.10—*19.10*; 17.10; 15.3—*20.3*; 22.3
23	Clive Road ...	39	27.9—*29.9*; 4.10—*4.10*; 4.10
24	Do. ...	33	27.9; 1.10—*4.10*
25	Raichore Street ...	Shed	28.9—*30.9*
26	Argyle Road	66	28.9—*18.10*; 16.10—*18.10*; 18.10; 20.10—*25.10*; 20.3—*30.3*; 21.5; 27.5
27	Do.	2	29.9—*4.10*; 6.10; 16.10; 17.10; 25.10—*28 10*; 27.10; 7.11—*8.11*; 19.11—*21.11*; 16.3—*20.3*; 1.4—*3.4*; 7.4; 13.4—*15.4*; 16.4—*17.4*; 18.4; 24.4—*25.4*

"The many members of the Scientific Missions I have taken round the city have all been astonished at three conditions in our city:

(a) The size of the buildings and the number of the people living in them.

(b) The density of the population.

(c) The cleanliness of the densely populated portions of the city."

To quote another paragraph in the report of the Health Officer:

"To show the pitiful condition in which the poor classes live let us enter a building in Khara Talao inspected by His Excellency the Governor. There is a ground-floor and a room above it. The length of the ground-floor room is 111 feet and the width 18½ feet. There is no means of ventilation on either side. In fact the room is a passage with a door in front between closed walls. We counted in this room 19 men, 20 women and 17 children. What a life! What can anything outside this room do for the people in their misery inside?"

The following are the notes made by the author of a morning's inspection in October 1897 in another district, and in which the houses were smaller and did not contain such large numbers of inmates as the chawls. It will be seen, however, that their lack of light and air was similar. "Met the Plague Committee at the Kama-tipuri District, where it had been decided to form some search parties to inspect the houses. Each search party was given a street and consisted of a medical man, an inspector, a native or European gentleman, a policeman, a man with a lamp, and another with a bunch of keys. There was one lady doctor among the party. The houses were taken seriatim, and each room carefully inspected and the inmates examined. The people took to the search very kindly, and there was no difficulty whatever experienced. Many of the people were out at work and their rooms locked. It was thought necessary to examine these and the man with the bunch of keys came into requisition. The houses in the Kamatipuri District are of a very bad type, being rather deep and two or three stories high, having shops in front and a long corridor passage from front to back. Into this dark corridor open small rooms which are windowless and enjoy neither light nor air. It is necessary to use a light before it is possible to say whether the room is occupied or not. Behind or sometimes in the centre of this corridor is the latrine for the house. The second story is as dark as the ground-floor if there is a third story. As the houses adjoin one another it is impossible to open out windows into the open air either for light or for ventilation, and the only remedy appears to be the pulling down of every other house, which will allow windows to be opened out into an open space and which will also secure ventilation. Two cases of plague and one suspicious case were discovered and sent to hospital."

In Cape Town plague broke out at a time when the town contained many refugees on account of the Transvaal war, and when **Cape Town.** a large number of natives had flocked into the town. It was among these and the poorest of the inhabitants that the plague first began to be epidemic. Cape Town for its size has a very large proportion of filthy slums and insanitary houses. The insanitary houses and areas were at the time overcrowded with a heterogeneous population, consisting of natives, coloured people, Indians, Arabs, and whites of almost every nationality. The natives coming direct from their kraals in the native territories to work in Cape Town, being unused to town life, are unable to adapt themselves to their new conditions and crowd together when permitted to an extraordinary degree. In one house from which some plague cases were removed 65 natives were secured as contacts, but over 30 escaped, making up a total of nearly one hundred persons living in a house which was by no means a large one. The poorer coloured people are as dirty in their habits as the natives; the Malays and Indians possess the habits of the Asiatic, and the poorer class, Portuguese, Italian, Levantine, and Polish Jews, which made up the bulk of the poor white, were almost as filthy as the others. It was accordingly among a poor and crowded population living in a very insanitary state in ill-ventilated, badly lighted and rat-infested houses that the plague acquired a hold upon the town. The majority of the whites attacked were foreigners. In one ward of the plague hospital out of 16 patients eleven nationalities were represented. The distribution of plague in Cape Town followed very closely the distribution of phthisis, the two diseases evidently finding in the insanitary houses and insanitary habits of the inmates excellent conditions for their propagation and spread.

Far worse from a hygienic point of view were the poorer class of houses in Port Elizabeth, where plague has continued to recrudesce annually since its first appearance in 1901.

The plague, now as formerly, is largely a disease of the poor, and perhaps falls proportionally more heavily than any other **Plague chiefly a disease of the poor.** infection on the lower strata of society. At one time it acquired the name of the beggars' disease, at another the poor plague, and at another miseriae morbus.

Dr Cabiadis in contrasting the immunity of Kerbela with the prevalence of plague in Hillah attributes the difference to the prosperous condition of the inhabitants of the former place[1], even the poorest class enjoying a meat diet, and to the spacious and well-aired houses, though the streets are narrow and crooked. He points out that Hillah is the very reverse of this; its houses are low, confined, and very imperfectly ventilated; they are, moreover, generally encumbered with a horse, with poultry, and with two or three buffaloes. These animals constitute the resources whence the lower classes of Hillah derive a livelihood by selling milk and eggs to the wealthier inhabitants, while they themselves limit their own nourishment to barley bread, dates, and onions, with sometimes fish in a putrescent state.

The following is a description of a Chinese village which lost nearly half of its inhabitants from plague in 1902[2]:—"Sua-bui is about an hour-and-a-half's sail from Swatow. The houses are clustered together, with a few lanes of some 6 to 8 feet in width and some passages not more than 4 feet intersecting the village. Fronting the lanes are shops and houses and entrances into court-yards. The shops are narrow, obtaining their light from the front. The houses in many instances are entered direct from the street and consist of one or more rooms and are usually devoid of other means of light than the doors; sometimes there is a small window of 1 foot in length by 9 inches in breadth. Other entrances give access to a small court-yard, around which are windowless buildings entered by separate doors. In fine weather the inhabitants when not out in the fields spend most of their time in the court-yard or the street. At the time of the visit the garbage was to be seen heaped up almost everywhere, being thrown out of the house and left to the disintegrating forces of nature and of the pigs and fowls. Pigs roved or lay about the lanes or were in the court-yard or in one of the rooms of the houses with the fowls. Calves and cows were usually tied in some corner of the lane or were in the court-yard. The drains were full of foul, putrefying black mud or stinking water which could get no outlet, being blocked with garbage. Streets, passages and court-yards were a mass of uncleanliness. The latrines, however, were well-built reservoirs, the faeces and urine being valuable, but the smell from them was extremely offensive. Several of the windowless houses

A Chinese village.

---

[1] "Supplement containing reports and papers on the progress of the Levantine Plague," by Mr Netten Radcliffe. *Ninth Annual Report, Local Govt. Board,* 1879–80.

[2] "Report on the causes and continuance of plague in Hongkong, and suggestions as to remedial measures." By W. J. Simpson, M.D., F.R.C.P., 1903.

were closed because their inmates had fled from them either to other villages or to the hills to escape from the plague which had been in the house. Among the congeries of badly-lighted, badly-ventilated, and filthy houses there were a few to be seen better built, better lighted, and cleaner. They were the exceptions and they had escaped plague."

It is an interesting observation that Macao though so near to Hong-

Macao.

kong remains comparatively free of plague after its first outbreak there. This immunity is attributed to the demolition of the buildings in some of the worst areas in which plague displayed great prevalence and malignity, and laying out in their place model areas containing sanitary buildings with an abundance of light and air in the rooms.

Social conditions connected with poverty, misery, deficient or ill-

Conclusion.

nutritious food and overcrowding, combined with the local conditions which are generally associated with these, such as insanitary dwellings, which are dark, damp, dirty, badly lighted, dilapidated, and harbouring rats and insects, are the factors commonly found to predispose to plague, and it is in a population living under these social and local conditions that plague usually commits its greatest ravages.

Wherever in towns there is the greatest overcrowding, the greatest crowding together of buildings on the smallest areas, and consequently the least amount of fresh air and sunlight in the dwelling-rooms, there plague finds a home from which it is difficult to be dislodged   Still it has to be recognised that insanitary conditions, although they render a locality a suitable nursery ground for the development or spread of the specific agent of plague, and cause the population to become susceptible to the disease, do not appear to be the only factors necessary to the production of an epidemic. They constitute a favourable soil, but before the plague germ can fructify to any great extent in that soil other factors must come into play; for instance seasonal influences possess a very marked controlling effect on the development and decline of plague epidemics. What these seasonal influences embrace and the conditions they produce are still subjects of speculation rather than of knowledge acquired by investigation, but it is certain that even with a soil receptive of plague by reason of its population living under insanitary conditions the plague germ once introduced is subject to seasonal and meteorological influences for its development and spread, and in different places it has to await these influences before it makes any marked progress.

CHAPTER X.

DIFFUSION AND MODES OF DISSEMINATION.

THERE are certain laws governing the diffusion of plague. The infection is greatly influenced in its development by season and other factors, but however much this may be it requires certain carriers for its dissemination.

The bacillary nature of the infection of plague permits of its transportability by means of certain vehicles. Living for a time in the human being or animal it attacks, the bacillus is carried wherever the human being or animal goes; moreover, capable as it is of life for a short time at least outside the animal body, it can also be transported on articles that have been contaminated with infected secretions. The infection is accordingly transportable by these vehicles, not only from house to house, but also from town to town and country to country. Plague prevalent in one locality may be carried to another locality or another country by infected human beings, by infected household effects, by infected merchandise, and by infected animals.

Plague is transportable, but requires certain carriers for its dissemination.

The infection is observed to travel generally by the most frequented trade routes. The pandemic of 1348 entered Europe *via* Constantinople and was brought to the coast towns of the Mediterranean by ships. It also came by Tiflis and Armenia into Asia Minor, and by the way of Mesopotamia into Egypt. In the subsequent prevalence of plague in Europe during the 14th, 15th, 16th, and 17th centuries the infection frequented the great trade centres. While Venice and the Italian States were the gateways for the commerce of the East with the West they were subject periodically to outbreaks of plague. The great trade routes from Venice to the north-west of Europe, to the Baltic, and to the North Sea were not by sea but by land, through Central

Plague travels by the most frequented trade routes.

Germany, and the infection was conveyed along these routes to the great commercial cities of the Hanseatic League, and from these spread in various directions. The Venetians were the first to recognise that the infection of plague could be transported from place to place, and were the first to introduce preventive measures against its introduction by ships. They instituted quarantine in 1484 and were particularly solicitous as to infection in merchandise.

In the existing pandemic the infection has been carried from infected localities over the seas to distant ports, from Hongkong to Bombay, Japan and San Francisco, from Bombay to Durban, from Rosario to Cape Town, from China to Mexico, and from Mexico to Peru, and many other distant places. As in the pandemic of 543 the corn-ships of Egypt carried plague to Byzantium, so have the corn-ships of modern times played an important part in the conveyance of plague to healthy ports. The infection also has been carried overland, as in India where most of the provinces have become infected. Sea-going ships and railways in recent times take the place of coasting ships and caravans of olden days. The trade routes have changed with maritime discovery and with improved methods of navigation, and coincidently with this alteration plague has been observed to be diverted from its former channels of extension. The Mediterranean towns have not, as formerly, been the first to be infected.

It is generally easier to observe the mode by which infection is carried from an infected locality to some distant place than to trace the various modes by which the disease is disseminated in an infected town. Instances are numerous of persons incubating or sick with plague fleeing from a plague centre, taking the infection into distant villages or ports, and there setting up new centres of the disease. The most dangerous types of plague for the dissemination of the disease in this way are the pneumonic and septicaemic; and it is not an uncommon occurrence for the inmates of a house to be one after the other attacked by plague after the arrival of a relative or friend who is either suffering from or falls ill within a few days with one of these forms of plague. Villages in China and India were frequently infected in this way.

Persons sick or incubating plague carry the infection to other localities.

For inland towns and villages, separated some considerable distance from an infected centre, human agency is the most commonly observed mode of dissemination from one locality to another. In an enquiry made by Captain James, I.M.S., into the source of infection of some of the

Punjaub villages he found that out of 63 villages no fewer than 47 or a percentage of 73 were infected by the arrival of infected persons, and much the same proportion probably holds good for other inland places. A similar experience falls to most investigators. Captain Browning Smith, I.M.S.[1], in a recent report on plague in villages in the Amritzar district, remarks that " in the great majority of villages infection could be traced to human intercourse between healthy and infected villages, and this is doubtless the manner in which the disease spreads from village to village, the usual history being that a person went to an infected village to visit relatives attacked with the disease or to be present at the funeral ceremonies of dead relatives; on return to the healthy village the person develops plague: the next step was the infection and death of rats in the infected and adjoining houses, followed by a rapid spread of the epidemic plague occurring in those houses and parts of the village in which rats died." This is the usual sequence except in pneumonic cases when infection takes place without the customary rat infection. The following two instances recorded by Captain Browning Smith may be mentioned.

(1) *Pneumonic plague.* At Munda Dina a Jullah returned from the infected village of Bagrian on 26th January, 1903, attacked on 27th January, died the same day, and fifteen members of the family died of pneumonic plague. The epidemic was pneumonic and only lasted a short time and did not spread, for the last case occurred on 8th February, 1903. No rats were seen dead during the epidemic.

(2) *Bubonic plague.* On 7th March, 1903, Mela a Jullah returned from Nagoke and was taken ill on the 13th, and died the same day of bubonic plague; rats began to die on 10th March, in the houses adjoining, and the first case after Mela occurred in them on 14th March. The epidemic, which lasted till 29th May and caused 174 cases with 144 deaths, was of the bubonic type.

It is not always persons ill or about to be ill with plague who create new foci of the disease in healthy localities. Healthy

Healthy persons sometimes carry the infection. persons from an infected house are able at times to carry the infection without being infected themselves. The infection in these circumstances appears to be carried on the clothes or personal effects of the traveller or refugee.

Major Anderson gives some specific instances of this kind to the Indian Plague Commission.

---

[1] " Report on plague and inoculation operations." By S. Browning Smith, Capt. I.M.S. *Indian Medical Gazette*, June, 1904,

"In Agashi the first local case occurred in the person of a Shimpi woman at whose house some friends from Bombay had come to live. None of these Bombay people were sick or were afterwards attacked. In Kelwa also the first local cases occurred in the persons of two Shimpis to whose house some Shimpis from Bombay had come five days before. These Bombay people were in good health, and after staying three days returned to Bombay.... At Versova a striking instance of the disease being carried by an apparently healthy person occurred. The first imported case at Versova occurred on 30th January in the person of a Brahmin who came sick from Bombay. The Brahmin schoolmaster of Versova visited this man while he was sick, and attended his funeral on 31st January. The schoolmaster lived in the village Talati's house. On the 2nd February the Talati's nephew who lived in this house was attacked by plague, while the schoolmaster himself was not attacked till the 5th of February.

"In Marol also the first case occurred in a house to which a number of people had come from Bombay to attend a wedding. These people were in good health and after staying some days they returned to Bombay in good health....

"Again, in the village of Madhan, an isolated case occurred prior to the outbreak there, in the person of a man at whose house a man from Bombay had come to live[1]."

In these cases the agent by which the infection is transported by the healthy person can only be a matter of conjecture. In other cases, however, the agent is definite enough. In one of the villages of

Infection transported and disseminated by infected clothes.

Fukien, South China, a girl brought home a bundle of clothes from a plague village. In a week or so most virulent plague broke out in the house and nine people died in that house alone[2]. Plague in 1900 was introduced into Durban from the Mauritius by infected clothing. A boy from the Mauritius, in order to avoid detention at Durban owing to quarantine, proceeded with his family to East London, from which port he afterwards embarked for Durban, landing there on April 1st On the 13th of May he unpacked part of his luggage and two days later was attacked with plague, dying on the third day of his illness.

In September, 1896, two Goanese sailors from Bombay were attacked by plague in London a fortnight after the ship's arrival, and at least

[1] *Report of the Indian Plague Commission*, Vol. v. chap. iii. pp. 106 and 107.
[2] *Appendix to the Report on the Causes and Continuance of Plague in Hongkong*, 1903. By W. J. Simpson, M.D.

37 days after leaving Bombay. It appeared to the Medical Officer of the Local Government Board who enquired into the circumstances that the probable cause of the infection was the wearing of clothes that during the voyage had been stowed away in one or other of the men's chests and only brought out after the ship's arrival in London[1].

A sweeper from Chinkoa, an infected village in the Punjaub, worked in Kulewal, in the house of a person who died of plague. The sweeper received as a present some of the patient's clothes. He took them home to his non-infected village and gave some of them to a neighbour. This neighbour was attacked by plague shortly afterwards and he appears to have been the first person who developed plague in Chinkoa[2].

Three men, some of whose friends had died from the plague in Bombay, arrived at Ahmedabad from that city and stayed for three days at the house of a relative outside the city wall. They then proceeded to Kadi, their village in the Baroda State, leaving some of their clothes behind them in the house at which they had stopped. Three days after their departure, plague cases occurred in the room which they had occupied. The three men were traced to Kadi, kept under observation, but remained quite well[3].

At another village, Akhada, some people returned from Bombay, bringing with them various goods and chattels. A few days later two of the friends with whom they were staying were stricken with plague. The visitors remained in good health[4].

The infection was introduced into Rajapur in the Ahmednagur district by a Marwari from Sirar, whose brother had died of plague and who presented the clothing of the deceased to a family of Mahars, of whom five caught the infection and died[5].

Many of the plague cases in the villages of China are attributed by medical men there to the practice of the Chinese wearing the clothes of persons who have died of plague. The same dangerous custom used to exist among the Mahommedans of Turkey and Egypt when plague

---

[1] *Twenty-sixth Annual Report of the Local Govt. Board.* "Report of the Medical Officer for 1896–97."

[2] *Report of the Indian Plague Commission,* Vol. v. chap. iii. p. 111.

[3] *Ibid.* and *Report of the Epidemic of Plague in the Bombay Presidency.* By J. A. Lowson, M.B., 1897.

[4] *Report of the Epidemic of Plague in the Bombay Presidency.* By J. A. Lowson, M.B., 1897.

[5] *A History of the Progress of Plague in the Bombay Presidency.* By Capt. J. R. Condon.

prevailed in these two countries and was considered to be a very potent means for the diffusion of the disease. Another example of transportability of plague infection in clothes may be cited. It is that of the epidemic at Eyam in 1665, when plague was imported from London during the month of September into this remote village away among the hills of the Derbyshire Peak. The village is 150 miles from London, not a great distance in these days of railways, but little accessible then.

Early in the month of September, when plague was at its worst in London, there was sent to George Vicars, a tailor, a box of clothes. He opened the box and hung the clothes to the fire and the account states he became violently sick and ill. On the second day he was worse, was delirious at intervals, and large swellings appeared on his neck and groin. On the third day the plague spot was on his breast and he died the following night. In the course of a year the plague thus introduced into the village attacked 76 families and destroyed 267 out of 350 inhabitants, or 79 % of the population[1].

The infection imported by infected persons or by infected articles of clothing may not be transmitted direct to man but may be and often is conveyed first of all to the rats in the house, these rodents being attacked with plague. In this way a new centre of infection is set up which later is transferred to man.

The infection conveyed to a new centre may affect rats before human beings.

A man lost his wife in Bombay from plague and 10 days later started for his native village near Hurnai, taking with him his wife's clothes. About a week after his arrival in his village, which until then was quite free from plague, the rats in his house and in its vicinity began to die, and shortly afterwards five of his relatives living in the house and who had never been out of the village were one after the other attacked with plague and died. Lastly the man himself was attacked with plague and later there was an outbreak of plague in the village.

Every epidemic causes a certain amount of uneasiness and alarm at its commencement, leading to flight of the inhabitants, but as the cases are not then numerous the infection has little chance of being imported into many healthy localities. Then as the plague is found to only slowly progress there springs up a feeling of security, the panic abates and the exodus, for the time being, ceases. Later a change in the progress of the epidemic, manifested by a sudden and rapid increase,

Additional risk of extension from an infected locality during the height of an epidemic.

[1] *Public Health,* p. 95. By William A. Guy, M.B., F.R.S., 1870.

leads to renewal of the panic on a more exaggerated scale and to a fresh flight of the inhabitants compared with which the first flight was insignificant. Crowds leave the infected locality. This time the infection among the refugees is much more disseminated. Large numbers leave with the infection on them, either already developed, developing, or about to develop into the most virulent types of the disease. The chances of sowing the seeds of infection in new places by human agency at this stage of the epidemic are therefore greater than at any other time. The greater danger attaching to the second flight appears not to be so much connected with the greater virulence of the disease, and hence its greater tendency to spread, nor because of the early cases in an epidemic being unable to create new centres of infection when transported to healthy localities in which the conditions are favourable, but because the later cases that flee to new districts in a rapidly rising epidemic are much more numerous and accordingly the chances of failure of engrafting themselves on new centres are fewer.

In the event of an outbreak of plague in a port the infection is not only carried inland to towns and villages by road and rail, but it is also carried by boats and ships to neighbouring and distant ports. At the time that plague was epidemic in Bombay, refugees were occasionally found ill on the principal roads leading from the city, also in the railway carriages and at the railway stations, where a system of inspection was instituted. Many towns and villages close to Bombay, and a few at a great distance, had cases of plague imported into them. Cases came by rail even as far as Calcutta. This repeats itself in connection with every new centre of plague: thus in 1902 no fewer than 176 cases were withdrawn from the railway trains at Jalarpet[1], the point where cases from the Mysore territory are received. The exodus from Bombay was by sea as well as by land, and boats and coasting steamers carried plague patients to neighbouring ports. When plague was epidemic in Canton the people who fled carried the infection into the villages far and near, many of them never reaching their homes but dying on the way; and those who fled in boats to Hongkong brought the infection into the Colony. The same occurrences repeated themselves in Hongkong, when plague became epidemic there, and were responsible for the infection of many of the ports of Southern China, for in the flight of the inhabitants on boats and coasting steamers the infection of plague was carried wherever they went. In one of these flights in 1901 in the course of five weeks no fewer than 160 persons were detected by the

---

[1] *Thirty-ninth Report of the Sanitary Commissioner for Madras for* 1902, p. 15.

Custom House Officers as suffering from plague on the steamers arriving at Canton from Hongkong, and 35 passengers were during the same time found dead of plague. These steamers were crowded with passengers and destined for short distances. In the case of long voyages greater care is usually taken to prevent sick persons from embarking, and there are usually not the same crowds leaving the infected port. Fewer cases consequently occur on these ships and there is less likelihood of sick persons carrying the infection to a distant port. Yet, though the chances are greatly reduced, ships from infected ports occasionally arrive after long voyages with persons on board suffering from plague. The illness is not among refugees, for of the latter, as a rule, there are none, but it is generally among the crew or sailors of the ship or, occasionally, a passenger is attacked. A few instances will suffice to exemplify the long distances the infection may be carried by ships. The s.s. *Bormida* arrived at Bombay in March, 1899, from Hongkong with a Chinese cook suffering from plague. The s.s. *Kilburn* arrived in Cape Town in 1900 from Rosario in the Argentine with the captain and several of the crew stricken with plague. The s.s. *Highland Mary* arrived in Liverpool in 1900 from Buenos Ayres after a voyage of 32 days with a seaman suffering from plague. The s.s. *Ben Lomond* arrived at London in 1900 from Cebu in the Philippine Islands after a voyage of 59 days with one of the engineers affected with plague. Almost every country which has commercial relations with infected ports can furnish instances of the arrival of ships with plague cases on board. A full account of those ships which arrived in England with cases of plague on board from 1896 to 1901 is given by Dr R. Low in the reports and papers on bubonic plague and issued by the Local Government Board in 1902.

The infection carried long distances in ships.

Next to the migration of panic-stricken people from infected centres movements of crowds from infected areas, whether it be of armies, pilgrims, coolies, or emigrants, facilitate the transport of infection. The spread of plague in Syria was frequently connected with the march of armies, which had become infected. The Arabian army in 639 is stated to have lost 25,000 men from the disease and to have been the means of spreading the infection. Two commanders-in-chief died of the plague, after which Abu Obeida removed his troops from the towns and distributed them in the highlands, with the result that the plague was successfully overcome. Similarly in Mesopotamia and Persia, the arenas so often of conflicts and of the marching and counter-marching

Transport of infection facilitated by the movements of crowds.

of armies, the infection was carried to and fro and epidemics set up in fresh localities. Later, infection was carried by the Crusaders who, in turn, had received the infection from the Saracens. The Thirty Years' War in Europe was a period of plague prevalence among the inhabitants of the countries in which it was waged, the different armies carrying the infection from place to place. In 1632, when the opposing armies of Wallenstein and Gustavus Adolphus, King of Sweden, numbering some 111,000 men, encamped close to Nuremberg, having a population of its own of 50,000 and which was considerably increased by refugees, plague broke out in July and in seven weeks 30,000 of the town inhabitants perished and each of the two armies is recorded as losing one-third of its effective strength. In the following year, 1633, Schweidnitz in Silesia suffered from the encamping of two armies in its neighbourhood. Of 24,000 inhabitants it is stated to have lost 16,000, *i.e.* two-thirds, while the Imperialist army lost 8000 out of 30,000 of its troops, or more than one-fourth, and the Swedes lost 12,000 out of 25,000, or nearly one-half[1]. Plague has, in more modern times, been spread by Turkish armies in Hungary and the region of the Balkans. The epidemic of Moscow in 1771, which cost that city 60,000 of its inhabitants, is attributed to infection being carried into the town by Turkish prisoners of war and Russian soldiers returned from the war then being waged between Turkey and Russia. M. Rocher in describing the spread of plague in 1870 and 1871 in the province of Yunnan draws attention to the infection being carried to different towns by infected troops.

It is not always infected persons or infected clothes that spread the infection of plague. In the South African War the immense transport required for feeding the army, and a portion of which was brought from infected countries, was the means of introducing the infection into the South African ports. Plague broke out at Cape Town and Port Elizabeth where fodder and grain, brought from Rosario in Argentina, Bombay, and other places infected with plague, were stored in large quantities. The infection was evidently imported with the produce, either by means of infected rats or infected material, which set up an epizootic among the local rats which in turn infected the inhabitants.

Transport of infection may be by vehicles other than infected persons or infected clothes.

For ships to be a danger to the port at which they arrive it is not

---

[1] *La Peste en Allemagne pendant la première moitié du dix-septième siècle.* Par E. Charvérat. Lyons, 1892.

necessary that plague rats on board ship should infect any of the crew or passengers on the voyage. Not infrequently, though some of the rats on board are infected, there is no human sickness on the ship, and *vice versâ*, when there are a few cases of plague on board among the passengers or crew there may be no infection of the rats. In the course of two months in one year the rats on 7 out of 14 ships arriving in Marseilles from an infected port were found to be infected. Kossel and Nocht also found dead rats on board two vessels arriving in port in which no human cases of plague had occurred, and there is one instance of a vessel, the s.s. *Rembrandt*, arriving at Bristol in which plague rats were discovered on board without any plague among passengers or crew. The risk to the port on account of the arrival of these ships was none the less dangerous because all the passengers were found to be in a good state of health. No special measures of prevention were taken at the Cape with regard to ships arriving from infected ports with fodder on board as long as there were no sick persons on board or no history of plague during the voyage. The practices pursued in regard to such ships were the same as elsewhere and were in conformity with the prevalent views at the time of human agency being not only the most important but the sole carrier of the infection, in contradistinction to the older and no doubt also exaggerated views of a couple of centuries ago that merchandise was the chief danger. It is becoming clearer every day that the doctrine of human agency as the only conveyer of infection on ships arriving from infected ports is incorrect, and that the modern view must be modified in the light of actual experience, which is that, notwithstanding the few cases of human plague detected among passengers from infected ports, yet there is the fact that plague spreads from port to port. It has to be recognised that different diseases have often different modes of dissemination, and that which may be true and applicable to one is not so to another. Some diseases, no doubt, are transportable on ships from one country to another solely by human agency, and by human agency is included not only sick persons but also their personal effects, but so far as plague is concerned it is in a different

Instances of infection being connected with cargoes and infected rats. Cape Town.

category and the infection can be transported by other means. It was in the great storage depôts and sheds in the docks at Cape Town and in the vicinity of the immense stacks of fodder in the neighbourhood of the wharves in Port Elizabeth that the rats began to die of plague, and it was subsequent to this rat mortality that the workmen connected with these shipments and storage depôts were first attacked with plague. In 1901 a quantity of military stores and merchandise which had been lying at Cape Town was taken by sea to Mossel Bay, a small town on the south coast between Cape Town and Port Elizabeth. Soon after the landing of the shipments the rats began

Mossel Bay.
to die in the neighbourhood of the landing jetty of Mossel Bay, followed by a number of cases of plague among the inhabitants, all of which were traced to rat infection. Apart from military operations plague may be similarly introduced under the

East London.
conditions of ordinary maritime commerce. In East London, South Africa, the first indication of infection was the death in February, 1902, of rats in a shed close to the wharves receiving goods from Durban where plague prevailed. The rat mortality from plague spread in the neighbourhood, after which there were cases of human plague associated with rat infection. Plague is credited with

Durban.
being re-introduced much in the same way into the port of Durban in December, 1902, when the rats in a limited area of the harbour frontage were attacked with plague, and a resident was soon afterwards attacked with plague on the premises where the rats were dying. On the 13th of November the s.s. *Kassala* brought a large consignment of Lucerne hay from the Argentine, a portion of which was delivered to the premises on which the rats first began to die. For the first two months the majority of the cases of plague were satisfactorily traced to infection in the shipping area and were principally associated with rat infection.

The part which merchandise takes in the conveyance of infection from one port to another is difficult to gauge. It is associated so closely with the rôle that the rats on board may play when plague-stricken, that the separation and consideration of the two factors apart from one another are seldom possible.

Theoretically it is not impossible for merchandise to carry infection, for the bacillus, once getting on to textile material, may live and retain its virulence for a considerable period, but there is no instance in which it has been absolutely demonstrated that merchandise unconnected with its usual association with infected rats has been responsible for an outbreak of plague. The detection by Kitasato of the plague

Osaka.
bacillus on cotton goods consigned to a mill in Osaka, in which plague broke out after receipt of the goods, shows that the danger may be a real one, though it is difficult to prove. The soiling of merchandise by infected rats may account for the fact that men employed in discharging cargo have fallen ill after sleeping

on bales or on empty sacks, and may also explain one of the means by which local rats become infected.

Dr J. S. Low[1], who was Medical Officer on plague duty in Cape Colony, cites an instance of plague being probably caused by handling infected goods. It was in Port Elizabeth, where a European had occasion to unpack a bale of goods at his warehouse, after it had come from the docks where many plague rats had been found. A rat, proved bacteriologically to have died of plague, was found among the goods, and four days after the man was attacked by plague. The only source of infection at all probable is stated to have been the handling of the infected goods, and Dr Low remarks that, had the bale gone up country, it is possible it might have furnished the first indigenous case at its destination.

The infection at Bhujpur, a village of Cutch, was attributed by the authorities to infected gunny bags, the plague breaking **Bhujpur.** out in the house of a Banniah who brought gunny bags from Bombay for sale. He was attacked on the 31st July, 1898, and two other Banniahs also who, it is said, bought gunny bags from him for the storing and export of grain. As there was then no communication with Bombay by sea owing to the monsoon, the Banniah had been in Bhujpur for at least two months before being attacked with plague. There is, however, the possibility of trade relation with Mandvi, where plague prevailed, and that Bombay was not the actual source of infection[2].

Bombay, Sydney, Oporto, Naples and other places are believed to have received their infection from infected rats on board of ships arriving from infected ports. In the majority of ports it has been observed that without any known entrance of sick persons, and without any history of illness occurring among recent arrivals, the first signs of the disease have been an outbreak of plague among the rats on the quays, or in the immediate vicinity of the docks, and that it was among the employees, where the rats were dying, that the first cases of plague were discovered.

Plague appears to have been imported in 1903 into Pisco, one of the ports of Peru, by a vessel bringing corn from Mazatlan, **Pisco.** where there were at the time many cases of plague. The epidemic among men was preceded by an epizootic among rats. In the middle of April many dead rats were found in the neighbourhood of the

[1] *Encyclopaedia Medica*, Vol. XIII. p. 562.
[2] *Indian Plague Commission*, Vol. II. p. 213.

Custom House, and the first individuals attacked, three in number, were employed as sweepers in that place. In the fourth case the infection had not this origin, but was probably acquired from one of the former, whom he had nursed during his short illness and whose dead body he laid out and accompanied from San Andres to Pisco[1].

Callao is suspected to have been infected in a similar fashion, but it

Callao. was impossible when the outbreak was enquired into to trace the origin of infection. Attention was first attracted to the fact that in the middle of April, 1903, numbers of rats were seen sick and dead in various parts of Callao[2]; first, in the mill of Santa Rosa; secondly, in the principal station of the English railway; thirdly, in one of the rooms of the municipal buildings; finally in the upper stories of the International Hotel. This phenomenon was noticed synchronously in these different places. In the mill of Santa Rosa an unusual mortality of rats was noticed for about 15 days, which produced an insupportable stench in the different floors and divisions of the establishment, including the garden, so much so, that in the room where the sacks were stored the odour became so offensive that before opening the door it was necessary to hold the breath and then to depart instantly in order to let in fresh air before entering. The number of dead rats in this mill was estimated at 300.

The first case occurred on the 28th of April in the person of Pedro Digueroa, an employee of the mill of Santa Rosa, who died on May 1st.

In the night of the 29th of April Emilio Klapp, also a labourer at the mill, was attacked, and died on the 6th of May. On the night of the 30th of April Pascual Novelli, a companion of the above, and on the 1st of May Miguel Cornejo, also of the mill, fell ill, and died on the 7th inst. On the 2nd of May Pedro Castro, a painter, who had worked at the mill from the 21st of April, fell ill with the same symptoms. On the 3rd of May Manuel Feubi, a Chinese cook employed by the overseer of the mill, was taken violently ill and died in 72 hours. The same day Samuel Gonzalez, also a labourer at the mill, fell ill and died after a prolonged struggle on the 29th of May. On the 4th, Juan Fernandez, and on the 7th, Alfredo Valela and Juan Ramirez, all employees of the mill, were attacked, and the first died on the 29th of May.

Thus in the course of ten days, *i.e.* from the 28th of April to the 7th

---

[1] "Gaceta de los Hospitales, Civiles y Militares," 15th Feb. and 1st March, 1904.

[2] "La Peste Bubonica. Informe presentado a la Academia Nacional de Medicina, por la Comision especial encargada de estudiar la compuesta por los miembros titulares, Dr Manuel R. Artoth, Dr Julian Arce, y Dr Daniel E. Lavoreria."

of May, ten employees of the mill of Santa Rosa fell sick, with 60 % of deaths amongst the attacked. The mill was closed on the 8th of May.

Further enquiry elicited the fact that suspicious cases of plague had occurred in Callao. In February or March of 1903 Cesar Silva, a servant of Mr Weiss, station-master of the English railway, fell sick with fever and double inguinal adenitis, without specific cause, and was treated in the paying wards of the hospital of Guadeloupe, whence he was discharged cured in about 20 days. At the end of March José Aguilard, employed at the station, was attacked with high fever and a glandular swelling in the left axilla, which suppurated and was opened, and had besides a painful swelling of the left inguinal glands. The Commission reporting on the outbreak regarded these two cases as being probably either Pestis minor or Pestis ambulans.

The plague at Asuncion, the capital of Paraguay, is stated to have **Asuncion.** been brought on a river steamer, the s.s. *Centauro*, to which at Montevideo bags of rice had been transhipped from the sailing vessel the *Zeir*, which in turn had received the rice at Rotterdam from a vessel arriving from an Indian port. On the *Zeir's* arrival at Las Palmas, dead rats were found among the sacks of rice, and afterwards on the voyage two sailors fell ill, one of them dying suddenly. During the voyage of the *Centauro* from Montevideo to Asuncion, dead rats were found on the ship, and three of the sailors died from diseases which were considered at the time to be pneumonia, typhoid fever, and pleurisy. A fortnight after the arrival of the *Centauro*, there was a mortality among rats in the custom-house premises at Asuncion. This mortality spread over different parts of the town, and was later, by bacteriological examination, established to be due to plague[1].

The plague at Unsie, a city in China, was traced by Dr J. P. Maxwell **Unsie.** to the arrival, from the plague-infected port of Swatow, of a boat on which there were plague-infected rats. About the middle of April of 1902, a junk with rats dying on board arrived at Unsie. Shortly after, rats began to die in that portion of the town which adjoins the quay, and on May 2nd or 3rd plague broke out in the house of a man who resided some 250 yards from the quay. Dead rats were found in the house about a fortnight previously[2].

Plague on board ship, while the vessel is in a plague-infected port,

---

[1] *Annales de l'Institut Pasteur*, No. II., 1901, p. 857.

[2] *Appendices to the Report on the Causes and Continuance of Plague in Hongkong*. By W. J. Simpson, M.D., 1903.

or after its departure from such a port, ascribed to the rats on the ship having become infected by some means, has happened sufficiently often for such an occurrence to be reckoned as one of the risks which is run by a ship lying in an infected port.

Inland towns sometimes owe their infection to the importation of rats infected with plague or rat-infected merchandise.

Inland towns sometimes infected by conveyance by railway of rats infected with plague or rat-infected merchandise. Especially has this been observed in Cape Colony. Graaf-Reinet, King William's Town, Kei Road and Burghersdorp were infected in this manner. Dr J. A. Mitchell, Assistant Medical Officer of Health for the Colony, reporting on these observations states that, during the first week of February of 1903, plague-infected rats were found in the railway station premises at Graaf-Reinet, that some time previously a large quantity of forage and military supplies principally from Port Elizabeth had been stored in the immediate vicinity of these premises, and that later an epizootic of plague occurred among the local rat population. Again, on the 7th March, four cases of plague were almost simultaneously discovered among the employees at the railway goods shed at King William's Town. No dead rats had previously been observed but during the disinfection of the premises several mummified rats and mice were discovered; owing to their condition it was impossible to determine the cause of death but there appears to have been little doubt that they died of plague. Plague-infected rats and several cases of plague were discovered later in different parts of the town. Again, a number of dead rats in a state of decomposition too far advanced to admit of a definite diagnosis being made as to the cause of death, were discovered in the railway premises at Kei Road, and four days afterwards a case of plague occurred in the station-master's wife. During the process of disinfection of the premises the carcases of a considerable number of rats dead of plague were discovered. In regard to Burghersdorp an apparently healthy rat was caught at the railway station and subsequently killed and examined. Bacilli apparently identical with those of plague were found on microscopical examination of the remains and the diagnosis of plague was subsequently confirmed by inoculation experiments. The railway premises were then disinfected but no dead or sick rats were discovered during the process. Subsequently a number of dead mice were found in forage stored near the railway station and specimens from these were found on examination to contain plague bacilli. Dr Mitchell makes the following pertinent remarks on this subject:

"A number of instances has been observed where live rats have come ashore from vessels or have been carried long distances by rail or otherwise in bales of forage, or in 'skeleton' or partially open crates. Sick rats are probably more likely to remain in a bale of forage or in a crate of merchandise during transport than healthy ones. Again, a rat suffering from plague may enter and die in a bale of forage or in a 'skeleton' crate and thus be carried long distances by sea or rail. The carcase remains infectious for a considerable period. On the arrival of the bale or crate at its destination, local rats are likely to investigate its contents, perhaps devouring the carcase of the dead rat and thus becoming infected. Or again, bales of forage or open or 'skeleton' crates containing fruit, hardware, or similar goods packed in straw or other material of a like nature, if stored at a place where plague exists among the rats, may be infected by their discharges, and if subsequently removed to another locality are liable to transmit the infection to the rat population of the latter. It is practically certain that plague infection has been conveyed inland to Graaf-Reinet, King William's Town, Kei Road, and Burghersdorp in one or other of these three ways."

CHAPTER XI.

MODES OF DISSEMINATION IN AN INFECTED LOCALITY.

IT is recognised that the pneumonic type of plague is distinctly and directly infectious. Medical men and nurses have frequently been attacked while attending on patients suffering from this variety of the disease, whereas it is rare for them to contract plague from patients suffering from the septicaemic or bubonic form. The sputum of a pneumonic plague patient teems with virulent bacilli which, in the act of coughing, may be transmitted a short distance through the air. Nurse Macdougall in Bombay attending to a patient suffering from pneumonic plague received, during a fit of coughing on the part of the patient, a particle of plague sputum in the eye, which next day set up conjunctivitis followed by swelling of the parotid and cervical glands and an attack of plague to which she succumbed. Surgeon-Major Manser of Bombay contracted pneumonic plague of which he died by attending a patient suffering from this form of the disease, and Nurse Joyce who nursed him was attacked on the evening of the third day by pneumonic plague and died in two days. Dr Mueller of Vienna and Nurse Pecha contracted pneumonic plague while attending on Barisch, the laboratory attendant who received his infection while working among the infected laboratory animals. In Cape Town, Miss Kayser, the lady superintendent of the Plague Hospital, contracted pneumonic plague from a patient, and after a few days' illness died; the day after her death her sister, who had nursed her, was taken ill and died of pneumonic plague.

The occurrence of pneumonic cases in a town is, as a rule, traceable to personal contact with patients affected with this form of the disease and the history is generally one of the disease spreading in the track of relations and friends who have visited, and who have come into close relationship with the patient. The source of pneumonic plague, although frequently, is, by no means, always derived from an antecedent case.

This is exemplified by the occasional cases of pneumonic plague which arise among persons in the laboratory. The history of most of these cases is that the persons attacked have been dealing with infected animals and the disease has most probably been contracted from these animals. The mode of conveyance of the infection might easily be the hand which has become infected by handling a plague-stricken rat and which has been accidentally raised to the nose, thereby infecting the nasal mucous membrane. It may be in such instances that the type of the disease in the infecting animals is pneumonic, but this has yet to be established.

To a similar source, viz. infected animals, may occasionally be traced the first in a series of pneumonic cases occurring in an infected locality, the first case generally arising in a house in which a large number of rats have died. The author has observed this in a number of cases. Once established as pneumonic plague the infection breeds true, for some time giving rise to pneumonic cases, but later it fails to reproduce itself in this form and is propagated as a septicaemic or bubonic type. The Indian Plague Commission[1] give in their report a genealogical table, constructed from material furnished them by Surgeon-Major Green of the Indian Medical Service, which exhibits the very remarkable power of pneumonic plague giving rise to pneumonic plague from patient to patient through no fewer than five consecutive series. The table is reproduced on page 212.

On the other hand experience shows that pneumonic cases give rise to bubonic cases both when contracted under the ordinary condition of natural infection and also under accidental circumstances such as a post-mortem. There are several cases on record in which, owing to an accidental wound in the hand when performing a post-mortem on a pneumonic case of plague, plague of a bubonic type has been contracted. There is a case also reported in which a patient delirious with pneumonic plague bit a compounder at Hubli on the thumb, who afterwards suffered from a mild attack of plague with an axillary bubo.

The infectivity of septicaemic and of bubonic cases which become septicaemic before death is not to be judged by the rarity with which medical men and nurses contract plague when attending such cases in hospital. If that were the standard the conclusion arrived at would be that the powers of infection were feeble instead of being as they are extremely potent. The

Septicaemic plague infectious.

---

[1] *Report of the Indian Plague Commission*, Vol. v. p. 91.

ORIGINAL SOURCE OF INFECTION IN THE HOUSE OF KAVIRAJ DWARKA NATH IN CALCUTTA.

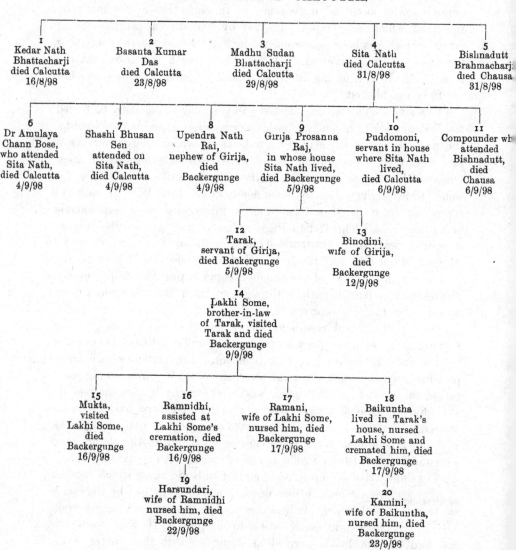

1 Kedar Nath Bhattacharji died Calcutta 16/8/98

2 Basanta Kumar Das died Calcutta 23/8/98

3 Madhu Sudan Bhattacharji died Calcutta 29/8/98

4 Sita Nath died Calcutta 31/8/98

5 Bishnadutt Brahmacharji died Chausa 31/8/98

6 Dr Amulaya Chann Bose, who attended Sita Nath, died Calcutta 4/9/98

7 Shashi Bhusan Sen attended on Sita Nath, died Calcutta 4/9/98

8 Upendra Nath Rai, nephew of Girija, died Backergunge 4/9/98

9 Girija Prosanna Raj, in whose house Sita Nath lived, died Backergunge 5/9/98

10 Puddomoni, servant in house where Sita Nath lived, died Calcutta 6/9/98

11 Compounder wh attended Bishnadutt, died Chausa 6/9/98

12 Tarak, servant of Girija, died Backergunge 5/9/98

13 Binodini, wife of Girija, died Backergunge 12/9/98

14 Lakhi Some, brother-in-law of Tarak, visited Tarak and died Backergunge 9/9/98

15 Mukta, visited Lakhi Some, died Backergunge 16/9/98

16 Ramnidhi, assisted at Lakhi Some's cremation, died Backergunge 16/9/98

17 Ramani, wife of Lakhi Some, nursed him, died Backergunge 17/9/98

18 Baikuntha lived in Tarak's house, nursed Lakhi Some and cremated him, died Backergunge 17/9/98

19 Harsundari, wife of Ramnidhi nursed him, died Backergunge 22/9/98

20 Kamini, wife of Baikuntha, nursed him, died Backergunge 23/9/98 conditions of home life under which plague generally occurs and the conditions of nursing in a small, ill-lighted, and badly-ventilated room by relatives and friends are in quite a different category from those existing in hospitals. Under the conditions of the home the general distribution of the plague bacillus in the blood, internal organs, and excretions in septicaemic cases renders them dangerously infective, especially when discharges are wiped away by the hands or with the clothes of the attendants. Plague bacilli escape from the body in septicaemic cases in the secretions and discharges of the mucous membranes, gaining an exit by the mouth and nostrils, bowels and kidneys. If the plague patient is not removed to hospital, secondary cases usually follow independently of other indirect means by which the disease may spread in a house.

Undertakers and those who lay out the dead are apt to contract the disease. In Hongkong many of the undertakers perished, and there is a general impression among the Chinese that the corpse is more dangerous than the patient. Attendance at funerals, especially when connected with feasting or ceremonial rites, is often dangerous, plague afterwards affecting those who have been present. Two of the earlier cases in the Glasgow outbreak of 1900 were traced to attendances on a "wake" on the occasion of a child and its grandmother having died of plague but whose deaths were certified to be " zymotic enteritis " and " acute gastro-enteritis[1]."

On the other hand bubonic plague which remains simple bubonic Simple plague is not directly infectious even under conditions of bubonic home life and it seldom affects the relatives and friends plague not directly in immediate and intimate association with the patient. infectious. It is by no means certain that bubonic cases, even of the Pestis ambulans type, are not indirectly infectious though the manner in which the infection leaves the body and the agency by which it spreads are still only matters of speculation. Captain James of the Indian Medical Service instances the village of Gobindpur in the Punjaub which he sets down as having become infected by the arrival of a boy suffering from Pestis ambulans. The person living next door to this boy in the same enclosure was attacked with a severe form of plague.

Among indirect means of dissemination of plague, infected clothes Dissemina- have a share. How large that share is it is difficult to tion by in- estimate; it probably varies in different epidemics and fected clothes. under different circumstances. The custom of removing

[1] "Report on certain Cases of Plague occurring in Glasgow in 1900." By the Medical Officer of Health.

as many articles as possible from an infected house is probably more common and more skilfully carried out among Asiatic people wherever they may be than among Europeans. It often happens that by the time the health officials hear of the death and arrive at the infected house, most or a great many of the portable household articles have disappeared. In Cape Town there was much secret disposal of effects when Malays were attacked, but the practice was not limited to them. It is remarkable how adherent the infection may remain among the different members of a family and its branches, the infection being discovered in many instances to be associated with the surreptitious disposal and removal, from house to house, of effects which have not been subjected to disinfection. It was noticed in India that the incidence on the Dhobies or washermen was exceptionally heavy.

Plague-stricken rats must also be included as one of the indirect modes of dissemination of the disease in a locality. The association of epizootics of plague among rats with epidemics of plague has already been referred to as having been observed in many important epidemics of plague. In fact as regards modern plague since 1894 there has been no great prevalence in any part of the world without also an epizootic among rats.

Dissemination by infected rats.

As opportunity for observation has arisen in the different epidemics in different places the part which this epizootic takes in the dissemination of plague has been discovered to be exceptionally powerful. Certain observers have gone so far as to declare that with the exception of pneumonic plague propagated by direct contagion all other forms of plague are disseminated by the rat. This is an extreme view which like many extreme views though containing much, perhaps the greater portion, that is correct, does not represent the whole truth. It is interesting to note that, though dogs and cats were considered to be dangerous both on account of their suffering from plague and their carrying infectious material on their coats, nowhere does the part which the rat has been observed to play in the dissemination of plague appear to have been recognised in the same light as during this pandemic. The phenomenon of rat mortality was taken as a sign of a coming plague or that plague was a soil disease and that these ground animals became first affected with plague, rather than that the rats themselves were dangerous.

Hankin and Simonds in 1898 summarised in the *Annales de l'Institut Pasteur* the facts which had then been observed, and came to the conclusion that rats played an important part in the dissemination of the disease. This conclusion was the same as that which had been arrived at by many with practical experience of plague. Since that time there has been ample opportunity of verifying its correctness.

The great influence which plague-stricken rats exercise in the dissemination of the disease comes prominently into notice in those towns and places where plague cases are removed to hospital with promptitude, and where the infected clothes are disinfected, and yet the epidemic continues to develop. Such has been the case in Cape Town, Port Elizabeth, East London, Durban and other towns in South Africa, and also in Brisbane and Sydney in Australia.

Special value attaches to the observations in South Africa and Australia. Special value attaches to the observations in South Africa and Australia, because the history of each case was more readily traceable than in Eastern countries. The spread of plague in the towns of South Africa and Australia was associated principally with the course of the plague epizootic among rats, the direct infection from human being to human being and the indirect infection communicated by infected clothes having been eliminated by the action of the sanitary administration.

In Cape Town not only were the first cases in the docks associated with the rat mortality and traceable to it, but the progress of the disease in its later phases was notably connected either with the movement of rats from infected centres, which resulted in the setting up of new foci of disease, or with the infection of rats in new centres by other modes than the migration of rats. As regards the latter mode, a block of houses was infected by bringing to one of its houses bales of goods from the docks. Whether these bales of goods contained infected rats at the time of their removal from the docks, or were infected in the docks themselves by the discharges from plague rats, it is impossible to say, but the conveyance of these goods to a healthy part of the town infected the local rats. On the discovery of infection of the rats all the houses but one were evacuated. The single exception was left because there was no available accommodation in the health camp. In a short time plague attacked the inmates of the house, while the others who had been removed to camp remained unaffected. In Cape Town it was possible, by bacteriological examination of the rats brought in from different parts of the town, to trace in a general way the course of the plague epidemic, for it corresponded with that of the epizootic.

The majority of cases of plague were traceable to infection from rats, dead or infected rodents being found at the residences and workshops of those attacked with the disease. The number occasionally found under the floors of infected premises was extraordinary, notwithstanding the absence of the signs of sick or dead rats on the surface of the premises. In one house there were as many as 105 rats discovered by the cleansing department, in another 52, and in the majority one to half-a-dozen. There were houses in which no rats were found and in many of these cases the source of infection was traced to other causes.

The same intimate association of plague-stricken rats with plague in man and the relationship of cause which the former bore to the latter were traced in Port Elizabeth, East London, Durban and other towns invaded with plague.

Two interesting features about the epizootic among rats in Port Elizabeth are worthy of mention. The first is that the epizootic has never been so severe as that which prevailed in Cape Town, and the second is that it has continued in a more or less sporadic form since its commencement. Similarly, the epidemic of plague has not been of a very severe character and has continued in a more or less sporadic form. There are evidently different degrees of severity and rapidity of diffusion of plague among rats as there are differences in this respect in epidemics of plague in different localities. Apparently when the rats are much infected and over a wide area in a locality, the epidemic in man is correspondingly wide and severe, but when the rats are only sporadically attacked the disease in man is also sporadic.

The history of the epidemics in Sydney in 1900 and 1901, and in Brisbane in 1901 and 1902, which agrees in many respects with that of South Africa, and which establishes both in time and place the close relationship existing between the incidence of rat plague and the subsequent occurrences of human plague, demonstrates the very important share which rat plague takes in the dissemination of human plague, and the very small part that human intercourse sometimes plays in the local diffusion of the disease.

In the Hongkong epidemic of 1902 hundreds of rats were daily examined bacteriologically, and it was found that the presence of plague-infected rats in a house or locality meant, sooner or later, if immediate measures of precaution were not taken, cases of plague in that locality or house, and that the dissemination of the plague by rats was even a more influential factor in the spread of the disease than its dissemination by man. By an examination of the rats it was possible to plot out the localities

Observations in Hongkong.

which were likely to remain healthy and those in which plague cases might be expected. It was observed in Hongkong that the rat plague would occasionally pass along a number of houses on one side of the street and then suddenly pass over to the other side. A similar phenomenon has been observed in different epidemics of plague in human beings, and there is reason now to suppose that the explanation of this peculiar course of plague is to be found in the movements of infected rats. To turn now to a few specific instances. In 1901 30 men were employed in Hongkong to collect rats, and no fewer than nine or 30 % died of plague, three others leaving the Colony sick. In a private firm of 30 coolies employed in sorting, and one of whose duties was to collect dead rats from the godown when required, five or 16·6 % contracted plague and died. In another firm rats were dying in the store-room and two men engaged in removing them were attacked with and died of plague. There are similar examples to these

Observations in India.

mentioned by Hankin and Simonds in the Bombay epidemic. Hankin records a case of this kind in a mill in which there were several thousands of workmen. Rats were noticed to die in large numbers; 20 coolies were employed to remove the dead rats; out of the 20 no fewer than 12 were attacked by the plague, while the rest of the workmen and others in the building remained healthy. Simonds also records an example of rat infection in two women caused by handling dead rats. The inhabitants of a village in the Punjaub were turned out of their village and placed in camp because of a commencing mortality among rats. While in camp two women were permitted to visit their home and found on the floor of their house some dead rats; these they picked up and threw into the street; they returned to camp and a few days later they were attacked with plague. Two instances placed before the Indian Plague Commission may be mentioned. Both were villages in the Punjaub and under the supervision of Captain James of the Indian Medical Service.

"The inhabitants of Mahlgahla, some 2500 in number, were placed in camp by Captain James, I.M.S., on account of an outbreak of plague which was confined to one special quarter of the village. This quarter having been disinfected without incident the disinfection of the rest of the evacuated village was taken in hand. In the absence of other available labour the house owners were here employed upon the disinfection of their own houses. As soon as they were set to work they came upon dead rats all over the village, in one case no fewer than 15 of these being found in a single room. Five days after the commencement of the work of disinfecting the houses, which had been free of plague at the time the village was evacuated, numerous cases of plague began to occur among the disinfectors. So severe was the outbreak of the disease among these (the resulting epidemic did not subside till 75 persons in all had been attacked) that the disinfection operations had to be suspended. The quarter of the village in which most of the disinfectors were attacked was the quarter most remote from that in which the original group of plague cases had occurred[1]."

The second case is the village of Chak Kalal, which was evacuated as a precautionary measure. "A few days afterwards owing to the downpour of rain a considerable number of the inhabitants returned to their houses. A number of rats (and these were shown by bacteriological examination to have died of plague) were found lying dead all over the village. Within a few days afterwards quite a considerable number of people contracted plague. It seems clear that the infection was here disseminated over the whole village as a result of the outbreak of plague in an epidemic form among rats[2]."

The agency by which plague is transmitted from the rat to man is

The agency by which plague is transmitted from the rat to man.
unfortunately still a matter of conjecture. Three modes have been suggested; one is by the parasites on the rat, a second is by food which has been contaminated by the saliva, excreta, and urine of plague-stricken rats, and a third is by inoculation of the foot or hand owing to an abrasion coming into contact with bacilli on the rat itself or on something soiled by the plague rat. It will only be necessary to deal at this stage with the first, as the others will be considered when treating of the channels by which the infection enters the human system. Of the

The flea theory.
parasites of the rat the flea is the most important, first because it is a blood-sucking insect, and secondly because it possesses the power of transferring itself from animal to animal. Many observers, the first being Ogata[3], have found plague bacilli in fleas taken from plague-infected rats, the bacilli remaining in the bodies of the fleas for some time after feeding on infected blood. The fleas themselves are apparently not injuriously affected by the bacilli. On this observation, coupled with the fact that fleas are frequently numerous on such rats, Simonds conceived the theory that the flea is the connecting agent

---

[1] *Report Indian Plague Commission*, Vol. v. chap. iii. p. 124.

[2] *Ibid.* p. 125.

[3] "Ueber die Pestepidemie in Formosa." *Centralblatt für Bakteriologie*, Vol. xxi. 1897.

between plague in man and the rat. When the rat becomes ill it is sometimes covered with fleas, which leave the body on its death and transfer themselves to other animals. It is in this transference of fleas from an infected rat to a healthy one or to man that Simonds explains the mode of dissemination between rat and rat and between rat and man. Nuttall[1] in subjecting these views to the experimental test, including both bugs and fleas, which he allowed to bite animals dying from plague and then immediately afterwards transferred them to healthy animals, was unable to produce a single case of infection.

The theory of Simonds rests on the view that plague is usually caused both in man and in the rat by inoculation of the infection through the skin, and on the aptitude of rat fleas for biting man. Both of these have been controverted. It is a fascinating theory, but it still requires much more evidence in its support than exists at present to place it on an absolutely firm foundation, and even then it by no means excludes other agencies.

Four species of fleas, Typhlopsylla musculi, Pulex fasciatus, Pulex serraticeps, and Pulex pallidus, have been found on rats, while two, Pulex irritans and Pulex serraticeps, have been found on man. The Pulex serraticeps is also commonly found on dogs and cats. There can be little doubt that the Pulices will bite man if they have the opportunity though it may be only on occasion that they do so. The fact that they do bite man has been observed by Tidswell[2] and by Gauthier[3] and Raybaud.

The only experiments hitherto made which appear to support the view that fleas from a plague rat may possibly cause plague in higher animals are those mentioned as having been made at Hongkong. They are, however, not conclusive in that the results obtained were solely clinical, the illness from which the monkeys suffered not proving fatal, and no examinations having been made to ascertain the presence or absence of plague bacilli in the organs of the monkeys.

On the other hand, the transmission of plague from rat to rat by the agency of fleas has been successfully accomplished by MM. J. C. Gauthier and A. Raybaud, who in five experiments were able to convey

---

[1] Nuttall, "On the rôle of insects, arachnids, and myriapôds as carriers in the spread of bacterial and parasitic diseases of men and animals." *Johns Hopkins Hospital Reports*, Vol. VIII. 1900.

[2] *Report of the Board of Health on a Second Outbreak of Plague at Sydney*, 1902, by J. A. Thompson, M.D., D.P.H.

[3] *Revue d'Hygiène*, xxv. p. 426, May, 1903.

the disease to healthy rats by the bites of fleas which had fed on a plague-infected rat.

Experiments also carried out in Bombay by Dr Elkington and Captain Liston of the Indian Medical Service were successful in conveying the disease by fleas from infected to healthy rats and from a septicaemic case of plague in man to healthy rats[1].

An interesting observation was made by Dr J. M. Clarke in regard to the immunity of a locality near which plague was prevalent. While plague continued at Iquique not a single case of plague originated in the interior immediately adjoining, which was on the Pampas and some three thousand feet above the sea, where the deposits of nitrate of soda are found together with immense salt beds, although there was a continual interchange of population whose habits were filthy, and sanitary measures unknown. It is suggested by Dr Clarke that the immunity might have been due to fleas not being able to live in the locality. By way of experiment a number of fleas were taken up and in less than one hour they all died.

Rats do not exhaust the list of rodents or other animals which may disseminate plague. It was a commonly accepted opinion in the 16th and 17th centuries that cats, dogs, pigeons and fowls spread the disease. Athanasius Kircher, after describing the manner in which the contagious virus adheres to bedding, linen, clothes, skins, carpets, leather, even to spoons, knives, tabletops, cups, shoes, belts, &c., adds that animals such as "cats, dogs, pigeons, fowls and the like, dwelling within the precincts of an infected house at the very first contact with the things infected take the contagiousness which breeds contagion; and even if, by a kind of contrariety of nature, they are not affected internally by it they nevertheless do carry it into the neighbouring houses and spread the plague they have caught throughout the city. Therefore, in time of plague, the slaying and extermination of dogs and cats and suchlike domestic animals is prescribed. Examples beyond all count show how great is the danger from such animals when a house is stricken by plague[2]." He quotes the case of a nun in Milan who, when the plague was beginning in that city, isolated herself from her companions and endeavoured to protect herself by fumigating and burning of scents in her chamber. On one occasion, however, having

In the 16th and 17th centuries cats, dogs, pigeons and fowls were believed to spread plague.

---

[1] *Australasian Medical Gazette*, xxII. p. 348, August, 1903.

[2] Athanasii Kircheri, E. S. J., *Scrutinium Physico-Medicum Contagiosae Luis, quae Pestis dicitur.* Rome. 1658.

to leave her cell, the door was left open and on her return she found a cat on the bed that had caught the plague elsewhere, which is believed to have infected the bed, which again infected the nun, who was attacked and died on the third day of her illness. It is remarked by Orengius, on whose authority the story is given, that the cats on the premises were killed and the nunnery after that was free from the contagion.

There are few old "plague orders" that do not attach importance to the destruction of dogs and cats. Dr Maunagetta in his "plague order" mentions that Dr Marsilius Ficinus, who reports on the plague of 1479 in Florence, states that plague was conveyed from infected houses to healthy ones by cats and dogs. Roderick von Casto made a similar observation during one of the plagues of Hamburg.

At Padua during an epidemic all the dogs and cats within a radius of 4 miles were destroyed in order to prevent the extension of the plague. In the London epidemic of 1543[1] the plague order enjoins among other things "that all persons having any dogs in their house, other than hounds, spaniels, or mastiffs, necessary for the custody or safe keeping of their houses, should forthwith convey them out of the city or cause them to be killed and carried out of the city and burned at the common lay-stall, and that such as kept hounds, spaniels, or mastiffs should not suffer them to go abroad but closely confine them."

In subsequent orders similar injunctions in regard to dogs, cats, and swine appear. At the height of the Marseilles epidemic it is recorded that no fewer than 10,000 dogs had been killed. Skeyne in 1568 remarks that if the domestic fowls become pestilential it is the sign of a most dangerous pest to follow. The Franks in Egypt and Syria, when shutting themselves up in their houses during the plague season, which used to be their custom, also shut up in cages their dogs and cats, and were careful to shut up all openings or holes to prevent any animal gaining access to the house from the outside. Any animal entering the house was immediately killed.

It was, moreover, held that insects were the means of conveying **Ancient belief in the possibility of insects conveying infection.** contagion. Dr Girolamo Mercurialis in the 16th century states that flies filled with the juice from patients as well as corpses passing into the neighbouring houses and tainting with their dirt, eatables, have brought the contagion upon such people as partook of them. Athanasius Kircher instances a case of infection caused by a hornet: "In the late plague of

---

[1] *History of Epidemics in Britain*, Vol. I. p. 314. By Charles Creighton, M.A., M.D., 1891.

Naples a nobleman was looking at something at the window when suddenly a hornet flew in and settled upon his nose and stinging him produced a swelling: gradually this grew and the poison creeping through his flesh within two days of catching the plague he died, most certainly from the contagious humour which the insect had sucked from a corpse."

From observations then made, when plague used to be prevalent in Europe and Egypt, it is evident the opinion was formed that animals and insects were able to spread the infection. That opinion has been confirmed in many respects by the experiments and observations of recent years. It has already been shown that fleas may be transmitters of plague infection from rat to rat. Ants, bugs, flies and mosquitoes have also at various times come under suspicion of being either active

Plague bacilli detected in ants, bugs and flies.

or passive agents in the dissemination of plague. Plague bacilli have been detected in ants, bugs and flies which have fed on or come into contact with plague material in an infected house, or in a mortuary, or in the laboratory.

An interesting case is reported by Calmette and Salimbeni in the Oporto epidemic of 1899 in which the lesion produced by the bite of a bug was the starting-point of an infection of plague[1]. The person attacked was bitten on the night of Sept. 21st by a bug on the left hand; the next day the hand and forearm were in a state of intense inflammatory oedema and at the site of the bite a large black areola formed, the centre quickly necrosing and the necrosis extending soon over the whole of the dorsum of the hand. On the same day the symptoms of plague declared themselves. On the 23rd September the temperature was 40° C.; there was delirium; the cervical glands were much engorged and painful, especially the right; the inguinal glands on both sides were slightly swollen and sensitive to pressure; a track of lymphangitis on right thigh and ecchymosis on the back of the right hand. On the 24th September the temperature was 38·5° C., pulse 120, tongue and lips fuliginous, respiration frequent and the patient sank into a state of coma which continued for three days, death occurring on the 27th September. The post-mortem of this case showed large necrotic ulceration on the dorsum of the left hand, a right femoro-inguinal bubo, which when incised exuded a dense and viscous chocolate-coloured fluid; general glandular enlargement and the usual appearances of a septicaemia.

---

[1] "La Peste Bubonique, étude de l'épidémie d'Oporto en 1899." Par A. Calmette et A. T. Salimbeni. *Annales de l'Institut Pasteur*. December, 1899.

It is established experimentally that animals of different species are
more or less susceptible to plague; among these are cats,
dogs, pigs, calves, sheep, poultry, monkeys, and squirrels
and snakes. Plague has also been discovered as occurring
by natural infection among cats in the Mauritius, Cape
Town and elsewhere, among dogs in China, among poultry
in Hongkong, among monkeys, squirrels and porcupines in
India, and in a wallaroo, pademelon, tree-kangaroo, Indian
antelope and wallabies in Sydney. There is reason, also, to
suspect the susceptibility of moles and bats. The rôle of all these
animals in the direct dissemination of plague in the existing pandemic
has not yet been proved to be of much importance. Possibly, as plague
becomes more diffused and endemic in the areas that it has invaded, the
natural infection to which these animals are subject may have a greater
opportunity of becoming more general, and the older observations as to
their power of disseminating the infection will be found to be correct.

The rôle of animals other than rats in the dissemination of plague not judged to be important from existing observations.

In regard to direct infection communicated by the cat an interesting
case occurred in the Cape Town outbreak of 1901. The Rev. Mr Gressley, who took up his residence in the Health Camp and voluntarily
performed the duties of chaplain, was attacked with plague under the
following circumstances: a cat of his became sick and after a few days
died; examination proved its illness and death to be due to plague.
One peculiarity of the bacillus, however, was its staining with Gram's
method. A few days afterwards Mr Gressley was attacked with plague,
his infection being attributed to the cat. Curiously enough the bacillus
in Mr Gressley's bubo also possessed the character of staining with
Gram's method.

The epizootic disease which affects the tarbagan marmot, a rodent
which is very common in the Transbaikal province of
Siberia, has already been stated to be communicable to
man. Although the bacteriological test has not been
applied yet the descriptions given by Dr Bieliavski and
Dr Rieshetnikof respectively leave little doubt that the
disease affecting these rodents, and which is liable to be communicated
to man, is plague.

The tarbagan (Arctomys bobac) subject to an epizootic much like plague.

Dr Clemow gives in the *Journal of Tropical Medicine*[1] a full and
interesting account of the disease, derived from the contents of two
articles published in the *Journal of General Hygiene and Legal and*

---

[1] "Plague in Siberia and Mongolia and the Tarbagan (Arctomys bobac)." By Frank
Clemow, M.D., D.P.H., *Journal of Tropical Medicine*, February, 1900.

Practical Medicine for April, 1895 (*Viestnik obshtchestvennoi Gigiénui Sudelnoi i Praktitcheskoi Meditzinui*), the official journal of the medical department of the Russian Ministry of the Interior.

The tarbagan is a rodent of about 26 inches in length, with a thick fur of a dull yellow colour, which is of a darker shading on the back and snout and round the lips and eyes. The animal builds large underground dwellings in which it hybernates from September to March. It is hunted by the nomad Buriats and by the Cossacks, its flesh being considered a delicacy for the table, but it is principally sought for on account of its fat, which is used for greasing straps, harness and other leather objects. In some years, and usually in the autumn, the tarbagan is attacked by an epizootic disease, the symptoms of which are as follows.

The animal becomes languid and ceases to bark; its gait is unsteady and sometimes under one shoulder a reddish tense swelling appears; if far from its home the animal may be unable from its dazed condition to find it, and readily falls a prey to its foes. Sometimes the swelling is absent or very small, and the Buriats, to determine whether the animal is diseased or not cut into the sole of one pad and if the blood is coagulated they consider the animal is diseased and give it to the dogs. Dr Clemow remarks that it is an interesting fact that neither dogs nor wolves contract the disease.

The disease in man which is believed to be contracted from this **The disease in man contracted from sick tarbagans.** epizootic disease of the tarbagan has the clinical symptoms of plague with its great fatality. The symptoms are severe headache, fever, vomiting, sometimes diarrhoea, but more commonly constipation, and pain in the arm-pit or groin with glandular swelling, which, however, is not always present, ending fatally as a rule in a few days. In the village of Soktui in August, 1889, in a Cossack family of ten persons a girl aged 16 years died of this disease after three days' illness, and her death was followed by that of three other members of the family. Then a relative took home some of the clothes and washed them, and in a few days was attacked with the disease and died. Five other members of this second family were attacked and died and only a child of five years remained unaffected; a young Buriat aged 10 years, who played with the children, also sickened and died.

It appears that the members of the family first attacked were occupied in catching and skinning tarbagans, and two years later one of the remaining six sons contracted the disease and died after skinning and removing the fat from a sickly looking animal. His death was followed by that of his brother, aged 5. At the same time in the town of Aksha a small outbreak took place, the first case being that of a man who, while away from home, had eaten some tarbagan flesh with some Mongolians. He sickened the day after his return and died three days afterwards. Five other members of the family were attacked and died. One of these was removed while ill to a neighbour's house, where two of the household afterwards sickened and died. The symptoms were high fever, giddiness, severe headache, red and flushed face with anxious expression, rapid and progressively weaker pulse. Some patients complained of oppression and pain in the chest with occasional dry cough, and the expectoration of a small amount of occasionally blood-stained sputum. The weakness and depression were extreme, but there was usually consciousness to the end. In some there was pain and swelling of the glands in the axilla or groin, while in others there were no glandular swellings.

In 1894 there was a severe visitation in Soktui in another Cossack family, which was caused by the head of the family, on his way to attend the court at Tzagan-Olui, carrying six tarbagans which his dog had caught and killed. The rapidity with which the animals were caught seemed to show that they must have been suffering from disease. He was taken ill two days after his return home and died three days later. His symptoms were headache, drowsiness, vomiting and diarrhoea. On September 14th the youngest son fell ill with the same symptoms, and had pain and swelling "in the arm-pits and groins." On September 15th a son, on the 17th the mother, on the 19th the grandfather, on the 29th the grandmother, on the 23rd the eldest daughter fell ill and died.

None of the villagers would go near the sick but they brought food and drink for them, which they placed at some distance from the infected house. The dead were buried by the survivors, who threw into the grave the clothes and linen of the deceased. Sixteen days after the last death the survivors went to the house of a relative after changing all their clothes in an out-house, burning their old clothes and putting on new ones provided by the relative.

The tarbagan is to be found in Eastern Europe, Siberia, Mongolia, and Tibet, but, as pointed out by Dr Clemow, there is no evidence to show that it suffers from the fatal epizootic described except in the Transbaikal province, and possibly in the neighbourhood of the Solenko valley in Mongolia.

PART III.

PLAGUE IN THE INDIVIDUAL.

CHAPTER XII.

MORBID ANATOMY AND PATHOLOGY.

IT is usually on the post-mortem table that the first case of plague is discovered. The characteristic appearance in a necropsy of plague is that of engorgement and haemorrhage associated with enlargement of the lymphatic glands and extravasations into the periglandular tissues of one or more groups of these glands. Nearly every organ participates more or less in the extravasation of blood from the veins.

Professor Frazer[1] (now Sir Thomas) points out that the vascular changes, and especially the pervading and characteristic tendency to extravasation of blood in almost every part of the body, are closely reproduced in the toxaemia caused by the organic poison secreted by the venom glands of several species of serpents, such as the black snake (Pseudechis porphyriacus) of Australia.

Pathological changes special to plague occur in the skin, lymphatic glands and the adjoining blood vessels, in the spleen, lungs, Skin. heart, liver, and kidneys. Decomposition of the dead body is not accelerated in plague unless in the mixed form when streptococci are present, then putrefaction may set in very early. On the skin there are often small haemorrhages chiefly on and in the vicinity of the bubo and on the head, arms, neck and shoulders; these haemorrhages contain plague bacilli. Haemorrhages are also found in the muscles, chiefly in those of the abdomen and of the temporal bones, as well as in

---

[1] *Report of the Indian Plague Commission*, Vol. v. Appendix ii. p. 436.

the muscles near the primary bubo; they contain polynuclear leucocytes and plague bacilli. Carbuncles, boils, vesicles, or pustules may be present on any part of the body. Epidemics differ much in this respect, some being distinguished for the comparative rarity of these skin manifestations, others for their frequency. They appear over intensely inflamed glands or in other regions of the body, and are local infiltrations of the skin and areolar tissue and contain plague bacilli and leucocytes. They vary in size, present at first a vesicular or blister-like appearance on the surface of the skin, but when the blister is broken there is underneath an ulcer with uneven surface of a reddish-yellow colour. Cut into, they are thick, hard and dense and haemorrhagic.

The condition of the lymph glands is peculiar to plague. There is
Lymphatic glands. no other infectious disease which shows a similar multiple inflammation of the lymphatic glands, together with haemorrhages, exudative infiltrations into the periglandular tissue, and presence of characteristic bacilli.

In the bubonic form the gland or group of glands affected are
External primary buboes. manifested externally as buboes in the region of the groin, arm-pit, and neck. The groin is by far the most frequent site, one or both sides exhibiting buboes. Occasionally there are buboes at the elbow and in the space behind the knee. The buboes vary in size and shape according to their situation, the number of glands affected, and the amount of haemorrhagic serous or serosanguinolent effusion from the glands into the periglandular tissue. At times the amount of effusion is small or absent, and only one or a few glands slightly swollen, then the bubo is small and easily felt. Most frequently the opposite conditions prevail. The effusion is extensive, the bubo is large and readily recognised. Then the connective tissue is infiltrated with blood or with a yellow gelatinous oedema, or with both, which mats together the haemorrhagic and much swollen glands and forms a swelling which may be the size of a man's fist. The exact limits of this tumour are often ill-defined owing to a surrounding oedematous condition. Between the above-mentioned extremes there is every gradation. Anatomically then the bubo consists of connective tissue more or less engorged or infiltrated with blood, or serum, or both, which forms a dense sanguineous gelatinous or oedematous mass in a state of inflammation in which is embedded one or more enlarged glands inflamed or haemorrhagically infarcted. On the boundaries of this hard and tense tumour there is often an extensive oedema. The colour of the bubo and the adjacent tissues will accord with the relative

15—2

amount of blood or exudative infiltration effused from the glands, the one being black and the other yellow. Much variety in coloration will occur according to whichever predominates. The mass will also exhibit different stages of inflammation, exudation, haemorrhagic infarction, suppuration and necrosis according to the intensity of the disease and the duration of the illness. The size of the separate swollen glands varies, being from that of a pea to that of a walnut. The enlargement is due to hyperaemia, inflammation, exudation and haemorrhage, and these processes obliterate more or less the distinction between cortical and medullary substance. The condition of the lymphatic glands depends largely on the time of death. In severe cases in which death takes place rapidly the glands may be of a purple or dark plum colour, and partially or completely infarcted haemorrhagically and exhibit on section a deep red-brown or blackish-red appearance. The haemorrhages with an exudative oedema may have broken through the capsules and infiltrated the surrounding periglandular tissue, matting together the separate glands which are in various stages of inflammation, and involving the neighbouring fascia, adipose tissue, muscles, vessels and nerve sheaths to a greater or less extent. In other cases the glands are red or violet or brownish-red in colour, moderately hard and with their capsules distended. On section the parenchyma may be of soft or firm consistence and of a granular mottled or marbled appearance, the medullary substance being profusely sprinkled or streaked with bright red extravasations of varying sizes. At the periphery of the gland there is frequently a fine granulation formed of yellow nodules, on which there is a ropy or viscid material. The exudation is not so haemorrhagic but of a sero-sanguinolent nature forming a yellow, gelatinous oedema mixed with blood extravasations. Commencing necrosis is evidenced by a greyish-yellow or mottled brownish-red and grey appearance. In later cases in which the disease is protracted to the 8th or 9th day, the parenchyma of the gland usually contains a yellow or yellowish-red pus, while the periglandular tissue may have improved in condition or is in a state of suppuration. In other cases there may be a general sloughing of glands and tissues.

The veins in the vicinity of the bubo, such as the femoral, axillary and jugular, participate more or less in the disease, being embedded in a yellow gelatinous mass containing extravasated blood. They are affected by the haemorrhagic infiltration and inflammatory exudations proceeding from the glands, and are thus often incorporated in the bubo mass forming

Veins in the vicinity of the bubo affected.

a part of the tumour. The haemorrhages and inflammatory exudations do not confine themselves to an infiltration of the tissues around the veins, but they penetrate into and between their walls so that when the veins are opened their inner surface shows large and suffused hae-morrhagic patches which become smaller, more isolated and punctated the further away they are from the bubo. By the haemorrhages into the walls of the veins there is established a direct communication between the glands and the veins.

Major Childe, I.M.S., was the first to point out this haemorrhage into the walls of the veins included in the bubo and the continuity of the extravasated blood in the gland, in the areolar tissue outside the gland and in the walls of the veins incorporated in the bubo[1].

This destruction of the walls of blood vessels, inside and outside the glands leading to haemorrhages, appears chiefly to be brought about by the plague bacillus and its toxines in the glands and in the exudative infiltration acting chemically on the minute vessels of the walls.

There may be other buboes in connection with the buboes in the groin, arm-pit, and neck. A bubo in the groin not infre-

Internal buboes.

quently extends through the crural ring into the pelvis and abdominal cavity, involving successively the glands, tissues, and vessels in the iliac and lumbar regions and forming one or more large tumours. The bubo possesses similar characters to the ordinary bubo, both as regards the degree of intensity and number of glands affected and as regards the amount of sero-sanguinolent infiltration and oedema into the tissues around them; occasionally the iliac glands show much more change and swelling than the inguinal. In some cases the chain of glands along the spinal column as far as the thoracic cavity and even up to the hinder mediastinal glands are extensively affected, or this condition may extend over to the glands of the other side of the body and there may be large buboes on both sides of the spine to the diaphragm. Similarly in an axillary bubo the chain of glands to the subclavian vein and to the neck may participate, while a bubo in the cervical region may extend down into the thoracic wall and affect the glands there and frequently to the axilla. These internal buboes like the external are characterised by altered and swollen glands, haemorrhages and oedema, and may be in a worse condition than the external ones, but the area involved and the acute inflammatory changes in the surrounding tissues are usually less, there being more of the yellowish gelatinous oedema than there is of the copious haemorrhagic infiltration characteristic of those buboes first affected. The glands may vary from

[1] Report of Major Lyons, I.M.S., President, Bombay Plague Research Committee.

the size of a pea to an olive, and on section display a considerable range in the degree to which they are affected, some being completely haemorrhagically infarcted, while others are of a reddish-brown, reddish-yellow, or straw-yellow colour. Of internal glands the mesenteric and retroperitoneal are frequently affected. This was very noticeable in the autopsies at Hongkong. They were generally dark red or purple in colour, of the size of a bean, and embedded in an extravasated mass of blood. The adjoining veins and lymph vessels were in these cases dilated and their walls suffused with blood.

There are other buboes which in contradistinction to those already referred to may be termed secondary, although they may not be preceded by primary buboes. They originate when the circulation is invaded in force by the plague bacilli, which are then carried by the blood to different glands in the body. This occurs either in consequence of the walls of the veins incorporated in the bubo becoming so damaged by the infiltration as to permit of a direct entrance for the microbes from the glands into the circulation, or it occurs in cases when the blood stream is directly infected and the bacilli multiply in the blood instead of in the lymphatic glands. In each instance the disease becomes septicaemic, that is, the blood stream becomes the agent for the distribution of the plague bacilli to the different organs and glands in the body. These secondary buboes may therefore develop in all regions of the body quite independently of the seat of a primary bubo, from which they differ in some very important respects. The glands are enlarged, but seldom larger than a bean or hazel-nut; they are hard and solid and of a pink colour; on section they are found to be engorged with blood; and the parenchyma is hyperaemic, soft, of splenic consistence and easily scraped off with a knife. In a later stage the soft, swollen, parenchymatous tissue is oedematous, with distinct greyish-red haemorrhages and softened areas: in still later cases the haemorrhagic infarcts occupy a considerable area within the gland, but do not go beyond the capsule, so that further than occasional oedematous condition of the surrounding tissues there is rarely any haemorrhagic or gelatinous infiltration to be seen connected with these glands.

The best description of the histological changes is given by Albrecht and Ghon[1], whose work in Bombay in this respect on behalf of the Austrian Government is of the most careful and minute character.

Secondary buboes.

[1] "Ueber die Beulenpest in Bombay im Jahre 1897." *Gesammtbericht der von der Kaiserlichen Akademie der Wissenschaft in Wien zum Studium der Beulenpest nach Indien entsendeter Commission.* Vienna, 1898.

The histological changes in the bubo are essentially those which are produced by the irritating and destructive action of the plague bacillus and its toxines. They appear to be first an inflammatory action on the cellular elements of the tissues, followed by necrotic and disintegrating processes

Histological changes in primary bubo.

which affect the capillaries and blood vessels, leading to haemorrhages and exudative infiltrations which favour a further destructive effect and a further spread of the bacillus. Wherever bacilli are to be found in large numbers, which is the case in a primary bubo, there, sooner or later, the tissues gradually break up, disintegrate, and finally form into masses of detritus. With the gland as the starting-point of the tissue changes in the bubo, the glandular tissue shows a more advanced degree of haemorrhages, infiltration of leucocytes and bacilli and necrotic degenerations than the periglandular tissue.

With the invasion of the bacilli, which may be aggregated in masses in the gland or extend throughout the whole gland, the parenchyma is either partially or completely disintegrated. Haemorrhagic extravasations take the place of the disintegrated portion of the gland, or it is crowded with polynuclear leucocytes showing a tendency to necrosis. There is also a very abundant infiltration of plague bacilli. The appearance is variable, depending on the amount of the haemorrhages, the infiltration of leucocytes and bacilli and the necrosis. With the complete or almost complete disintegration of the adenoid tissue, the normal structure of the gland disappears and the separate parts are indistinguishable. The leucocytes are in such masses that they give the appearance of a purulent infiltration. In the infiltration itself there is a granular disintegration of the nuclei as well as of the leucocytes, the detritus extending over large areas, or the outline of the cells may be more or less retained, but the nuclei have disappeared or are indistinct. The necrosis is generally most marked in the central portions of the gland, while the haemorrhages and infiltrations of leucocytes and bacilli are to be best seen at the periphery. The bacilli in the region of the necrotic portions assume more or less the degenerative forms to be found in other parts. In fresh pus there is to be found in addition to polynuclear leucocytes numerous fully degenerated cells and débris of cells and nuclei. The walls of the vessels and capillaries that have resisted the disintegrating process are thickened and dilated, while the others which have given way and from which the blood has poured out are in all stages of necrosis, some consisting of mere shreds and detritus. The blood is coagulated and forms a network both within and without the vessels, or is broken up into débris. In this network or débris are nuclei of cells, disintegrated leucocytes, and plague bacilli. The capsule of the gland is broken in places by the extravasation of blood and infiltration of the periglandular tissue with bacilli and leucocytes, and its fibres are torn, swollen or destroyed so as to be indistinguishable from the affected glandular and periglandular tissues. The infiltration of the surrounding connective and adipose tissue, when not haemorrhagic, is essentially cellular and contains polynuclear leucocytes in different stages of disintegration, and large numbers of plague bacilli. The oedema, on the other hand, is either homogeneous or finely granular in character. In some cases there is not much haemorrhage or cellular infiltration into the connective and adipose tissue, but merely oedematous fluid swarming with plague bacilli. The lymphatic vessels in the vicinity of the disintegrated glands are usually much dilated, being filled with lymph cells and masses of plague bacilli mixed with a few white and red blood corpuscles. The walls of the vessel are thinner, but there is rarely any great change in them, though occasionally they are filled with bacilli and leucocytes or are necrotic and so disintegrated as to form detritus-like masses.

In the secondary buboes or those infected by plague bacilli conveyed to them by the circulation the changes in the glands are **Histological changes in secondary buboes.** not nearly so pronounced. The parenchyma is uniformly hyperaemic, the capillaries and vessels being distended with blood in which will be found plague bacilli in varying numbers; the fibrous capsule of the gland remains intact, the lymphatic vessels and lymph channels are distended with lymph cells, and the sinus is much distended, its cells being swollen, pale, granular, or fatty. Within the sinus are often polynuclear leucocytes and red blood corpuscles, frequently arranged around vessels or smaller haemorrhages. Sometimes the sinus is gorged with blood or there are necrotic centres with granular disintegration of the cell nuclei.

In buboes which have healed before the process of necrosis or deep-seated suppuration has begun, complete resolution takes place, leaving only a slight but general thickening of the capsule of the parenchyma of the gland, of the blood vessels, and of the connective tissue.

The most characteristic feature of cover-glass and sectional prepara- **The plague bacillus.** tions from primary buboes is the enormous number of plague bacilli which are to be seen. Even when necrosis of the gland has set in, and there are few bacilli in the cover-glass preparations, the cultures furnish many colonies of plague bacilli.

The more typical-shaped bacilli are usually to be found in the peripheral portions of the periglandular tissues, whereas the degenerative or involution forms are generally in those parts of the bubo most affected, where the plague bacilli have destroyed the tissues, and which correspond with the gland. The plague bacilli are generally extracellular, and it is only in the most recent infiltration that they may be seen within the leucocytes. In secondary buboes, however, the plague bacilli may be seen within the swollen or desquamated endothelium of the capillaries and lymphatic vessels. In a cover-glass preparation the size and form of the bacilli correspond with the histological changes in the bubo. At an early stage the typical short, thick rod forms with rounded ends, often exhibiting a capsule, are the most numerous. They may be single, in pairs, and in short chains, and stain deeply at the poles with carbol-fuchsin, borax methyl-blue, Loeffler's methylene blue, or other aniline dyes. The number of bacilli taking on the bi-polar staining is very noticeable. In later stages the bacillus tends to lose its plump appearance and assumes much variety in shape and irregularity of size. There is to be seen coccoid, globular, spherical, bladder-like, tadpole, and sickle-shaped forms, which differ much in their staining properties, some of them staining but faintly, others only at the margin of the circumference or on a portion of the rim, and others remaining colourless.

It is not infrequent to meet with a mixed infection in plague, and in these cases the pneumococcus may be found with the plague bacillus; or the streptococcus or staphylococcus may be associated with it.

It frequently happens that when a cover-glass preparation shows numerous plague bacilli mixed with only small numbers of streptococci, diplococci, and staphylococci, the cultures do not show plague bacilli. This occurs not only with cultures from glands and buboes, but also with cultures from the spleen and liver in which plague bacilli are distinct and numerous in smear specimens. Sometimes when only a few bacilli, or perhaps none, are seen on the cover-glass preparation, cultures may show colonies of plague bacilli. It is important, therefore, as pointed out by Albrecht and Ghon[1], when it is a question of doubtful diagnosis, that both cultures and cover-glass preparations should be made, and they should be supplemented by inoculation of animals.

Another important point is that though the bacillus is often not to

---

[1] "Ueber die Beulenpest in Bombay im Jahre 1897." *Gesammtbericht der von der Kaiserlichen Akademie der Wissenschaft in Wien zum Studium der Beulenpest nach Indien entsendeter Commission.* Vienna, 1898, p. 508.

be found in a suppurating bubo, yet suppuration does not necessarily destroy its vitality. It has been found in cases of this description in man and also in animals. The Austrian Commission first drew attention to this[1]. In this connection two cases are mentioned by Dr Choksy[2] of Bombay, in which iliac buboes were opened through the abdominal wall on the 48th day of illness, and the pus was found to contain plague bacilli in an active state and capable of growth when cultured.

Plague bacilli are not only present in the buboes and adjacent tissues, but in septic cases they are also present in the blood, in the glands, in the lungs, liver, kidney, in the bone marrow, in the bile, in the urine and faeces, in the peritoneal fluid, and in fact in every organ and secretion of the body.

The spleen is enlarged and congested, having the capsule distended,
Spleen. of a light grey opacity and sometimes marbled with hae-morrhages. On section it is seen to be much engorged, is a deep red, chocolate-brown or purple colour, and has a granular appearance. The Malpighian bodies are swollen and engorged, the substance may be fairly firm or friable and soft, or it may be almost diffluent.

Histologically the changes in the spleen are similar to those in the lymphatic glands, and consist of haemorrhages, inflammations, infiltration of leucocytes and bacilli, and necrosis. The infiltration of the pulp and blood spaces with blood, polynuclear leucocytes and epithelial cells, renders the spongy structure of the spleen indistinct. The Malpighian corpuscles remain intact. The trabiculae are mostly swollen.

Small necrotic centres are frequently to be seen surrounded by numerous plague bacilli. They are formed by the coagulating and disintegrating action of the bacilli, and are composed of the débris of the disintegrated walls of the blood vessels and the detritus of coagulated blood. Plague bacilli have been found in the spleen of a patient who died on the 52nd day of illness[3].

The pericardial cavity usually contains a large quantity of blood-
Circulatory stained or straw-coloured fluid. Ecchymoses occur on the
system. pericardium and endocardium. The heart muscle is pale, soft, and friable, and is in a condition of cloudy swelling or fatty degeneration. The right side is usually distended with dark red blood and coagulated to form soft clots, or is in a semi-fluid condition. On

---

[1] "Ueber die Beulenpest in Bombay im Jahre 1897," p. 510.
[2] *The Treatment of Plague with Professor Lustig's Serum.* By N. H. Choksy, M.D., 1903.
[3] H. Albrecht u. A. Ghon. "Ueber die Beulenpest in Bombay im Jahre 1897," p. 532.

the valves may occasionally be observed haemorrhagic growths. The blood itself is in a state of leucocytosis of the polynuclear variety, and generally contains plague bacilli. It has very little tendency to coagulate and remains fluid. It is usually of a very dark colour. The great veins of the thorax and abdomen are distended with dark blood, and there is a general distension of the veins and smaller blood vessels, accompanied by large and small haemorrhages. Haemorrhages are, in fact, one of the characteristics of the disease. There are haemorrhages in nearly every organ of the body, on the serous and mucous coats of the cavities, and in and around the specially affected lymphatic glands. The plague bacilli and their toxines appear to have a peculiar coagulative and necrotic effect on the walls of the smaller veins and minute capillaries, leading to exudations.

The veins of the trunk when cut open display numerous small punctated haemorrhages which, the nearer the veins approach the vicinity of a bubo, become haemorrhagic patches of considerable size. It has already been stated, that the walls of large veins in the region of primary buboes are much affected. In those veins which are embedded in the sero-sanguinolent, gelatinous, or haemorrhagic infiltration, and which are thus subjected to the solvent action of the plague bacillus and its glutinous toxines, the outer walls become destroyed, and the tunica intima exhibits large haemorrhagic and suffused patches with erosions. In the event of perforation taking place through the intima, the copious haemorrhagic and oedematous effusions crowded with bacilli find their way into the blood stream: microscopical examination shows that the coats of the venous walls are separated by masses of blood, that the endothelium is taken off or has disappeared, and that plague bacilli are present in great numbers. Venous haemorrhage of this kind only occurs as a rule when the lymphatic glands are in an advanced state of change.

The mucous membrane of the larynx, trachea and the large bronchi
The respiratory system. exhibit a more or less catarrhal condition. In some cases of cervical bubo or in tonsillar plague the exudation may extend to the glottis, causing oedema of one or both folds of this organ. The effusion presents the same yellowish jelly-like appearance characteristic of oedema in the vicinity of the bubo. Microscopically it consists of homogeneous, finely granular fluid containing leucocytes, red corpuscles and plague bacilli.

In all forms of plague the lungs are congested and oedematous, and on section a sero-frothy mucus exudes from them. There are small

haemorrhages into the lungs and more or less extensive pleural haemorrhages in the region of the diaphragm, on the chest walls, and on
the surface of the lung. Microscopically the vessels of bronchi, lung
tissue and pleura are distended with blood, plague bacilli are to be seen
in the lung oedema, and especially wherever there are haemorrhages.

In the pneumonic form of plague first described by Childe[1], which
is of a primary character and usually unaccompanied by buboes, and in
the pneumonic form of a secondary nature with buboes, the lungs are the
seat of a well-marked disseminated broncho-pneumonia. In pneumonic
plague, in addition to the great engorgement and oedema of the lungs
which exist in other forms of plague, the bronchi are inflamed and
haemorrhagic, and filled with a blood-stained frothy mucus, and the lung
tissue contains numerous pneumonic patches scattered throughout its
substance. These patches vary in size from a pea to that of an egg, and,
when superficial, are raised above the surface, forming small tumours; the
pleura over them generally shows signs of inflammation and is covered with
a fibrinous exudation. They are of a deep red, pink or reddish-grey colour,
solid, airless, and sink in water, and they are separated from the surrounding crepitant lung tissue by a distinct ring of engorgement. The patches
are lobular in type, and as a rule are distinct, but they may be confluent so as to form large areas or even affect the whole of one lobe
and exhibit the appearance of that of a croupous pneumonia. In these
cases the consistence of the part is friable, the colour is of a chocolate
hue, and on pressure there exudes from the lung a prune-coloured
liquid rich in plague bacilli. The bronchial glands are engorged,
swollen, and are often haemorrhagic. Microscopical examination of the
pneumonic patches shows the alveoli to contain catarrhal epithelium,
leucocytes, blood cells, granular débris, and fibrils of destroyed septa,
together with a homogeneous coagulated mass of oedematous fluid and a
large number of plague bacilli occasionally mixed with pneumococci and
streptococci. The bronchioles and bronchi are also full of plague
bacilli, which during life appear in the sputum; portions of the patches
may have undergone necrosis. The fibrinous exudation in the pleura
contains plague bacilli. The patches in secondary pneumonia are frequently of the nature of small metastatic infarcts.

There is an interesting record of a post-mortem made by Dr
Thomson on plague in the Great Plague of London. It was evidently
of the pneumonic type; it is that of a dissection of a young man who

---

[1] Report by Surgeon-Major Lyons, I.M.S., of Bombay, President of the Plague Research
Committee.

died of plague. It is recorded that "the superficies of the lungs were stigmatized with several large ill-favoured marks, much tumefied and distended, the inward part being pertunded with my knife a sanious dreggy corruption issued forth and a pale ichor destitute of any blood[1]."

Dr Thomson was himself attacked with plague the next day after the dissection, but recovered and got up on the 8th day; he, however, had a relapse. Three other persons were attacked in his house but all recovered.

Liver. The liver may be enlarged or normal in size .and engorged with blood, but the parenchyma is generally pale, soft, and friable and in a state of cloudy swelling or fatty degeneration. Yellow necrotic patches are often seen in its substance, and especially on its upper surface. On microscopical examination the capillaries are seen to be distended and may show colonies of plague bacilli with leucocytes, both of which are particularly numerous in and near the yellow necrotic patches, as well as in numerous ecchymoses, which may be often seen on the surface of the liver and on the glissonic capsule.

The gall-bladder has its mucous membrane not infrequently studded with small multiple haemorrhages, which sometimes joining give it a dark, marbled appearance. These minute haemorrhages may extend into the mucous membrane of the bile-ducts. Plague bacilli are in these haemorrhages as well as in the bile.

The pancreas may be congested but is otherwise normal in appearance.

Alimentary canal. The mucous membrane of the pharynx and oesophagus are generally congested and inflamed and the seat of petechiae. The tonsils may be normal but sometimes they are swollen and haemorrhagic, presenting on section the mottled appearance seen in buboes. In some cases the tonsil may be surrounded by an oedematous infiltration, extending into the palatine arch or to the glottis. In other cases both pharynx and tonsil may be covered by a pseudo-diphtheritic dirty-yellowish membrane which undergoes necrosis. This destructive process is due to infiltration of plague bacilli, often mixed with other pyogenic microbes. In connection with this condition of the tonsils the lymph glands of the neck are generally affected and plague bacilli are to be found in the sputum.

It may be here pointed out that in a number of experiments on

---

[1] "Loimotomia on the Pest," by George Thomson, M.D., 1666.

animals already mentioned, in which plague was produced by feeding with plague bacilli, the pharynx and cervical glands were much affected.

Small punctate haemorrhages occur in the stomach and intestines in the mucous coat, and extravasated blood is occasionally to be found in the stomach. At times the haemorrhages in stomach and intestines may be extensive and the mucous membrane intensely inflamed and covered with mucus. In these cases there is an infiltration into or oedema of the sub-mucous coat. The solitary glands and Peyer's patches are often congested and swollen, the patches being denuded of their epithelium and sometimes ulcerated. Ulcerations may occur on the ileo-caecal valve. In the haemorrhages are plague bacilli. There are extravasations into the mesentery. The mesenteric and retro-peritoneal glands sometimes show much swelling, inflammation, and haemorrhagic infiltration. This was more frequent in Hongkong than elsewhere. There, not infrequently, were observed extensive extravasations of blood in the mesentery, and in the majority of cases more or less enlargement and inflammation of the mesenteric glands, which varied from a white to a purple colour, and were sometimes surrounded by a sero-sanguineous infiltration similar to that of an external bubo.

The connective tissue around the kidneys is frequently infiltrated The urinary with a large mass of extravasated blood of a tarry colour. system. The kidneys are swollen, purplish in colour, and with the surface dotted with petechiae. The stellate veins are visible, the capsule usually adherent, and the kidney substance pale and soft from parenchymatous and fatty degeneration. The cortical portion is the most affected, being studded more or less by yellow necrotic foci, attaining at times the size of a pea. These foci contain a very large number of plague bacilli and polynuclear leucocytes.

Sometimes the glomeruli are swollen and the capillaries may have undergone necrotic changes. There are haemorrhages into the mucous membrane of the pelvis, and occasionally these are so extensive as to break through the mucous membrane and pass into the ureter, coagula of blood being then found in the pelvis of the kidney, the ureter and bladder. Plague bacilli are to be found in these haemorrhages; the ureter besides containing coagulated blood has on its mucous membrane petechiae. The bladder is generally contracted, and its mucous membrane the seat of numerous small haemorrhages which contain plague bacilli. Owing to the haemorrhage in the kidneys and along the urinary tract the urine as a rule contains plague bacilli.

The suprarenal capsule may be normal although engorged, or it may be the seat of necrotic centres.

The cerebral membranes are congested and the venous sinuses **Nervous system.** engorged with blood. Petechiae or ecchymoses may be seen in the dura mater. There may be extravasation of blood or effusion of serous fluid into the cavity of the arachnoid or under that membrane. The cortex of the brain may be in a state of congestion, while the substance of the brain shows an unusual number of red points in it indicating increased vascularity. It may also be oedematous, but beyond slight softening of the tissue there appears to be no marked lesion in the brain substance. The spinal cord when examined is found to be congested.

Bubonic plague, judged by the pathological changes observed in the **Conclusion.** dead body, is a disease both of the lymphatic and vascular system, on which the plague bacilli and its toxines when brought in contact with them in large numbers and quantity exercise an inflammatory, coagulative and necrotic effect. The microbic agent and its toxines thus acting lead to enlargement of the external and internal lymph glands, necrosis of their substance and often haemorrhage or infiltration into the surrounding tissues, to dilatation of the veins and capillaries, to destruction of their walls, to haemorrhagic extravasations into nearly every part of the body, to enlargement and engorgement of various organs, and to metastatic parenchymatous degeneration in the liver, spleen, and kidneys. Pneumonic plague differs from bubonic in having these changes more concentrated on the lung tissues and its lymphatic system than on the other lymph glands of the body.

AUTOPSIES.

Malay girl, aged 7 years. Nothing on skin. On making an incision into skin over inguinal region, *left inguinal gland* found to be the size of a large Brazil nut; surface haemorrhagic on one portion. On section upper half dark maroon or coffee colour, lower half dark grey with streaks of haemorrhage passing from the surface to the interior. Around the gland a large amount of haemorrhagic infiltration extending well above Poupart's ligament and also down to nearly one-third of the upper part of the thigh, matting together in its fibrinated tissue a number of maroon-coloured glands. The oedema extends beyond this infiltration. The infiltration and oedema of the left inguinal glands extend to the iliac glands inside the abdomen which are also haemorrhagic and coffee-coloured, but there is no extensive oedema around these iliac glands; the right iliac glands healthy.

The right *inguinal region* enlarged but not so much as the left; periphery of gland haemorrhagic, the central portion being greyish in colour. Left and right *lungs* not pneumonic but coffee-coloured. The *spleen* enlarged, elastic and much engorged. Plague bacilli in *glands, lungs*, and *spleen*.

Malay girl, aged 12 *years*. Taken ill with fever and difficulty of breathing, and pain in the abdomen, was ill for 3 days, no buboes. Died suddenly; diagnosis, inflammation of the bowels.

Post-mortem. *Glands* in both groins slightly enlarged and haemorrhagic. Fat of right groin blood-stained. *Femoral vein* deeply congested. Glands in iliac region congested. Glands of mesentery enlarged and of a maroon appearance. *Small intestine* inflamed and congested. *Lungs* not patchy, but with one lobe on either side deeply congested and full of a prune-coloured juice. Plague bacilli found in the *lungs, glands*, and other organs of body.

Hindú, male, aged 28 *years*. Fell ill on 17th July. Admitted to hospital on the evening of the 21st.

History. On 17th July, evening, was suddenly attacked with vomiting accompanied with fever and very bad headache. About the same time he felt a stabbing pain in the left groin and noticed that a swelling was there. The next day he was very prostrated and almost unconscious.

Present state. Is in great agony. Pulse cannot be counted. Temperature 101·1° F.; typical plague tongue, surface covered with yellowish-brown coating with small red points in it. In left femoral region a bubo, size of a large hen's egg. Skin over bubo red and much infiltrated. Patient died one hour after admission.

Post-mortem. Skin in femoral region haemorrhagically discoloured. Bubo size of a hen's egg; on section there oozes out a bloody oedematous gelatinous fluid; the periglandular tissue of a gelatinous nature with a great infiltration of blood. All the *lymphatic glands* of this region matted together forming one large bubo, which on section is of a dark violet colour; lymphatic glands in right region are swollen and form small separate buboes. All the lymphatic glands in the body are swollen and congested. On opening chest *lungs* contract normally, lungs oedematous: interlobular ecchymoses. In left lung·on section a few small rose-coloured patches; on pressure a red-yellow fluid devoid of air oozes out. Over the *heart* numerous ecchymoses. Heart small, valves and openings normal. *Spleen* very much enlarged. Capsule of spleen very distended. On section the pulp is swollen and friable. *Kidneys* slightly enlarged. On section surface shows swollen cortex, discoloured and with indistinct picture. *Liver* enlarged, structure indistinct. *Stomach* normal. Mucous membrane of *ileum* very much injected, but no ulcerations. In *fossa iliacum* a recto-peritoneal bubo of walnut size on right side; *mesenteric glands* swollen and congested.

Bacteriological examination. Numerous plague bacilli in direct preparations from bubo and glands on right side, blood, and spleen. All give pure cultures.

Hindú, male, aged 25[1]. Admitted on March 6th and died the same day. History unknown.

Post-mortem next morning.

Well-developed, well-nourished body. Rigor mortis almost disappeared, no petechiae visible. *Conjunctivae* injected, mucous membrane of the mouth pale. Under Poupart's ligament, near the median line, a lymphatic gland larger than a hazel-nut can be felt.

No oedema of the lower extremities. The skin of the soles much fissured; no exterior injuries perceptible. The *lymphatic glands* in both submaxillary regions the size of beans, and on section dark red and juicy. Both *tonsils* enlarged, on section exhibit many yellow spots; the left side is infiltrated with a soft medullary substance, and is very juicy, dark red, and sprinkled with yellow. The mucous membrane of the pharynx is reddish-violet and swollen, the mucous membrane of the epiglottis is much reddened and swollen. The follicles at the base of the tongue reddened and enlarged; numerous punctiform ecchymoses in the larynx and at the root of the tongue. *Lungs* congested, and on section frothy and slightly oedematous. *Pericardium* contains a small amount of clear serous fluid, epicardium dotted with ecchymoses size of millet seeds; *heart* normal in size, fibrinous coagula, left side parenchymatous, pale and soft. The mucous membrane of the trachea and the large bronchia somewhat reddened. The lymphatic glands at the bifurcation as large as beans and infarcted. *Alimentary canal* not pathologically changed. *Liver* soft, but normal in size; on section moderately haemorrhagic, flecked with yellow; generally brownish-grey, the outlines of the lobes obliterated. The gall-bladder filled with dark bile, mucous membrane thin and yellowish-brown. *Spleen* very soft, and dark red on section; pulp oozy, stroma not increased, follicles recognisable in

[1] Case extracted from the Report of the Austrian Plague Commission,

parts. *Right kidney* somewhat enlarged and congested on section; cortex swollen, sprinkled, and striped with greyish-yellow and red, well bordered off from the pyramids, the periphery of the latter being injected with vivid red. Condition of *left kidney* similar. Both renal pelves normal. The *bladder* filled with yellowish urine, its mucous membrane whitish. The *deep inguinal lymphatic glands* at the interior femoral ring on the left side the size of hazel-nuts; three lymphatic glands about the size of beans in their vicinity. The connective tissue round the latter, and round the iliac vessels, is wet with gelatinous material, and sanguineously infiltrated, as is also the vicinity of both ureters. There are numerous confluent dark bluish-red haemorrhages in the wall of the *left femoral vein,* composed of smaller haemorrhages about the size of millet seeds, and which infiltrate almost the entire intima of the region. The *superficial inguinal lymphatic glands* of the left side considerably swollen, moderately hard, protruding on incision, haemorrhagic and congested, and infiltrated with yellow spots.

1. Three forms of bacteria are found in cover-glass preparations of the left tonsil, but not in very great numbers. A long, slender species of bacillus is most prominent, and ovoid or longish forms of typical plague bacilli are present in somewhat less numbers; they take bipolar staining well, and most lie singly, more rarely as diplobacilli. The third species, present in least numbers, is formed as a minute rod, likewise with bipolar stain, and which resembles the smallest diplococcus. No plague colonies are visible in the cultures, but there are numerous colonies of the coli group and the spore-bearing rodlets.

Bacteriological condition.

2. A haemorrhagically infiltrated cervical lymphatic gland from the left submaxillary region exhibits, microscopically, typical plague bacilli in fairly large numbers, lying singly or as diplococci, and of roundish or oval form; in addition to bacilli exhibiting good bipolar staining there are paler, ovoid, and large, roundish, inflated forms.

The cultures are contaminated and are therefore not used.

3. Numerous plague bacilli are exhibited microscopically in the juice of the spleen; they mostly lie alone, being of round, oval, or longish form, with bipolar stain, or are only stained faintly, and of various forms.

The cultures exhibit numerous plague colonies exclusively.

4. Cover-glass preparations of a haemorrhagically infiltrated superficial inguinal lymphatic gland of the right side exhibit copious masses of plague bacilli in the same form and order as 3, but the degenerative forms are more numerous; every form is present, even the large inflated

forms, of which frequently only the outlines are stained (annular forms).

On using Pittfield's mixture no distinct capsular appearances are seen, but one may observe a faintly tinted violet area in a number of bacilli; this area is more or less distinctly bordered, or there may be an unstained area which is bordered off by a stained contour.

The cultures exhibit very numerous colonies of the plague bacillus, and 6 colonies of the unknown species of bacillus (contamination).

1. *Enlarged superficial lymphatic gland from the left inguinal region.* Only isolated follicles in the cortical layer are left
Histological condition. of the parenchyma, also a few septa of the connective tissue closely infiltrated by polynuclear leucocytes, and numerous small and large vessels full of blood, the walls of which in places are closely infiltrated by leucocytes.

The enlargement of the gland seems mostly to have been caused by enormous masses of plague bacilli, which infiltrate it entirely in connected masses, cutting into the vessels in all directions and including relatively few leucocytes. In between there are small haemorrhages in all directions, often round vessels with entirely homogeneous walls. These (veins, arteries, and lymph vessels) often contain numerous polynuclear leucocytes and numbers of bacilli.

The fibrous capsule of the lymphatic gland infiltrated by copious round-cell and bacillar infiltration, so that there is no sharp border between the gland and its vicinity. In the latter also enormous numbers of bacilli and copious confluent haemorrhages are found. The adipose tissue, especially, appears to be so closely infiltrated with bacilli in parts that its meshes seem to be surrounded by broad lines of bacilli. Only slight nuclear atrophy or cellular disintegration. The plague bacilli only stain slightly with methylene blue, and particularly where they lie close together in large masses exhibit pronounced coccus forms (separate ones being remarkably large). They are situated extra- and intracellularly. There are no other bacteria, and only very little fibrine is perceptible.

2. *Lymphatic gland* from the left side of neck (fossa submaxillaris) about the size of a bean. The gland exhibits extensive hyperaemia, the numerous capillaries and small vessels being quite full of blood. There are only a few isolated extravasations of blood. The sinuses somewhat dilated, and in them, here and there, single red blood cells and polynuclear leucocytes in moderate numbers are seen. Attention is immediately arrested by the size of the endothelial cells and their nuclei

which belong to the fine lymph channels of the sinus and cover the follicles and rays of medullary substance, and which almost entirely fill the sinus. They are frequently of epithelial-like form, having either one or several faintly stained nuclei with several nucleoli which appear to be round or lobulate.

The endothelium of the blood vessels is also large, with large pale nuclei. In sections stained with alkaline methylene blue, plague bacilli are seen, more or less abundant in number, in each of the numerous blood vessels; they are in diplococcus form, and are always adjacent to or within the endothelial cells. Only a few isolated groups are found in the sinus.

3. *Sections through the left tonsil* exhibit the same condition generally as that of the gland described above: extensive hyperaemia with increase of the polynuclear leucocytes; in addition, well-defined bordering off of the adenoid tissue from the surrounding connective tissue, and healthy epithelial covering. No haemorrhages.

Here, also in almost every dilated blood vessel, there are large or small agglomerations of plague bacilli; adjacent to the endothelium, or, doubtless, also within it. There are small groups consisting of only a few bacilli in the adenoid tissue and always in an intracellular position. The cells surrounding them are large endothelial cells that are unfilled collapsed blood or lymph capillaries.

4. The histological examination of somewhat *enlarged follicles at the base of the tongue* shows the same results. The so-called germinal centre is copiously infiltrated with polynuclear leucocytes. The condition as regards the plague bacillus is also analogous.

5. *Spleen* exhibits histologically a very copious infiltration of polynuclear leucocytes in the region of the pulp, as well as severe hyperaemia. Many pulp cavities remain intact and filled with blood, the endothelium cells very large; in those parts where there exist sanguineous infiltrations of the pulp, they are mixed irregularly with the extravasated blood. Follicles frequently remarkably small, and free from bacilli. The spleen substance is infiltrated with enormous masses of plague bacilli, which are sometimes intracellular. At some places there are isolated, long, thick rods (saprophytes) which stain well with methylene blue. Trabeculae somewhat spread, faintly coloured, and having irregular granulations in parts; their nuclei likewise very pale.

6. *Kidney.* The epithelial cells of the renal cortex, particularly the tubuli contorti, either large and unshapely as if swollen, with faintly coloured nuclei, or without nucleus, in which case the borders can hardly

be distinguished or are entirely obliterated and contain drops of fat of various size. In the interior of the tubules numerous indistinctly granulated masses stained with eosin. The capillaries in part greatly dilated and there are small extravasations of blood between the tubuli in the interstitial connective tissue. The glomeruli large; sometimes filled with blood; the separate capillary loops dilated. The nuclei of the epithelia of Bowman's capsule very numerous and large. No particular changes in the renal pyramids. Small groups of plague bacilli to be seen in the dilated capillaries of the glomeruli and of the connective tissue interstices of the cortex.

In this case the infection, doubtless, originates from that region of the skin appertaining to the left inguinal group of lymphatic glands. At this side the deep-seated inguinal lymphatic glands in the region of the interior crural ring are considerably altered, there are copious haemorrhages, especially in the wall of the large veins, and there is also the typical gelatinous yellowish oedema.

Conclusion.

Microscopically the liver and kidneys exhibit distinct signs of degeneration; the spleen is acutely swollen. Excepting those haemorrhages in the region of the primary bubo no others are discoverable.

The microscopical examination exhibits the enlargement of a superficial inguinal lymphatic gland principally induced by enormous bacillary infiltration and, in a far less degree, by the increase of the polynuclear leucocytes and by haemorrhages.

The swelling of the lymphatic apparatus at the neck is caused by being swamped by plague bacilli. They are present in the lumens of the vessels and are frequently demonstrable in their endothelial cells. Whereas, therefore, we first of all observe intensely active hyperaemia in the fresh metastatic glands infected through the circulation, we also find increase of the polynuclear leucocytes in the dilated sinus, and germinal centres, and a remarkable swelling of the lymphatic endothelia and the cells of the sinus, with swelling and lobulation of their nuclei.

The acute splenic tumour is caused by hyperaemia, enormous infiltration of bacilli and leucocytes permeating the organ evenly, and proliferation of the endothelium of the pulp cavity.

Extensive fatty degeneration is found in the kidney, especially in the epithelia of the tubuli contorti; this is sometimes increased to complete nuclear atrophy. The glomeruli are large, often quite full of blood; there are isolated haemorrhages in the interstitial tissue. Plague bacilli are discernible everywhere in the capillaries.

Bacteriologically, the case is proved to be one of pure plague infection.

Chinese. " An adult male, aet. 25, brought to the public mortuary for examination[1]. The body was found in a deserted house. The corpse was that of a well-nourished man. The skin had the cyanosed appearance met with in plague. On superficial examination *the case looked like one of small-pox*, vesicles and pustules being scattered over the face, shoulders, arms, body, and legs. The caretaker of the mortuary, who has had a large experience, pointed out the case as one of small-pox. An eruption covered the skin. Papules, vesicles, and pustules were present side by side. They were numerous over the neck, back, shoulders, back of arms, ventral surface of the abdomen, the extensor surfaces of the thigh and the buttocks.

"The papules were fewest in number. They were small, never larger than a pea, raised above the general surface of the skin, and surrounded by extravasated blood.

"The vesicles varied in size, they were occasionally umbilicated, apparently ran together, contained turbid serum containing a few plague bacilli and were also surrounded by a discoloured area of skin due to blood extravasation. The pustules were the most numerous. They also varied much in size. One was present on the shoulder which resembled an ordinary boil. Their bacteriological contents were subject to considerable variation. Plague bacilli were found in what appeared to be the most recently formed pustules. In others, which were evidently more advanced, no plague bacilli were found, ordinary pyogenic micro-organisms being present. There was no question of small-pox.

" A bubo was present in the right groin, which contained plague bacilli.

" Plague bacilli were also found in the heart blood and spleen.

" This case was interesting from several points of view, namely :—

    1.   The bubonic nature of the case.

    2   The presence of a generalised skin eruption.

    3.   The nature of the eruption being papular, vesicular, and pustular.

    4.   The presence of the *B. pestis* in the erupted foci.

    5.   The absence of any apparent lymphatic connection between the eruption and the bubo.

    6.   The likeness presented by the case to small-pox."

---

[1] *A Research into Epidemic and Epizootic Plague.* By William Hunter, Government Bacteriologist, Hongkong, 1904.

The following are brief notes of some post-mortems, made for diagnostic purposes, on persons who died during prevalence of plague.

Indian, male. Large bubo in right groin, skin over bubo plum colour; on section gland shows dirty yellowish colour with fleshy patches and haemorrhagic streaks. Glands embedded in haemorrhagic clots and oedema. Plague bacilli present.

Malay, male. Right inguinal bubo (leg flexed and abducted on post-mortem table). Much oedema of subcutaneous tissue in region of groin. This extends up on the anterior abdominal wall for about 3 inches. The subcutaneous fat is marked with petechiae. Glands large, dark brown in colour, and surrounded with blood-stained oedema. Smears swarming with typical bacilli.

European, male. Glands in groin not enlarged. No bacilli. Right lung adherent slightly; lower part of upper and all lower lobe in a state of grey hepatisation, very friable. On section dirty brown fluid poured out; air had been entering to some extent the affected portion; there was some gelatinous exudation between the lower part of lung and diaphragm. Smears contain *B. pestis*. The immediate cause of death was a large ante-mortem clot in left side of heart.

Malay, female. Glands in right femoral and inguinal region enlarged, very dark in colour. Smears from same contain many typical bacilli. Lungs large, pneumonic (early stage) portions in both bases, *B. pestis* in smears. Spleen large, very soft. Kidneys soft and congested. Suprarenal glands dark in colour and congested around.

Coloured, female. Femoral and inguinal glands on right side are much enlarged, the inguinal being congested and haemorrhagic. No organisms found in the glands on microscopic examination. There had been great haemorrhage from the nose and mouth just previous to death. Lungs pneumonic, several patches and full of blood. *B. pestis* present in the pneumonic patches. Liver cirrhotic, spleen large, but no bacilli present.

European, female. There is a mark purple in colour, like a bruise, over left femoral region, a distinct swelling being noticed, soft and boggy to the touch, no enlarged gland can be exactly made out. On section it is seen that much haemorrhage has taken place into the subcutaneous and intermuscular tissue, the glands are much enlarged and soft, almost black in colour and completely surrounded by extravasated blood. Smears made from glands and blood surrounding them swarm with *B. pestis*.

Greek, male. Glands in groins small, pink, not haemorrhagic. Pericardium filled with clear yellow fluid, a few petechiae on outer surface. Base and lower lobe of left lung quite solid, pleura tense, on section a dark, thick, blood-stained and prune-juice fluid, sticky in character, exudes. The surface of the section mottled and streaked with haemorrhages much like gland. No pleurisy. Right lung also pneumonic and solid. Typical *B. pestis* present in great numbers.

Malay, female. Glands in left groin enlarged; upper half of largest gland deep red-brown in colour, the lower part only pink. Much oedema around the glands. the oedema extending for about 3 inches on to the abdominal wall on the left side. *B. pestis* present in great numbers in smears from glands and spleen.

CHAPTER XIII.

CHANNELS OF INFECTION.

It is a well-known fact that the glands draining a pigmented or tattooed cutaneous area are blackish in colour. It is in view of this

Infection through the skin direct to the lymphatics. fact, and of the further fact that microbes which gain access to the lymph channels through the skin are obstructed in the nearest groups of glands and affect them by their pathogenic action, that the occurrence of primary buboes in the inguinal and axillary regions in most cases of plague has given rise to the conception that the most frequent mode of entrance of the infection is through the skin direct to the lymphatics. According to this view the plague microbe, having reached the lymphatic vessels distributed in the skin, is conveyed by them to the lymph glands, which, becoming affected, form the buboes in question. At this stage no bacilli are to be detected in the blood in the majority of cases, and it is not until a direct communication is opened between the infected glands of the bubo and the walls of the adjoining veins, by the coagulative and necrotic action on the tissues by the plague microbe and its toxines contained in the bubo, that there is an entrance of bacilli in great numbers into the general circulation. The entrance of the bacilli into the blood in septicaemic cases is explained by the weak screen which the lymphatic glands are able to furnish against the penetrative energy of a virulent microbe. The explanation is not a very satisfactory one. The limitation which narrows down the entrance of the microbes to the vascular system by the path of the lymphatic vessels is of too restrictive a nature, even when the infection has taken place through the skin.

The anatomical distribution of the superficial lymphatics with their collecting trunks converging to the inguinal and axillary regions certainly affords facilities for the absorption of the infection, in the case of an accidental wound of the skin, if the infection does not pass direct into the blood stream.

Instances occur in nearly every epidemic in which medical men **Post-mortem wounds.** contract plague through a wound or abrasion in their hand which has been infected while performing a post-mortem on a plague case. Aoyama in Hongkong in 1894, Sticker in Bombay in 1898, Evans in Calcutta in 1899, and Pestana in Oporto in 1900, may be mentioned among the many that have become infected in this way. In such cases the first visible sign of disease is usually an axillary bubo, the plague bacillus having found its way to the group of glands draining the area subjected to the inoculation. Sometimes there are clear signs of lymphangitis proceeding from the seat of inoculation to the affected glands, sometimes there is a vesicle at the site of infection without any further local reaction, as in Sticker's case, while at times there is no positive evidence to be gathered by any visible local reaction as to the exact site of the entrance of the plague bacilli, although that site is known from the circumstance of the wound. Aoyama, who scratched his left hand at one post-mortem, and his right hand at another post-mortem four days after, suffered from a bubo in the left axilla without lymphangitis, and with a well-marked lymphangitis on the right arm. This power of the bacillus to enter the **Power of the bacillus to enter the system through a small lesion in the skin without producing a local reaction at site of inoculation.** system through a small lesion in the skin without producing a local reaction at the seat of the inoculation is noteworthy, for, apart from accidental woundings of the skin at post-mortems, the seat of inoculation in natural infections is seldom traceable, not more than 5 % showing any visible signs of the infection having entered through a wound. So remarkable is this fact that there are some physicians who hold the opinion that the skin is not the most frequent channel of infection, but that the bacillus is taken into the lungs, or alimentary canal, enters the general circulation and multiplies in the blood, or selects the glands in the groin, arm-pit, or neck for its multiplication. Small-pox can, like plague, be produced by inoculation, but it is contended, and reasonably so, that inoculation of the small-pox virus is not the most frequent mode by which the natural small-pox gains an entrance into the human system. In plague there may be an eruption of vesicles which contain plague bacilli over different parts of the body, which can only be considered as a manifestation of a general disease and not as a local infection. Phlyctenules of a vesicular, pustular, carbuncular, or furuncular nature are occasionally to be observed on the hand or arm when there are axillary buboes, and on the foot or leg in inguinal buboes; but on the whole the appearance of such or of other signs is rare. The phlyctenules contain plague bacilli, and are usually ascribed to the bite or sting of an infected insect.

There are now a number of cases recorded of direct infection caused by the bite of a plague-stricken rat. A case of infection by the bite of a sick rat is reported by Dr Francis Clark, the Medical Officer of Health for Hongkong. A man employed as a turncock was bitten on the left thumb and some two or three days later the arm became swollen and painful. The man died in some 9 or 10 days, his illness not being reported. On post-mortem examination two small wounds were found on the ball of the left thumb, the left hand and fore-arm were much swollen, and in the left axilla there was a brawny, oedematous swelling, in the midst of which was an enlarged haemorrhagic gland; a smear preparation from this gland showed numerous typical plague bacilli[1].

It has been observed that disinfectors and others exposed to the infection appear to be less liable to be attacked when wearing boots. The explanation of this may be that the boots protect the feet which have lesions on them from coming in contact with infectious material, or that they protect them from the bites of infected insects. The experiments already referred to in another part of this work show that infected fleas are capable of infecting healthy rats and possibly monkeys with plague, that these same fleas will attack man when they are hungry, and it is reasonable to suppose that their capacity to cause plague in animals extends to man. It has also been observed that oilmen appear to enjoy exceptional immunity from plague, which has been attributed to the protection afforded by the oil to the skin. It used to be a common practice for oil to be employed as a protective against plague.

Sometimes a prick or scratch with an infected instrument may introduce the infection direct into the blood vessels of the part and thence into the circulation, and then the bacilli may lodge in a group of glands more remote than that receiving the lymph from the wounded part. For instance at Oporto in 1900 Professor Levi of Stockholm had the front part of his left fore-arm accidentally scratched by an infected knife while he was performing a post-mortem. The wound was immediately washed and bathed with a solution of sublimate and lysol. In 40 hours a sudden pain was felt in the left groin together with general malaise, and in

Infection through the skin direct to the blood vessels.

[1] "A Report of the Epidemic of Bubonic Plague in Hongkong for the year 1900." By the Medical Officer of Health for the Colony.

8 hours a femoral bubo developed at the seat of pain. In this case there was no screening or arrest of the bacilli until they reached the inguinal region, and the route by which they arrived at this group of glands could not have been through the lymphatic system. The selection of the inguinal region for the bubo when the infection entered the system through the skin of the fore-arm is noteworthy. A similar direct blood infection may take place when the inoculation of the bacillus is effected by the bite of an infected insect. It is possible also for a blood infection to occur by the direct connection which sometimes exists anatomically between the lymphatic vessels and veins, and occasionally arteries in the thoracic, axillary and inguinal region. These direct connections between the lymphatic and circulatory systems have been shown by Dr Leaf to exist[1]. He points out that some of the smaller arteries in the thoracic region open directly into lymphatic trunks; that direct communications are found to exist between arteries, lymphatic vessels and veins in many regions of the body; and that the portal, axillary, internal iliac, and the azygos veins all directly communicate with the lymphatic system. It is evident that if, under these conditions, one of the systems becomes infected, there is an opportunity of the infection spreading to the other system, and it is by no means a *sine quâ non* that the blood stream is only infected after the lymph glands in the bubo have broken down, even in those cases when the infection travels along the lymph channels.

The frequency of septicaemic cases, amounting in some epidemics to at least 50 and 60 % of the cases, indicates that the plague bacillus can obtain ready access to the blood, and this without any greater injury to the glands in the inguinal or axillary regions than that to other lymph glands in the body. The similar condition of all the lymph glands of the body points to some other entrance of the bacillus into the system than through the inguinal or axillary glands.

That infection can and often does take place through the skin there is no manner of doubt, but when this mode of infection occurs it is not established that the plague bacillus reaches the inguinal or axillary regions only by the lymph channels. It is not even established that the skin is the most frequent channel of infection.

The preponderance of inguinal buboes among people with bare feet was held at one time to be proof of infection through the skin of the feet. Among people that go about barefooted cracks and abrasions on

[1] "On the Relation of Blood to Lymphatic Vessels." By C. H. Leaf, M.B. *Lancet*, March 3rd. 1900.

the feet are common, and this fact was used as an argument in support of this mode of infection. But the same preponderance of inguinal buboes occurs among Europeans when booted, and in most epidemics, in whatever part of the world they may occur, inguinal buboes are the most frequent. Further, in cases of primary bubo of the inguinal or axillary region, the bubo is not always the first symptom of illness. There may be shivering, fever, prostration, and general illness for a day or several days before there is any appearance of a bubo. The order of symptoms is such as to be suggestive that during the period of incubation and earlier stage of the disease the bacillus is already in some part of the vascular system, and only later selects the group of glands for its bubonic manifestations. It is possible that in some cases in which the buboes appear to be the first manifestation, infection of the inguinal or axillary glands also takes place from the blood, these groups of glands possessing a selective power for the plague bacilli in the blood. This view has certain facts in its support. Plague microbes have been found in the blood in mild types of the disease when large quantities of blood have been employed for the examination. They have also been found in the blood, so far as Hongkong is concerned, in every variety of the disease there. The detection of the bacilli was made by taking thick films of blood, washing out their haemoglobin, and then staining. The method is the same as that adopted by Ross for detecting the malarial organism. By this method plague bacilli have been discovered in the blood before the onset of the fever or the appearance of buboes, during the progress of the disease and during convalescence.

The fact of the bubo frequently making its appearance several days after the onset of the illness favours the view just *Older view is* enunciated, and which was held by older writers, viz. that *that plague* plague is primarily a general disease, and that the affection *is a general* *disease, and* of the glands, internal or external, with the eruption of *that the bu-* the bubo or buboes, is a local manifestation of the disease *boes are its* *local mani-* similar to that which appears in the skin eruption in *festations.* small-pox, scarlet fever, and measles. It is based on the general experience that the glands in all cases of plague are more or less affected. This view is contrary to that commonly accepted to-day, which considers the bubo to be the primary local lesion, the toxines from which become absorbed and give rise to the general symptoms. The whole question still appears to be a moot point and is by no means yet settled. Neither view adopted exclusively explains the different types of plague. In the early days of the Bombay epidemic when the latter theory was formulated, it was a rare occurrence to detect plague bacilli in bubonic cases except a short time before death, but now at least 45 % of the cases received into hospital contain plague bacilli in their blood. The latter percentage more nearly approaches the results obtained by Kitasato, Wilm, and others in Hongkong, where in the epidemic of 1894 and the recurring outbreaks since then plague bacilli have been found in the blood in more than 80 % of the cases. It is evident that plague may differ in its character at different times in one locality as well as in different localities, and that the absence or presence of certain characteristics in an epidemic does not justify denial or positive assurance of their existence in another. At the same time that which appears obvious in one epidemic may receive considerable modification when viewed from the experience derived in another epidemic.

Inoculation through the mucous membrane is another mode of infection. The mucous membrane is more liable than the skin to slight abrasions, and the passage of infected food over its surface probably subjects it to a more frequent exposure to the risk of infection than even any part of the skin. Not infrequent channels of infection are the mouth and the tonsils, giving rise respectively to submaxillary and cervical buboes; this has often been proved experimentally. Monkeys, pigs, calves, sheep, rats, hens, ducks, geese and pigeons contract plague by feeding on food which has previously been infected. The monkey is the nearest approach to man of the animals experimented on, and plague-infected food certainly gives plague to the monkey. The plague is often of a septicaemic type with no particular enlargement of the glands of the neck, while sometimes there is a very distinct affection of the tonsils and glands of the neck. The facility with which the lower animals contract plague by feeding is in favour of man contracting it often in the same way. In Hongkong the mesenteric glands were often swollen and extravasated and the condition of the stomach was very haemorrhagic; the morbid appearances seemed to point to a primary infection of the glands, but in those cases in which the glands were not specially affected the fact does not exclude infection from the alimentary canal, in that if it is admitted that a septicaemic case of plague may be caused by an infection through the skin without any primary buboes or any visible sign of solution of continuity the same conditions may apply to the infection passing through an intact mucous membrane. Plague bacilli placed on the mucous membrane of the nostrils and tonsils will pass

Infection through the mucous membrane.

through these membranes although there may be no lesion. The situation of the blood vessels above the lymphatic network in the alimentary canal may allow of the direct entrance of the bacillus into the circulation. On deducting these cases in which the cervical glands appeared to be primarily infected the usual type of plague caused by feeding animals with plague material was the septicaemic. On the other hand it is necessary to point out that in Natal, where plague has never reached epidemic proportions, experiments by feeding carried out after the plague season failed to produce plague in animals[1].

The presence of plague bacilli in the intestinal contents, mucus of the mouth and urine, of about one-third of the rats infected with plague subjects the food which may be exposed over-night in an infected house to considerable risk of contamination. With food that has still to be cooked the danger is small, but with food that has already been cooked and which will be eaten cold the danger of infection is great. It is of small importance what part of the alimentary canal takes up the infection.

In Hongkong plague-infected fowls were discovered in the markets, and it was pointed out by Dr Atkinson, the Principal Medical Officer of Health of Hongkong, that it is the custom of many of the Chinese to use the uncooked entrails of fowls as a sort of relish, and to eat fowls only half-cooked, preferring them in this condition. Under these circumstances the danger attendant on eating plague-infected poultry is a real one. In 1903 Dr Hunter discovered plague bacilli in two samples of rice taken from a house in Hongkong.

Cervical buboes may be caused by infection derived from the skin, or from the mouth, or tonsils, or nostrils. Buboes in the cervical region in Chinese patients have been traced to mothers sucking the open buboes of their children. Unless there is a clear history it may be difficult to say from the appearance of the tonsils and pharynx which is the source of infection, because these often become affected by extension of the pathological changes from the cervical glands. Similar inflammatory and diphtheritic appearances may sometimes be seen in the tonsils in cases in which the infection has obtained access to the blood and when the buboes are inguinal or axillary. Plague bacilli may be found in the sputum whenever the tonsils and pharynx are much affected, whether due to a local infection, or to an extension from the cervical glands, or to a general infection.

[1] *Report on the Plague in Natal*, 1902–3. By Ernest Hill, Health Officer for the Colony.

In 1897 a Bombay nurse at the Parel Hospital received in the eye a particle of sputum coughed up by a patient suffering from pneumonic plague. Although the parts were carefully washed conjunctivitis set in the next day, which was followed by a swelling of the parotid, a bubo below the ear on the affected side, and death. A similar case occurred in Hongkong.

Another mode of infection is by the respiratory tract. The local infection of nostrils, pharynx, or mouth may extend into the lungs and set up the pneumonic form of plague, or the bacillus may gain an entrance direct into the lungs by the inspiration of infected material producing bronchitis and pneumonia. In the latter mode of infection there is no primary bubo of the neck. There is no cervical bubo when the broncho-pneumonia of plague is experimentally caused by the intratracheal injection of cultures of the plague bacillus. Pneumonic plague has also followed subcutaneous injection of animals with plague material from pneumonic plague, so that it is apparent that primary plague pneumonia may be produced in some cases by the plague bacillus entering the lungs from the general circulation. It appears to be a case of selection of the lungs instead of the glands of the groin, arm-pit, or neck. In this connection some of the cases of plague caused by post-mortem wounds have resulted in plague pneumonia, and it is a curious fact that those cases which have arisen from laboratory infections, and which are generally attributed to direct infection from animals handled, were of a pneumonic type.

Infection through the respiratory tract.

The secondary pneumonia of plague is caused by an infection from the general circulation sequent either to a septicaemic case or to the haemorrhagic extravasation of a bubo into a vein. In pneumonic plague the specific bacillus is often associated with the diplococcus pneumoniae, which may in some pneumonic patches be exceedingly numerous and in greater numbers than the plague bacillus.

Mixed infection.

Mixed infections, except in the lung when the diplococcus pneumoniae is associated with the plague microbe, appear to be generally due to the entrance into the blood of other micro-organisms through the ulcerated mucous membrane of the mouth and tonsils.

During life the mode of exit of infection will depend on the type of the disease and the condition of the patient. In the bubonic type in its earlier stages, in which the primary bubo appears to be the result of the plague bacillus

Mode of exit of infection from the body.

reaching the affected glands by the lymphatic channels, the infective agent is limited to the glandular or periglandular tissue and only finds an exit externally when the bubo suppurates. At the stage of suppuration bacilli are often not to be found in the pus, and it is only towards the periphery of the necrosed tissue that bacilli, not infrequently of an involuted form, may be discovered. The rounded forms which are very common may be mistaken for micrococci, and the bladder-like forms are apt to be overlooked because of their not staining well. There is, however, much variation in both the number of bacilli and the duration of their vitality in suppurating buboes. Generally the bacilli are rapidly destroyed, and few or even none may be left to escape to contaminate dressings and bed-clothes, but occasionally they retain their vitality for a long period and remain alive so long as any pus or necrosed tissue remains.

In cervical buboes in consequence of the involvement of the mucous membrane of the mouth and pharynx and of the tonsils, plague bacilli may escape by the mouth in the sputum and saliva. Similarly bacilli may appear in the sputum when the tonsils or glands of the mouth are primarily infected. As boils, vesicles, pustules, haemorrhages, and other eruptions on the skin which occur in plague usually contain plague bacilli, any detachment, rupture or breach of the epidermis over these will allow of the escape of plague bacilli. Should the bacilli find their way in considerable numbers from the primary bubo into the general circulation, which is a common occurrence a short time before death, then the avenues of exit become similar to those of a plague case which is septicaemic from the commencement.

In a septicaemic case all the secretions and excretions except the perspiration may contain the plague microbe, and the infectious agent may consequently appear in the sputum, saliva, urine, and faeces, and in haemorrhagic discharges. In the pneumonic cases there are usually enormous numbers of bacilli in the sputum. In the dead body the bacillus is usually in all the fluids of the system and will escape with any sanguineous discharges that may dribble from the cavities.

Closely connected with the mode of exit of the infective agent from the body is the duration of vitality of the bacillus in convalescent patients. In simple bubonic cases in which there is no secondary pneumonia or other complication, and in which the buboes resolve themselves and there are no bacilli in the blood, the infectivity is practically *nil* and need not be considered, but where the buboes suppurate the duration of the presence

The duration of the infectivity of convalescents.

of the bacillus varies so much that no set time can be placed upon it, and the only method of ascertaining freedom of infection is to examine microscopically and make cultures of the pus. In cases of doubt it may be advisable to inoculate an animal. There are occasionally cases of indolent buboes with late suppuration, and in these the vitality of the bacillus may be prolonged for a very lengthened period. Thus two cases are mentioned by Dr Choksy of Bombay, in which iliac[1] buboes were opened through the abdominal wall on the 48th day of illness and the pus was found to contain plague bacilli in an active state and capable of growth when cultured.

Kitasato isolated plague bacilli from the blood of convalescents, and this observation has been repeated and confirmed in Hongkong, but it is not determined how long they may remain in the system. The Austrian Commission[2] found plague bacilli in the spleen of a patient who died on the 52nd day, which points to the possibility of a patient retaining the infection for a long time.

Dr Gotschlich[3] records three instances of convalescents from pneumonic plague, which were treated in the hospital at Alexandria, showing bacilli of a virulent type in their sputum for considerable periods after they were apparently well. In the first case the bacilli retained their virulency to the 76th day of the patient's illness and the 42nd day after rising from his bed. In the second case the bacilli in the sputum were virulent on the 35th day after the onset of the disease, and 6 days after the patient had so far recovered as to leave his bed. In the third case the bacilli were isolated from the sputum up to the 41st day from the commencement of the illness and 19 days after the patient had left his bed.

The importance of a bacteriological examination of the sputum is obvious in order that patients shall not be allowed to mix with healthy persons while they are still in an infective state, and that due precautions shall be taken to disinfect the sputum as long as it contains plague bacilli. This question of the duration of the infectivity of patients who have been ill with plague requires much more investigation than it has yet received.

. The best mass of evidence collected on the length of the incubation

Incubation period of plague. period of plague is that recorded by the Indian Plague Commission[4]. Information regarding 71 cases is given, together with the references derived from the records of

[1] *The Treatment of Plague with Professor Lustig's Serum.* By N. H. Choksy, M.D. 1903.

[2] H. Albrecht u. A. Ghon. *Ueber die Beulenpest in Bombay im Jahre* 1897, p. 532.

[3] *Zeitschrift für Hygiene und Infectionskrankheiten*, 1899, xxxii. p. 402.

[4] *Report of the Indian Plague Commission*, Vol. v. cap. iii. p. 78.

segregation and evacuation camps. The cases are divided into three classes.

Class I. Group A, cases in which there is a history of a direct inoculation of infective material, and Group B, cases where there is a history of the patient having come specially into contact with infection on a particular occasion. In both groups there were cases in which the incubation period could not have been longer than 24 hours and other cases in which it extended to 5 days. The average length of the incubation period was about 3 days.

Class II consists of cases in which there is a history of the patient having been in contact with infection on and after a particular day. The data gathered for this class confirm those of Class I in placing the period of incubation between one and five days.

Class III represents cases in which plague developed after removal from infected surroundings. Out of 753 cases noted, 15 or 1.9%, developed plague after the 10th day. It is stated, however, that these later cases may have contracted the infection after removal to camp.

It is not the shortest period of incubation that is the most important for preventive measures, except it be a question as to whether a person exposed to the infection should be inoculated and the possibility or probability of the disease coming on before the prophylactic has had time to act. The extreme limit of the incubation period is however of the greatest consequence as forming a basis for practice in regard to the length of time required to segregate persons who have been exposed to infection, or to isolate crowds of emigrants or coolies from an infected country before their admission to one which is not infected, or to declare when a person who has been exposed to infection is safe from attack. In the vast majority of cases 6 days may be considered to be the extreme limit of the incubation period, but there is a residuum in which 10 days, fixed by the Venice Convention, are needed to cover the incubation period. There are very exceptional cases in which the period of incubation appears to have extended to 12 and even 14 days. But these are rareties and, except when dealing with emigrants and coolies in large numbers, they may be disregarded. The Paris Convention of 1903 has fixed a period of 5 days for isolation of persons from plague-infected ships, and which may or may not be followed by surveillance of not more than 5 days.

CHAPTER XIV.

CLINICAL FEATURES.

PLAGUE was formerly classified according to the mildness or severity
of the disease as Pestis Minor and Pestis Major, and
Pestis Siderans or Pestis Fulminans. Pestis Minor included cases which were of a mild character and ended in
recovery. Pestis Major comprised the more severe cases.
Pestis Siderans or Pestis Fulminans embraced those cases that were
rapidly or suddenly fatal. Other terms, such as bubonic, haemorrhagic,
and nervous, were employed to designate the more prominent features
that presented themselves in particular cases.

Different classification or types of plague.

The classification now adopted is one which is based more or less on
the particular system of the body invaded in force by the plague
bacillus, and plague is divided into bubonic, septicaemic, and pneumonic, according to whether the glandular, circulatory, or respiratory
systems are mostly involved. Other types, such as cellulo-cutaneous
or carbuncular, intestinal and cerebral, have been described. They are
applied to cases in which some symptom or symptoms are more pronounced than usual. A separate classification of these atypical cases
only unnecessarily complicates matters and will not be followed here,
though it should be mentioned that such modification of symptoms
has to be borne in mind from a diagnostic point of view. Even the
three accepted types are artificial distinctions useful to draw attention
to the different garbs in which the disease may present itself, and in
the case of the pneumonic variety, which is highly infective, valuable
from an administrative point of view in that it is desirable the cases
should be immediately isolated; but they are, after all, only different
manifestations or degrees of the same disease which in its main features
has a common likeness. The type with buboes is the most common,

ranging from 70 to 80 per cent. of the cases. Typical cases of each variety may be met with in every epidemic but they very frequently run into one another. Thus the bubonic form may become septicaemic, the septicaemic may develop buboes or pneumonia, and the pneumonic may become septicaemic or bubonic or both.

The disease also in its varying types may range from a mild to a severe attack, from a prolonged illness to death within a few hours, and it may have many of its symptoms absent or run an irregular course. The cases met with in China and India presented very considerable differences from those in South Africa, and it was difficult to realise at first that the patients were suffering from the same disease. The frequent presence of great mental aberration and of typhoid symptoms in the former contrasted with their comparative absence in the latter. It is probably variations of this kind which lead to such different observations in different places as regards the mode of infection, the variation in types, the liability of animals to disease, and the degree of infectivity. There are few diseases which present a greater variety of manifestations.

Plague may, for descriptive purposes, be broadly classified into plague with buboes and plague without buboes. This distinction is only a clinical one, for in all forms of plague the lymphatic glandular system, although it may not be detected during life, is found in post-mortems to be more or less affected. This is even the case in the pneumonic form. Superadded to the symptoms peculiar to the several varieties of plague, such as the appearance of buboes in bubonic plague and the affection of the lungs in pneumonic plague, and the sudden and intense prostration in septicaemic plague, there are certain symptoms in plague which are common to every variety. They are, the peculiar expression of the face, the characteristic appearance of the tongue, the intoxication or perturbation of the nervous system, the halting speech, the staggering gait, and the great prostration. These will be referred to later on.

Plague with and without buboes.

The incubation period of whatever type the disease may be varies generally between a few hours and five days, it being rarely longer. Cases have been recorded with longer periods, but it is often difficult to dissociate from them the possible exposure to infected clothes or infected animals at a date later than that which is believed to be the time of infection. Still the evidence at present existing does not exclude the possibility of the period of incubation being prolonged occasionally to 12 or 14 days.

Incubation period.

Premonitory symptoms are seldom observed. They, however,
Premonitory symptoms. occur in some cases and more in some epidemics than in
others. They usually consist in loss of appetite, languor,
low spirits, frontal headache, furred tongue with red tip and edges,
nausea, vomiting, diarrhoea, giddiness, weakness in the limbs, and pains
in the loins. These may continue for one or two days when the period
of invasion sets in, the symptoms of which vary according to the severity
of the attack. Perhaps the most remarkable characteristic in connection with plague is the difference in the onset and progress of the
disease in different cases. On the one hand no disease except cholera
manifests in its severer forms so rapid a development of its symptoms
and overwhelms or prostrates the patient to the verge of death in so
short a time. On the other hand it may take a most leisurely course.

In the mild variety of the bubonic form, which corresponds to the
The benign bubonic or Pestis minor. *Pestis minor* of the older classification, there is, in addition
to the phenomena already mentioned as occasionally met
with as prodromata, ill-defined or well-defined fever, pain
and tenderness in the groin, arm-pit, or neck, with the appearance at
the seat of pain of a glandular swelling or bubo, tender to pressure
or on movement of the parts, general debility, slight congestion of the
eyes, and slightly thickened speech. This is the acute form, which may
only last a week, the symptoms disappearing after the patient perspires.
The bubo terminates in resolution, suppuration, or induration. The
patient may not take to bed or at most is confined to it for only a few
days. In the more chronic form, which may last two or more months,
the bubo or buboes are indolent and they may undergo a slow process of
suppuration and sloughing, constituting a serious drain on the general
health of the patient, producing anaemia and extreme debility.

In the severe variety of the bubonic form, which often includes
The grave bubonic or Pestis major. septicaemic and pneumonic cases, and which is usually
described under *Pestis major*, the invasion of the disease
is as a rule sudden and pronounced, the onset being abrupt,
apparently without warning and frequently coming on when the person
attacked is at work. The disease is often fully established in a few
hours or at most in one day. The symptoms consist of shiverings or
tremblings, with fever of a remittent type, hot and dry skin, flushed
face, injected eyes, nausea and vomiting of mucous and bilious matter,
diarrhoea, severe and splitting frontal headache, depression, great giddiness, staggering gait when walking, as if intoxicated, quickened pulse
and respiration, stabbing pains in epigastrium, back and loins, white-

coated tongue, which is red at the tip and edges, mouth and fauces dry, and intense thirst. These symptoms differ little from those which characterise the onset of any specific disease, and have nothing to distinguish them at this early stage unless they are associated with glandular enlargements in some region of the body. If a bubo appears it is usually ushered in by intense pain in the groin, arm-pit, or neck, which is increased by movement or pressure. The pain at first is so severe that the attention of the patient is mainly directed to it, all other symptoms being considered insignificant compared to the suffering experienced in the gland affected. The pain is followed by a swelling which constitutes the bubo, and which, small and tender at first, consists of a single gland or a group of inflamed glands, the outlines of which are easy to define, but later cannot be differentiated. The bubo may remain small, hard and tense, or it may increase in dimensions and form a brawny, boggy oedematous swelling the size of a man's fist or that of an orange. It may reach a large size in a few hours or it may take several days for its full development. Gangrenous pustules may also accompany the bubo or appear later on different parts of the skin, and petechiae may be seen in some cases before death. If there is no bubo, the symptoms may be those of pneumonia or of extreme nervous prostration and muscular weakness, and instead of the face being flushed it may be pale and the temperature not much over 100° F. As the disease progresses the headache and vertigo increase in severity, the fever rises or continues at its maximum, the eyes assume a more suffused, congested, and sunken appearance, the face is drawn, and the expression is either anxious and denotes suffering or it is fixed and vacant. There is much restlessness, with an uncontrollable desire to wander about aimlessly to some other locality. Profound depression, great prostration, and an overpowering sense of fatigue set in. Ordinary consciousness is retained, but even with apparently perfect consciousness the mental condition is one of hébétude or drowsiness. The intellect loses its keenness and responds slowly to outward stimuli. Questions are answered slowly, the words or sentences being articulated in an embarrassed and hesitating manner, each syllable being pronounced slowly, indistinctly, and with difficulty, or the speech is staccato in character and uttered in a hurried and irritable tone. Cerebral derangement may occasionally be absent even at a later stage, but usually increasing disturbance of the nervous system quickly follows, evidenced by protracted sleeplessness or greater drowsiness, which may alternate with delirium, or by a drowsy and lethargic condition which merges into profound coma. The delirium may be of a quiet, noisy, furious, or terrifying kind; it is often of a muttering kind with restlessness and picking of the bed-clothes; but it may be violent and there may be much difficulty in keeping the patient in bed. The whitish coating of the tongue turns after the second or third day to a brown or reddish-brown colour, while the tips and edges remain red. The tongue, which was moist, now becomes dry, and sordes appear on the lips and teeth, the urine contains albumen, and the abdomen swells. The respiration becomes more frequent, accompanied by dyspnoea and cough. The pulse, which is soft and easily compressible at the onset, becomes intermittent, dicrotic and thready and difficult to count, and there is a tendency to collapse, the patient's extremities becoming cold and clammy. Concurrently pneumonic complications are apt to arise.

The patient may die from the disease in 48 or 24 hours or even less,
Causes of death.
with all the symptoms fully developed, or death may be delayed to any time between the third and seventh day or later, but it usually occurs between the second and sixth day, and generally takes place from heart failure; it may, however, be brought about by exhaustion or collapse caused by haemorrhage, or by asphyxia by pressure of the buboes and surrounding oedema on the respiratory organs, or by involvement of the lungs, or by coma from the poisonous effect of the toxines on the nervous centres.

After the sixth or seventh day the patient's chances of recovery are
Progress after the sixth or seventh day.
much increased, and in favourable cases the fever decreases, the skin perspires, the tongue becomes moist, the pulse stronger, and the expression natural. The temperature is usually normal about the tenth day. Once convalescence begins, which may be on the sixth or eighth day, the progress may be rapid or it may become tedious and protracted, and the patient may not be well for six to ten weeks or longer. Sometimes the symptoms do not improve on the sixth or eighth day. The tongue remains dry, reddish, cracked, and with a dark coating, the teeth and lips retain their sordes and a typhoid condition develops. The abdomen becomes more swollen, the diarrhoea, if any, is more obstinate, and the motions are foetid; the pulse continues frequent and irregular, the respiration laborious, the skin alternates between dryness and a state of perspiration, the sleep is disturbed and unrefreshing, and the patient lies in a condition of apathy and stupor. The buboes suppurate and discharge an offensive serous fluid, and it is not until the fifteenth or twentieth day that there

are any signs of convalescence, or it may happen about this time that the patient's strength gives way and death ensues.

The severest forms of plague are those that are classified as the septicaemic and pneumonic varieties; they correspond to the Pestis siderans or malignant form of the older writers, and generally prove fatal before the eruption of buboes.

The septic variety of plague is a virulent type, in which the
Septicaemic lymphatic glands usually show no special enlargement
plague. during life and consequently the bubo is absent, but after death the glands are found to be generally affected, being somewhat enlarged and much congested. In this form of plague the bacilli invade the blood in large numbers and are easily detected. The chief characteristics are the rapidity with which nervous and cerebral symptoms supervene and their intensity. The patient is profoundly affected by the amount and strength of the poison received, which appears to concentrate itself on the central nervous system. The attack begins with trembling and rigors, intense headache, vomiting, and high fever. At times the depression of the vital powers is so great that there is no power in the patient for reaction, and the temperature does not reach 100° F.; the countenance is pale and the expression apathetic or depicts intense anxiety. Extreme nervous prostration, weakness, drowsiness, restlessness, hurried and panting respiration, small and full pulse, tympanitis, delirium, picking of the bed-clothes, stupor and coma quickly follow on. The evacuations are involuntary, the patient becomes cold, and dies on the first, second, or third day. In these cases there may be bleeding from the nose, kidneys, and bowels. If there is any reaction, as is sometimes the case, the pulse becomes stronger, the face flushed, the eyes congested, and on the third, fourth, or fifth day buboes may appear simultaneously in the groin, arm-pit, or neck.

In pneumonic plague unaccompanied by buboes, and in which the
Pneumonic primary localisation of the disease is in the lungs, the
plague. illness commences with a rigor, general malaise, severe headache, nausea, vomiting, and pain in the limbs, followed by fever varying in range from 102° F. to 105° F., a sense of constriction across the chest, difficult and hurried breathing, cough and expectoration. In other cases a few days may elapse before the lung symptoms develop. Consciousness is generally not disturbed. The sputum, at first watery and frothy and tinged with blood, generally becomes more profuse as the disease advances, but less aërated. Sometimes it is scanty and consists of small pellets of congealed blood. The sputum has not the glairy

viscid, rusty character of that of acute pneumonia, though on the clothes it may be mistaken for this.   Physical examination does not reveal signs of sufficient gravity to account for the severity of the symptoms.   On auscultation the stethoscopic signs may be those of lobular pneumonia; moist sounds and crepitation may be heard over the pneumonic patches, but there is seldom marked dullness at the base or at the spots where crepitation is detected, and however hurried the breathing and quick the pulse may be there is not that disproportion between the pulse and respiration ratio which obtains in acute pneumonia.   The lung symptoms and cardiac distress rapidly grow worse, delirium supervenes, there is gradual failure of the heart's action with or without coma, and death with a cyanosed aspect occurs on the fourth or fifth day or earlier.   This form of plague, besides being the most infectious, is the most fatal. In cases which recover or linger for some time buboes are likely to appear, and in some cases the pneumonia and buboes may occur simultaneously at the commencement of the illness.

In each of these forms the symptoms more or less common are Characteristic   subject to many modifications.   The Pestica facies changes symptoms.   during the illness, being dependent on the state of consciousness of the patient, on the kind of delirium, on the severity of the headache, and on the degree of giddiness which forms part of the symptoms.   Many have injected eyes, a distressed aspect of countenance, the eyelids slightly closed and the mouth slightly open; some wear an expression of pain.   As a rule the countenance in the early stages depicts anxiety and distress, and in the later stages resignation and apathy.   The resigned, listless, and apathetic countenance is apt to deceive the physician, causing him, unless experienced in the disease, to entertain the opinion that the patient is better, whereas it is due to relaxation of the facial muscles from partial loss of nervous power and is not an improvement, but a sign of gravity and danger.   With delirium the face is flushed and the expression may be one of distraction, anxiety, terror, or menace, the patient being wild with excitement; the eyes are red, congested and sunken, and the conjunctivae are injected.   In a state of stupor the expression is gloomy, depressed, apathetic or vacant, the mouth is half open and the patient has the appearance of being under an hypnotic and yet unable to sleep, the eyes remaining wide open or half closed, glassy, vacant, and lustreless.

The tongue is generally swollen, indented, and is protruded with difficulty in a tremulous or jerky manner; it is coated on the surface with a creamy-white fur with angry looking papillae showing through, and the tips and edges are clean and red. Later the coating on the surface of the tongue is dry and has a mother-o'-pearl or glistening appearance; and later still it forms into a yellowish or reddish-brown or black crust and resembles that seen in typhus and typhoid fever. The lips, teeth, and gums become covered with sordes. The plague virus evidently produces a progressively intoxicating effect on the nervous system, which displays itself with varying degrees of intensity in different ways on different constitutions. In some there is insomnia, in others wild delirium, in others stupor, in all more or less loss of coordinating power over the voluntary muscles and dulling of the senses. The staggering gait and the inability to coordinate the movement of the hands are very characteristic symptoms. There is no paralysis of the limbs, but from the physical weakness, vertigo, and toxic impression on the nervous system the voluntary muscles are not completely under the command of the patient. The speech is also peculiarly hesitating, stuttering, thick, lisping, indistinct, and monosyllabic, often like that of a drunken man. The memory is confused, and in answering questions the patient forgets half the sentence or syllable of the word which he began to utter. It has happened that a plague patient with these symptoms has been taken to the police station under the supposition that the speech, staggering gait, and confusion of mind were due to drunkenness.

The general clinical features of plague in its different forms

Symptoms considered in relation to systems affected. having been described, some of the important symptoms with the system affected may now be more fully dealt with.

Temperature. *The temperature* is not characteristic; it rises in the bubonic form to 103°, 104° F. or may be to 105° F. or to 106° F., and may reach its highest on the evening of the first day and continue at its maximum, but more usually it gradually rises, reaching its maximum on the evening of the second or third and sometimes, but seldom, on the fourth day, an intermission of a degree or more frequently taking place during a part of the day. On the third, fourth, or fifth day the temperature usually falls 2 or 3 degrees or more, continues at this low temperature for a few hours or a day and then rises again, reaching nearly the same or a greater height than that of the previous evening. This primary fall in temperature is sometimes ascribed to the effect of medicines, but it is a feature which is common to many cases of plague when left to their natural course. With this secondary rise, especially if higher than the first, the symptoms increase in gravity and the patient is in a perilous condition.   If this stage is successfully passed through, the temperature again falls the next day, and then by successive evening exacerbations and morning remissions steadily comes down by degrees to normal or sub-normal, which may be reached on any morning between the sixth and eleventh day.   In simple bubonic cases of a mild character the temperature may fall to normal as early as the second or third day ; on the other hand the occurrence of complications or the eruption of buboes may cause great irregularity in the temperature and completely obliterate the more or less typical primary and secondary rise with the apyrexial interval.

Little is to be gathered as regards prognosis from the temperature ; generally the higher the temperature the graver are the symptoms ; and the later the first curve terminates the more likely is the secondary reaction to be moderate.   Fluctuating temperatures may mean nothing, but if simultaneously with the fall of temperature there is a considerable rise in the frequency of the pulse, the conjunction is, as a rule, unfavourable.   A sudden fall of temperature with a collapsed condition of the patient usually indicates a fatal issue ; on the other hand, a fall of temperature by degrees between the fifth and seventh day may be looked upon as favourable.   Sometimes the temperature is low and becomes subnormal.

Occasionally there may be no fever during the illness, which may merely consist of indisposition, coated tongue, headache, slight giddiness, and a bubo in groin, arm-pit, or neck.   The illness is such as not to confine the patient to bed, but is often protracted and sometimes terminates suddenly in death.

In septicaemic plague the temperature is usually high at the commencement, remains high, and runs an irregular course.   In the most severe cases of the septicaemic type the temperature may not rise above 100° F. or less in the early stage, and it is only if the patient lives long enough for reaction to set in that there is any considerable rise in temperature.

In pneumonic plague the temperature is high and usually runs an irregular course.   It may continue high to the end or fall suddenly before the patient's death.

The Charts taken from Surgeon-Major Lyon's Report on the Plague in Bombay, and from Dr J. A. Lowson's Report on Plague in Hongkong, and from some Cape Town cases will show the general character of the temperature in plague.

J.G.G.(E) L. FEM. BUBO SUPPURATED REC.

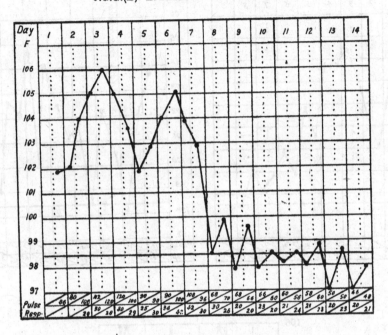

P.S.(H) L. FEM. BUBO SUPPURATED REC.

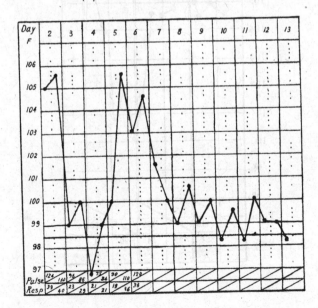

A.K.H.(M)   Left Axillary Bubo.

W.(E)   L. Fem. Bubo Resolution Rec.

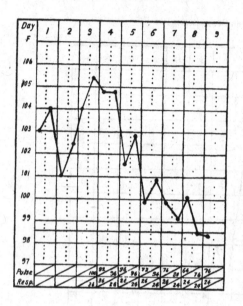

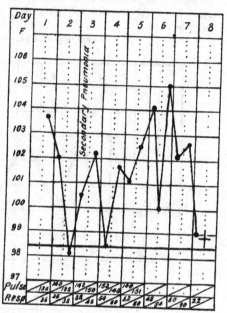

Right Femoral Bubo.

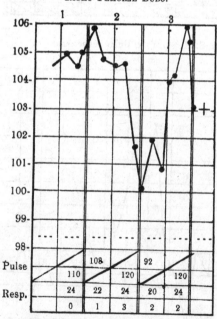

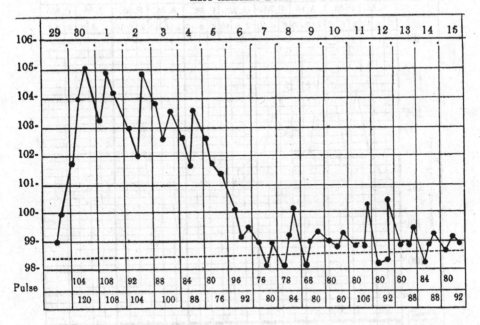

LEFT AXILLARY BUBO.

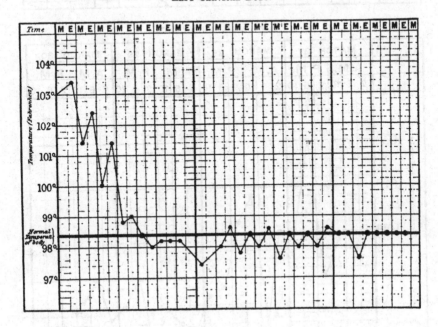

LEFT CERVICAL BUBO.

M.K. PNEUMONIC PLAGUE.

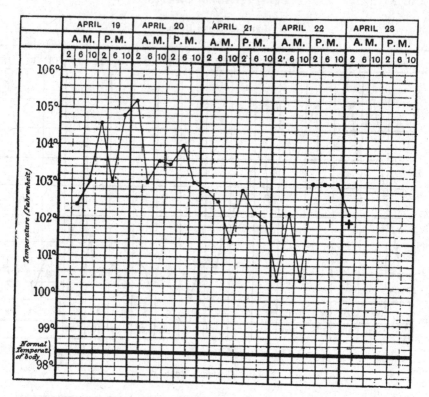

G.D. SEPTICAEMIC PLAGUE.

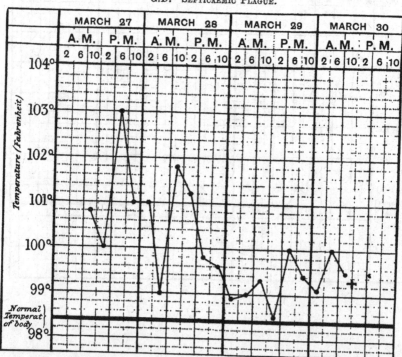

Contemporaneously with the fever, or before, or soon after its appearance, in some cases several days, and in rare cases a week or more later, intense pain is felt in one or more of the glandular regions of the body, generally in the femoro-inguinal, axillary or cervical region, or occasionally in the epitrochlear or popliteal space. At the seat of pain one or more of the glands is noticed to be swollen and to be specially tender on pressure. In the next 12 hours or in a shorter time the swelling rapidly increases in size and a bubo is formed. Sometimes more than one region is affected, and often groups of glands on the same course of lymphatics become successively infected. As a rule only one region of the body is affected, though in a small percentage of cases buboes may appear of a bilateral or multiple character in any part of the lymphatic glandular system. The bubo may be completely formed in a few hours, but more frequently its full development takes from one to five days.

Lymphatic system buboes.

The bubo or swelling consists of one or more inflamed and swollen lymphatic glands with a sero-sanguinolent or haemorrhagic effusion into the periglandular tissue, which, while matting together the neighbouring glands into a hard mass, also infiltrates the tissues around and renders them firm and oedematous. The periglandular tissue like the glands becomes inflamed. The effusion may be profuse or scanty. In cases which prove rapidly fatal the glands may remain hard and painful without any palpable periglandular infiltration, but the usual course, if the patient lives long enough, is extreme pain, swelling of the gland or glands, effusion, and the formation of a distinct bubo.

Contents and condition of buboes.

The discovery of the plague bacillus in the blood in nearly 45 % of the cases of plague admitted into hospital in Bombay in recent years, and the still greater percentage in Hongkong, would seem, as already stated, to indicate that the older views were more correct than the modern, and that the bubo in most cases is only a local manifestation of the disease already in the blood. Every extravasation whether on the skin or elsewhere contains plague bacilli.

The fact of the bubo frequently making its appearance several days after the onset of the illness is also in favour of plague being primarily a general disease, the affection of the glands with the eruption of the bubo or buboes being a local manifestation of the disease as much as the skin eruption in small-pox, scarlet fever, or measles. This view is contrary to that commonly accepted to-day, which considers the bubo to be the primary local lesion, the toxines from which become absorbed and give rise to the general symptoms.

The smaller the bubo usually the more fatal is the attack. The
Size.　　　　　size of the bubo depends on the number of glands
affected and the amount of effusion matting the inflamed
glands together and infiltrating into the surrounding tissues. When
the effusion is small the bubo may be no larger than an almond
and the affected glands may be distinctly felt, but when the quantity
of periglandular fluid is large it may be the size of a man's fist
or larger; then the outline of the glands is not to be discovered by
palpation. The bubo is usually of an oval or round shape and of uneven
surface owing to the conglomeration of affected glands. At first
moveable from surrounding structures it becomes adherent and immoveable, it is somewhat doughy or boggy to the touch on the surface
and of a hard consistence in the deeper tissue. The skin over the bubo
loses its soft and loose texture, becomes thickened, appears smooth and
tense, and is sometimes reddened or of a dusky hue from inflammatory
action. On the surface of the bubo may be haemorrhages, carbuncles or
blisters, and the skin covering the bubo may become gangrenous.

Pain.　　　　　Pain, tenderness, and swelling are the general characteristics of the bubo. The pain may be dull and aching
or sharp and stabbing, and is independent of the size of the bubo. The
smaller the size of the bubo the more painful is it likely to be. Much
of the pain disappears as the swelling increases in size. Sometimes
there is no pain, and the bubo when lying deep is only detected by the
tenderness caused by pressing over the part. Sometimes there is neither
pain nor tenderness and the bubo can be handled without causing any
Tenderness.　　　inconvenience to the patient. Tenderness on pressure
over the region of the glands is useful in a confirmatory
sense when the glands are small or lie so deep as not to be felt, but
absence of tenderness does not always mean no affected glands. Sometimes the tenderness is so acute that pressure over the bubo will cause
wincing and moaning from pain even when the patient is in a comatose
condition. In the acute stage of development if the bubo is cut into
it will bleed freely and the swollen glands will present a brick-red or
purple colour. At a later stage a similar incision will usually show
yellow or blood-stained pus.

The bubo in its natural course terminates by suppuration or by
Termination.　　sloughing, or it subsides by resolution, becoming dispersed
and absorbed, or it indurates and remains as a hard lump

for an indefinite period. In the event of suppuration, if the case is an uncomplicated one, the process begins after the seventh or eighth day without any rise of temperature, the skin over the infiltrated area becoming inflamed, and is completed in the course of ten or twelve days. The suppurating bubo heals in the course of a week to a month, leaving a large scar, more or less varying in size according to the amount of sloughing which has taken place. The healing process may, however, not be completed for six weeks or two months or longer. Indolent buboes, especially those in the iliac regions, may not suppurate for long periods. Choksy records a case of a bubo of this kind being opened on the 48th day of the patient's illness[1].

When the suppuration is accompanied as it may be by much sloughing, either of the bubo or of the bubo and the infiltrated tissue around it, large cavernous ulcers with rugged and indurated margins may result, laying bare the muscles, nerves, and blood vessels of the part and forming deep and unhealthy looking wounds which take a long time to heal and which are a heavy drain on the patient's strength. These large sloughing excavations, which are at all times dangerous, are specially so when they occur in the pelvis in connection with iliac buboes.

The pus in mild cases is healthy and presents no unusual characters, but in the more severe cases it varies much, sometimes being offensive and serous, at other times being chocolate colour and like wine lees and mixed with coagulated blood.

If the bubo ends in resolution the periglandular infiltration decreases, the outlines of the glands get more distinct, the glands lose their tenderness on pressure, the skin becomes softer, and beyond a slight induration and possibly a pigmenting of the skin there is little trace of the inflammation to which the glands and their surroundings have been subjected.

The situation of the buboes in order of frequency in the external
Situation. glandular region is the same in every country where plague occurs, whether the inhabitants wear boots or not. The most frequent seat for them is the inguino-femoral region, the next is the axillary, and the next the cervical.

A patient suffering from an inguinal bubo usually lies in bed with
Inguinal   the thigh flexed to relieve any pressure on the painful
buboes.   swelling. In the inguinal region the bubo may occupy a horizontal or vertical position, according to the group of glands

[1] *The Treatment of Plague with Prof. Lustig's Serum.* By N. H. Choksy, M.D.

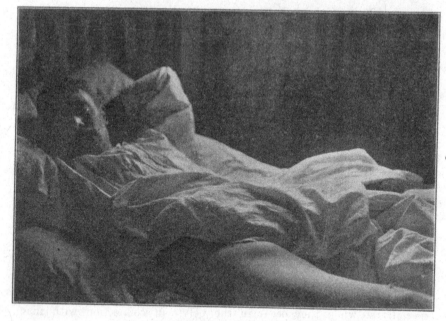

Inguinal Bubo.

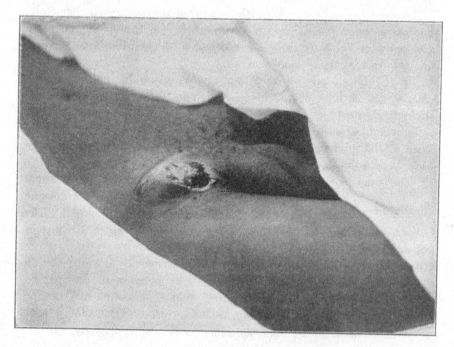

Inguinal Bubo.

that may be specially affected in Scarpa's triangle. The vertical set of glands below Poupart's ligament are the most frequently affected. The swelling may be small or it may be as large as an orange, and the oedema of the surrounding tissues may extend as far as the knee or well on to the abdominal wall. The figures on p. 276 show the kind of buboes most commonly met with in the inguinal region. Only one groin may be the seat of a bubo or both groins may be affected. The bubo in the inguinal region not infrequently extends into the iliac region, affecting the chain of glands and lymphatics in the abdominal cavity and forming a hard tumour to be felt through the abdominal wall. This iliac bubo is painful on pressure and may attain large dimensions. Sometimes these iliac buboes occur without any very noticeable enlargement of the inguinal glands, and may if situated on the right side be mistaken for the results of typhlitis or appendicitis.

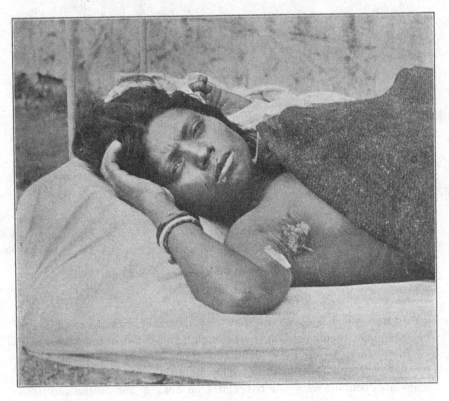

Axillary Bubo.

Patients with axillary buboes usually lie on the back with the affected arm held away from the side. In the axilla the bubo often occludes the axillary space and obliterates the outline of the margin of the pectoralis major. The exudation may become much greater than that accompanying inguinal buboes, and may extend over the side of the chest down to the loins and upwards to the shoulders, and even to the side of the neck. The result of this extensive sero-sanguinolent effusion is the formation on the side of the patient of

Axillary
buboes.

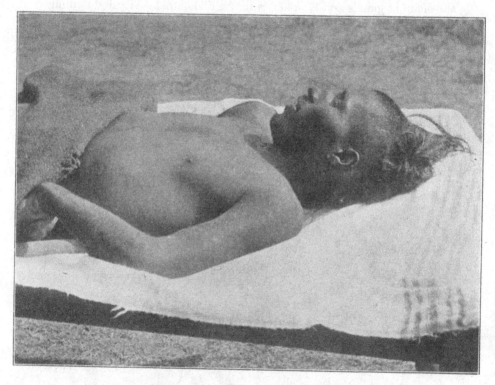

Left Axillary Bubo with Infiltration into Chest,
Shoulder and Arm.

a hard mass which is apt to interfere very materially with the respiratory movements or become a dangerous slough. Incision does not lessen the swelling, there being little exudation from the wound, which soon becomes dry and heals readily. The fluid that does exude does not coagulate spontaneously but coagulates on heating and on the addition of nitric acid. Axillary buboes with extensive exudation usually end fatally. Sometimes an axillary bubo will cause swelling of some of the cervical glands. It has been observed that axillary buboes are frequently associated with septicaemic and secondary pneumonia.

Buboes of the cervical region may be under the jaw or at its angle,
Cervical   in the neck and in the tonsils. The swelling in these
buboes.   situations may be small, and the disease run an ordinary
course, or it may be so great as to place the patient in imminent danger of suffocation. The oedema may extend down below the clavicles or to the chest and into the axilla, or upwards to the face and head, or inwards into the soft tissues with consequent pressure on neighbouring organs.

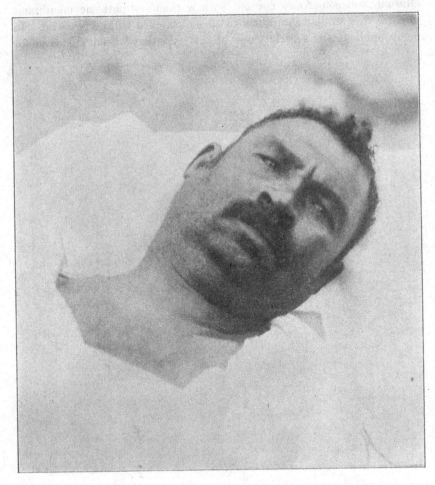

Cervical Bubo.

The trachea is subjected to more or less pressure and the glottis is apt to become oedematous. In these cases the patient lies down with head thrown back or sits up in bed, breathes hurriedly and with difficulty, the respirations being wheezy and stridulent, and the pharynx more or less fixed and immobile during inspiration, the voice is nasal, there is much difficulty in opening the jaw and the sputum contains blood and plague bacilli. The lips and cheeks may become cyanosed or the face may be pallid. Patients suffering from this form of the disease, which is generally tonsillar in its character, with the mucous membrane of the tonsils, pharynx, and larynx highly inflamed, infiltrated, with serous effusion, and sometimes covered with a pseudo-diphtheric membrane, present very similar symptoms to those attacked with diphtheria. In many epidemics the early cases of this type have been mistaken for

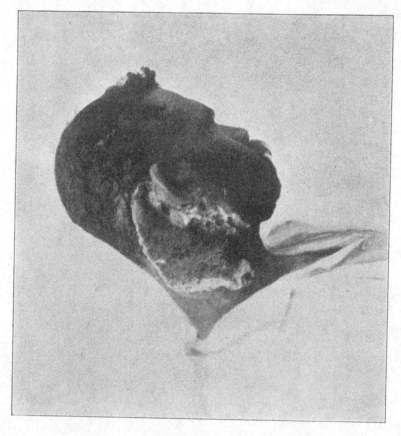

Cervical Bubo.

diphtheria. This was the case in Bombay, where some of the earlier cases of plague with swollen cervical glands were diagnosed as diphtheria. The sloughing of the skin over cervical buboes reminds one of what was seen in cases of scarlet fever when the cases were more malignant than they are at the present day.

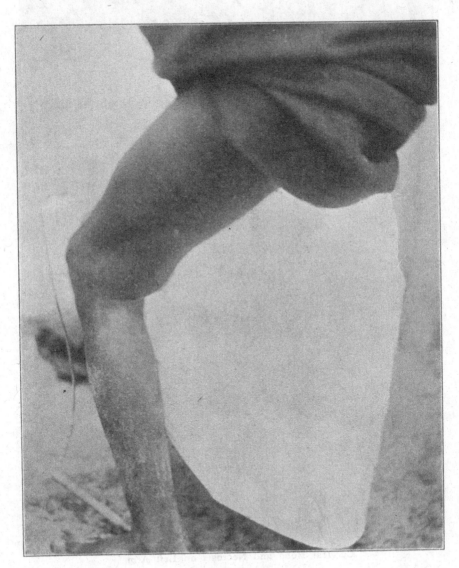

Popliteal Bubo.

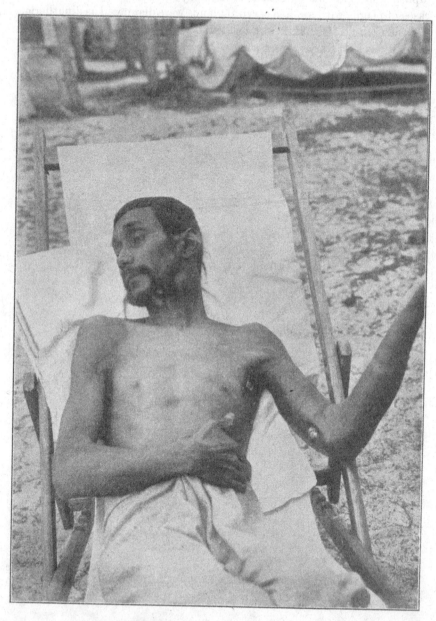

Cervical Bubo and Necrosis on Left Arm.

Buboes occasionally occur on other sites than those mentioned; in fact they may be found wherever glands exist. The most common of these unusual sites are the epitrochlear region and popliteal space, but the glands of the breast, testicle, or other parts may be exceptionally affected with buboes.

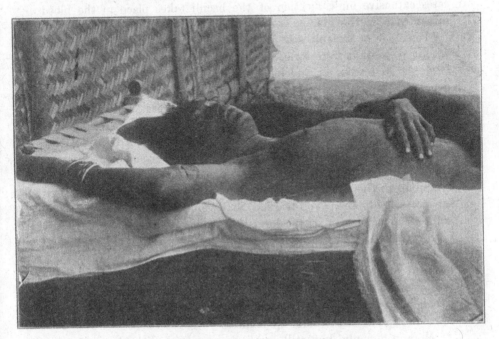

Supra-trochlear Bubo and Necrosis on Arm.

Multiple buboes may also occur either in regions in close proximity

Multiple buboes. to the primary bubo or in distant regions, or contiguous buboes may appear almost simultaneously. In the first case it is generally held that the pathological evidence indicates the passage of the bacillus to the other glandular group by the chain of glands and lymphatic vessels connecting them, or by the oedema formed from the first affected gland. Contiguous buboes most frequently occur in the femoral inguinal and iliac regions and often within a few hours of the onset of the disease. Although clinically these are all that are discernible the post-mortem examination usually shows buboes, haemorrhages and swollen glands in the deeper tissues of the thoracic, abdominal and pelvic cavities. In the case of buboes occurring simultaneously in such distant parts as the groin and axilla it is accepted that they can only be caused by bacilli being carried by the blood stream to the affected glands. In severe septicaemic cases however the glands of the whole glandular system of the body are affected, but they do not pass the stage of engorgement and slight swelling and clinically are not readily recognisable in the groin, arm-pit, or other region. In these cases extensive multiplication of the bacilli takes place in the blood rather than in the glands.

Petechiae of variable size and pustules forming necrotic patches, or

The skin.
Petechiae.

what were formerly called carbuncles, may appear on the buboes or independently of them. The petechiae are generally over buboes or on the abdomen, but they may be found in other parts of the body, such as the face, neck, breast, and extremities. Larger ecchymotic patches are occasionally seen. The petechiae and ecchymotic patches probably correspond to the tokens in the Great Plague of London which appear to have been a common feature in fatal cases. Neither petechiae nor ecchymoses have formed important symptoms in the different epidemics of the present pandemic, but they are occasionally seen well-marked in severe cases before death. In addition to patches of dark-coloured petechiae or ecchymoses there has been occasionally an eruption of pustules. The pustules on the skin may be of a variable nature, and in some cases of plague they have been so numerous as to raise a doubt as to whether it was not a case of small-pox that was being dealt with. This, however, is exceptional, but it is possible that this pustular form of plague was more common in some of the older epidemics.

More commonly, but still rarely as compared with the epidemics

Gangrenous
pustules or
carbuncles.

of former days, there is a slight eruption of a few pustules or carbuncles in the course of the disease and after the appearance of the bubo. They may appear in any part of the body and at any period of the acute stage of the illness. The pustules usually commence as ecchymotic or petechial spots, having the appearance of a flea-bite and with the same burning sensation in them ; these ecchymotic patches rapidly increase in size and then rise in the form of blisters with or without umbilication, while the circumference becomes hard, swollen and inflamed. The blisters contain at first a clear, serous fluid, which is later dark, sero-sanguinolent or haemorrhagic ; and in the contents are plague bacilli. The blisters soon break and show at their base a moist, bluish-red, inflamed and angry-looking circular or irregular patch, which at this stage may dry up and go no further, or the inflammation may extend to the subcutaneous tissue, causing a circumscribed or diffuse swelling, the centre of which begins in a few hours to necrose, forming a leathery-looking scab. From this centre the necrosis spreads rapidly to the periphery. The result is the formation of indolent ulcers more or less deep or superficial with hard and red overhanging margins. The necrosis may stop when the patch has reached a circumference of one or two inches, which is the usual limit, but in some cases it may continue to spread to the diameter of even eight or twelve inches, laying bare the muscles, the nerves and blood vessels, and even the bones, and sometimes causing severe haemorrhage. The slough is thrown off by suppuration and the drain on the strength of the patient is proportional to the size and number of ulcers formed by these gangrenous pustules. They may occur in all parts of the body, the largest having been noticed in the gluteal and

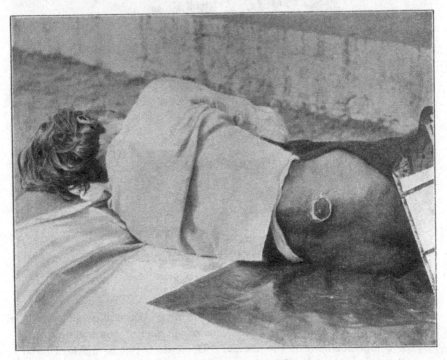

Right Inguinal Bubo and Necrosis or Carbuncle on Loin.

scapular region. Choksy has observed[1] that the mortality of plague cases in which these cellulo-cutaneous necroses occur is less than the

[1] *The Treatment of Plague with Prof. Lustig's Serum.* By N. H. Choksy, M.D.

bubonic type without them. A similar observation was made in Egypt in the epidemic of 1834–35, in which their occurrence was considered favourable. In the latter epidemic the so-called carbuncular variety appeared only at the middle and decline of the epidemic when the

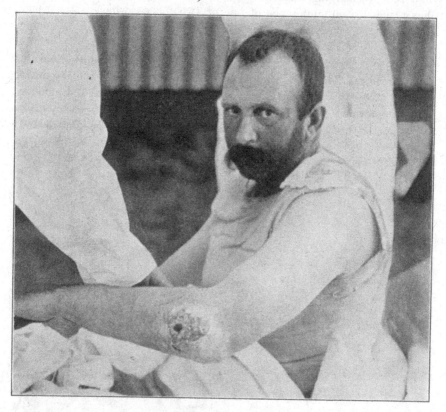

Carbuncle or Necrosis.

type of the disease was less fatal. In a small percentage of cases a single pustule on the wrist or ankle or other part of the body appears at the commencement of the disease. If on the wrist or ankle, a bubo usually occurs in the axilla or inguinal region of the same side. In such cases the mortality is less than in those in which an eruption of pustules manifests itself during the course of the disease. Plague bacilli with pyogenic organism are to be detected in the early stage in the pustules single or multiple.

Next to the eruption of buboes the most characteristic symptoms **Nervous** are those connected with the nervous system. Most of **phenomena.** these have already been mentioned, such as at the commencement of the illness the great depression, severe headache, giddiness, staggering gait, and stammering speech. The headache is usually frontal, though it may not be confined to any special part, and is not infrequently general. It is sometimes dull but more commonly acute in character. Restlessness and a desire to wander from one place to another are often exhibited in the early stage. Sleep is only obtained in snatches and is unrefreshing. As the disease progresses the disturbing effect of the toxines manifests itself on the intelligence in a marked degree, though this is not always the case. There are cases in which the patient remains conscious, rational, and with speech unaffected to the last, not an uncommon occurrence in primary pneumonic plague. Mental clearness is, however, the exception, but it sometimes occurs. It is of no special prognostic value. Heaviness, drowsiness, confusion of ideas and a state of hébétude, alternating with delirium of a low muttering or excited nature, are the most characteristic mental conditions. They come on early in the disease. The delirium may be continuous or only present at night, or it may be absent, and the patient remain in a semi-conscious condition. There are all transition stages of mental condition, from that in which the patient is easily aroused and answers questions slowly but with difficulty in a somewhat hesitating and stammering manner, to that in which he is in a state of stupor, with all the senses dulled, difficult to arouse, and if he answers it is in a muttering, indistinct and almost unintelligible manner, like that of a drunken man. There may be complete aphasia, the patient being unable to speak from paralysis of the laryngeal muscles. The dumbness may continue during convalescence and sometimes after recovery. The sense of taste may be perverted or lost during the illness. The delirium has already been described as being noisy or of a quiet character. It may be so violent as to necessitate the patient being put under restraint in bed to prevent self-injury or escape from the sick-room; sometimes it is accompanied by suicidal or homicidal tendencies and by hallucinations of a terrifying nature. The acute forms of delirium are more frequent than the low muttering variety. At the later stages hyperaesthesia of the skin, tremors, twitchings and spasms of the muscles of the face, neck, limbs, abdominal wall or chest, with convulsive seizures of the body, occasionally mark the strong irritating and toxic effect of the virus on the nervous system. On the other hand the action of the virus may be that of an hypnotic;

then, instead of gesticulations and incessant talking, the patient lies with fixed gaze, indifferent to surroundings, with facial muscles relaxed, powers of articulation lost, and in a state of mental and physical inertia. If the patient recovers the improvement is at most very gradual, and at times there may remain as sequelae a state of dementia, aphasia, or ataxia, which may be temporary or, rarely, permanent. One of the features of plague in those that recover is that the cerebral and nervous disturbances from which they have suffered are mostly functional in their nature, and do not commonly cause any permanent injury.

A feeling of oppression is frequently experienced over the praecardial **Vascular** regions. In mild cases of plague there may be no devia- **system.** tion of the pulse from normal, but in the more or less severe cases weakness soon displays itself, and in proportion to the severity of the nervous phenomena, the pulse shows signs of a tendency to heart failure produced by the paralysing effect of the plague toxines. In connection with this are the frequency of the pulse and the rapid fall in arterial tension. Even on the second day the pulse rate will rise to 120, 130, or 140. At first full and somewhat frequent the pulse soon becomes feeble, rapid, intermittent and dicrotic, and, at last, in cases likely to be fatal, so thready that it is impossible to count. Sometimes heart failure may suddenly occur without any sign of collapse. Sudden exertion, such as sitting up in bed or getting out of bed, may be the immediate cause of heart failure, but this may happen also without any such strain on the heart's action.

Lowson gives three sphygmographic tracings of the pulse in plague which are here reproduced. Two are of the radial pulse and one of the femoral, the first radial tracing showing the dicrotic pulse, the second radial and femoral illustrating the anacrotic pulse preceding failure.

His description of the tracings is as follows:

"The pulse which at first is full and bounding becomes (usually in from six to thirty-six hours) dicrotic and fairly easily compressible at the wrist. The accompanying tracing shows such a pulse where the dicrotism, although not extreme, is well marked.

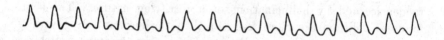

"Intermittency is often noticeable in this second stage of the pulse and becomes more marked as the third stage develops, when it becomes anacrotic and almost like the pulse of aortic insufficiency, there being no rebound wave at all, nor the slightest trace of it by sphygmograph in a well-marked case. In addition it is at this period very easily compressible, and the actual range of movement of the vessel is very limited at the wrist, whereas in the larger vessels the upheaval is usually well marked, slight pressure at the femoral being sufficient to arrest the pulse. The following tracing of the radial pulse is taken from a patient at this stage, there being no pressure on the sphygmograph button except its own weight.

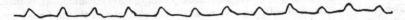

"This patient was a very lean man, and consequently a tracing of his femoral pulse could be easily obtained as the vessel passed over the brim of the pelvis. With slightly over an ounce of pressure (enough to visibly diminish the range of movement) the accompanying tracing was got.

"From this anacrotic stage gradual or sudden failure may set in, unless there is a general improvement in the case. The pulse generally becomes fast and running and scarcely perceptible or if perceptible it is generally intermittent. On the second day if a thin patient was naked one could usually see the femoral arteries beating at a distance of several yards, and this was equally true of the other large arteries. Often this large movement was to be seen in the vessels in the neck, axilla, or groin, and yet at the radial or posterior tibial arteries the pulse was hardly perceptible."

The sounds of the heart are usually clear but feeble. The blood contains, as the disease advances, an increasing number of **The blood.** leucocytes of the polynuclear kind, and at the later stages a short time before death large numbers of plague bacilli may be detected in the blood in bubonic cases, while in septicaemic cases plague bacilli are in the blood at an early stage. According to observations recently made in Hongkong, plague bacilli may be present in cases of plague during the initial stage, even before there is any marked rise in temperature or before the disease manifests itself in the septicaemic or bubonic form. The histories of four cases are given in which plague bacilli are shown to be present in the blood at a very early stage. A fact like this may account for the severity of the disease among the Chinese, whereas in European races and others the bacillus cannot at present readily multiply in the blood and selects in preference the lymphatic system. In the Bombay epidemic of 1896 there were few septicaemic cases compared with the number in later epidemics, while in the South African and Australian epidemics septicaemic cases were conspicuous by their absence.

Case No. I[1]. F. A., admitted to the Government Civil Hospital on the 17th March, 1903, complaining of severe diarrhoea. Temperature on admission, normal. The blood was examined with negative results. The character of the stool was loose, bile-stained and foul-smelling. Nothing characteristic was found in the stool when examined microscopically. The number of stools on the day of admission was 6. On the 18th 4 stools, on the 19th 4 stools, and on the 20th he had 2 stools. All the stools were of the same character as described. The temperature was still normal on the 20th. On the evening of the 20th it suddenly rose to 102° F. The diarrhoea was still present. On the 21st the evening temperature was 103° F., diarrhoea still present. On the 22nd the temperature was 103° F., diarrhoea small in amount. The blood was examined by the method recommended by Ross for malaria, and a number of oval, bipolar-shaped micro-organisms were found. These were regarded as plague bacilli, and the patient was removed to Kennedy Town Hospital. Here he complained of severe headache and sleepiness. The tongue was thickly furred, and in general the patient presented all the signs of severe plague infection. No bubo developed. *He went through an extremely severe attack of plague of the septicaemic type.*

Case No. II. S. S., a police constable, was admitted to the Government Civil Hospital on 3rd June, 1903, complaining of vomiting and diarrhoea of a day's duration. On admission the dejecta were found to be watery, bile-stained, and foul-smelling. The tongue was furred. The temperature was 100° F. The blood was examined by Ross's method, and large numbers of bacilli identical with the *B. pestis* were found. On the strength of this, the patient was removed to the Infectious Diseases Hospital; where *a severe and typical bubonic plague developed.*

Case No. III. T. K., a Chinese police constable, was admitted to the Government Civil Hospital on the 4th March, 1903, complaining of severe "colic," vomiting and constant watery diarrhoea. The bowels opened twice soon after admission, and the dejecta were watery and brownish-yellow in colour. Nothing abnormal was found in the stools. The patient looked very pinched, ill, and somnolent. The temperature was 99° F.

On the 5th the temperature was still 99° F. The patient was very sleepy and dull. He complained of severe headache. The tongue had become thickly coated. The diarrhoea was still profuse and of the same character. The blood was examined as in other cases. Bacteria morphologically identical with the *B. pestis* were found. He was removed at once to Kennedy Town Hospital where *he passed through a typical attack of plague of the bubonic type.*

[1] *A Research into Epidemic and Epizootic Plague.* By Wm. Hunter, Government Bacteriologist, Hongkong, 1904.

Case No. IV. H. T., a Chinese coolie, was admitted to the Government Civil Hospital on the 16th March, 1903, complaining of cramps in the abdomen, headache, vomiting and diarrhoea. On admission the temperature was 100·8° F., the tongue was foul, headache was constantly complained of, and vomiting and diarrhoea continued severe. Nothing abnormal was found microscopically in the stools. They had the usual naked-eye appearance. During the first 24 hours after admission the patient had 22 stools. The blood was examined as in other cases and organisms identical with plague bacilli found. He was transferred to Kennedy Town Hospital and *developed into a typical case of septicaemic plague with no bubonic formation.*

The appetite varies, being sometimes lost and at other times almost
The digestive ravenous. Intense thirst is, however, a more constant
system. symptom. The characteristic condition of the tongue at
the different stages of illness has already been referred to. The soft palate, fauces, and pharynx are inflamed, the tonsils swollen and may be covered with a diphtheritic coating. Patients may complain of burning, dryness and rawness in the throat. Vomiting preceded by nausea is one of the initial and most frequent symptoms: occasionally it may continue during the whole acute period of the illness. The material vomited after the digesta is a watery fluid, bilious or dark like coffee-grounds, and sometimes containing blood.

Constipation is the usual condition at the onset but diarrhoea may supervene later or even begin with the illness. The evacuations are usually very foetid and of a yellow or bilious colour. Sometimes they are dysenteric in character, blood, mucus, and epithelium appearing in the stools. Occasionally the diarrhoea is of such violence as to suggest cholera. These intestinal symptoms have been observed in India and China. In Hongkong Wilm[1] noted that in 20 % of the cases in which no external buboes were formed the intestinal symptoms were so predominant that the illness had to be regarded as an intestinal affection. Post-mortem examination of these cases revealed enlargement and inflammatory changes in the mesenteric and retro-peritoneal glands, and congestion and dilatation of the blood and lymph vessels between the affected glands and the intestine. A similar but milder form of visceral plague has been observed in Egypt by Valassopoulo[2].

Captain Höjel[3], I.M.S., first drew attention to the occurrence in the Bombay epidemic of a type of the disease in which abdominal symptoms

[1] *Report on the Epidemic of Bubonic Plague at Hongkong in the year* 1896. By Staff-Surgeon Wilm.

[2] *La Peste d'Alexandrie en* 1899. Par le Dr A. Valassopoulo, 1901.

[3] *Report of the Bombay Bubonic Plague Research Committee* by Surgeon-Major Lyons, I.M.S., President of the Bombay Research Committee.

predominated. In this form there were pain and tenderness in the epigastric region, pain in the back, abdominal tension, enlargement of the liver and spleen, and low nervous symptoms similar to those met with in enteric fever, accompanied in some cases by the appearance of petechiae on the abdomen and lower part of the thorax resembling the rash of enteric fever. Peyer's patches were found after death to be slightly raised, oedematous and congested, the solitary follicles as large as a hemp seed, but there was no enlargement of the mesenteric glands.

The urine is scanty, high-coloured, sometimes smoky, acid, and of The urinary system. varying degrees of specific gravity; it contains albumen in the majority of cases, but is deficient in chlorides, urea and uric acid. In grave cases there may be haematuria, or there may be suppression or retention in the one case owing to cessation of secretion, in the other to loss of power of the functions of the bladder, necessitating the employment of the catheter to draw off the urine. Plague bacilli are present in some cases[1].

The respiration in the milder cases or at the commencement of Respiratory system. those which become more serious may remain unaltered or only slightly accelerated, but with the severer forms and as the disease advances the condition of the respiration becomes an important feature in the disease. Oppression and tightness across the chest are experienced, the breathing is laborious, the respiration increased in frequency, rising to 30, 40, 50, and even 60 per minute; the breathing is hurried and difficult, the dyspnoea being due to a gradually increasing oedema of the lungs, which causes much distress to the patient. Cough is generally present. The sputum is scanty and viscid at first and later purulent, and in simple cases without blood. Auscultation and percussion may reveal signs of congestion of the base of the lung and a more general catarrh, or of nothing specially abnormal. In some cases there is bronchitis and secondary plague pneumonia as complications. Clinically there is nothing to facilitate the recognition of secondary pneumonia save a decrease in the respiratory murmur, some slight crepitant rales, and the rapid deterioration in the condition of the patient.

Complications and Sequelae.

The complications of plague are mainly those connected with the Complications. respiratory system, such as bronchitis, oedema of the lungs, and secondary pneumonia; occasionally pleurisy and pneu-

---

[1] *Austrian Report.*

mothorax may be met with. The first three may be viewed rather as an extension of the infective process to other parts of the system at a later stage of the disease, and from this aspect they form but a part of the disease. On the other hand there are plague cases with severe constitutional disturbances without these respiratory troubles. In-

Eye diseases. flammatory affections of the eye are not infrequent complications of plague; these may range from a simple inflammatory state to one which is accompanied by ulceration of the cornea, by copious haemorrhages, and in some cases total destruction of the eyesight.

Marasmus is another complication which occasionally sets in during the period of convalescence. It usually ends in death.

Marasmus and chronic plague. The patient becomes emaciated, feeble in mind and body, unable to take food, gets into a typhoid condition, and gradually sinks. This state may be caused by secondary infections of a pyaemic nature, in which streptococci and staphylococci play their part, or by the intense toxic effect of the plague virus.

Closely connected with this marasmus condition is another in which the disease runs a chronic course from the commencement. The patient may walk about notwithstanding a certain amount of indisposition and catarrh and yet succumb later to the disease, and be found the subject of abscesses containing plague bacilli in the lungs, liver, and spleen. This chronic type closely resembles that found in the lower animals.

Indolence of buboes, sinuses connected with buboes maintaining chronic discharges, and sloughing of buboes or of gangrenous pustules can hardly be classed as complications though they materially protract the duration of the illness and sap the strength of the patient. Abscesses and boils may also appear in different parts of the body and contribute to a retardation of recovery.

In pregnant women the most important complication is that of abortion, which in the majority of cases is fatal to mother

Pregnancy. and child. The danger of plague under this condition both to mother and child has been observed in every epidemic, ancient and modern. Exceptions may occur in which one or other or both may live, but they are rare.

Choksy mentions arthritis as being a common complication of cases of plague coming under his observation in Bombay[1]. He

Arthritis. describes it as appearing generally during convalescence

---

[1] *Report on Plague at Arthur Road Hospital, Bombay.* By Khan Bahadour N. H. Choksy, M.D.

and being ushered in with feverish reaction, the temperature rising slowly after having been low for a considerable time, accompanied by swelling and effusion into the joints. It ran a more or less acute course, and the joints principally involved were the shoulder, elbow, wrist, knee and ankle. Malaria, beriberi, cholera, relapsing fever, pulmonary phthisis and syphilis are diseases which have at times Concurrent been observed to coexist with plague. There is probably diseases. no disease that may not accidentally coexist with it, but these being the most common in India and China, where plague has been epidemic, the conjunction has been met with most frequently.

None of them give any immunity against an attack of plague. In the Hongkong plague epidemic of 1902, when cholera also prevailed as an epidemic, the two diseases were occasionally observed in the same person. The same has been noted in India. In Bombay during the prevalence of relapsing fever, cases of plague were seen in which, in addition to the plague bacillus isolated from the patient, the spirillum was observed in the blood.

Plague may occur in a patient suffering from malaria, or malaria may supervene in the course of an attack of plague. In these cases the malarial parasite may be found in the blood, and the plague bacillus in the bubo, in the sputum, or in the blood.

Of sequelae the most important are affections of the nervous system. Sequelae. Aphasia, ataxia, and dementia are the most common; happily they are generally of a temporary character though they may be permanent. Parotitis may also occur. Blindness also follows some of the destructive injuries to the eye, while the sloughing associated with buboes or pustules may injure important blood vessels and cause dangerous haemorrhage. Gangrene of the limb has also been observed in some rare cases.

Second attacks, though rare, do occur sometimes. It is now and Second again difficult to distinguish them from relapses which attacks. also occur occasionally. But this only happens when the second attack closely follows the first. Three cases of second attack are recorded as having occurred in the first epidemic at Bombay[1]. One was a European lady who was attacked at Hongkong in June, 1894, with a cervical bubo from which she recovered at the beginning of August. She was again attacked with plague at Bombay in December, 1896, with a femoral bubo which resolved without suppuration. The second attack was milder than the first.

[1] Report of the Health Officer for Bombay for 1896.

The second case was that of a native in Bombay, the details of which are as follows :—

First attack.   October 30, 1896.   Mahomed Allybux Kadirally (age 53), Samuel Street, No. 197, second-floor.

3rd day.   Left parotid bubo, size of a pigeon's egg, tender.   Pulse 150; respiration 44; temperature 105.   Shivering, delirious (bubo second day).   40 minims of medretine given and 10 minims of liq. hydrarg. perchl. every 2 hours.   Calomel gr. 2 stat.   Ice to the head; 2 powders given.

October 31.   Restless, 3 motions.   Temperature 103; pulse uncountable; respiration 56; bubo more painful and tender.   Delirious. Medretine given.   Phenacetin and soda salicylate every 2 hours, as necessary.

November 1.   Pulse 180; respiration 44; temperature 103·5.   Delirious; sleep disturbed; right lung congested.   Had one motion.   Had 3 powders and medretine given, 2 oz. in 24 hours.   Mixtures, stimulants and expectorants.

November 2.   Bubo enlarging and painful; pulse 130; respiration 40; temperature 102·2.   No headache; lung clear; had one motion. Treatment same.

November 3.   Temperature 101; pulse 132; respiration 33.   A little better.   Medretine given every 2 hours, and ext. carnis and rum every 4 hours.

November 4.   Temperature 102·2; pulse 144; respiration 40; bubo subsiding; right parotid gland appears tender; medretine every 4 hours; ext. carnis and rum every 4 hours.

November 6.   Temperature 100; pulse 140; respiration 40; lungs a little congested.

November 8.   Temperature 99; pulse 128; respiration 36.

November 15.   No fever; bubo suppurated; pulse 112.

Second attack or recurrence.   December 2.   Temperature 105; respiration 40; pulse 144.   Very delirious, and starting in bed.   Over left parotid gland much swollen and very tender.   Liq. hyd. per m. 15 every 2 hours.

December 3.   Temperature 104; respiration 60; pulse 100.

December 4.   Temperature 104; respiration 40; pulse 102; delirium less.

December 5.   Temperature 100; respiration 40; pulse 100; delirium less.

December 6.   Doing well.

The third case was Mr C. T., "an Inspector in the Bombay Customs House, a Bania by caste, age 27, who was attacked first in February, 1897; temperature rising to 105 and a gland in the left femoral region becoming enlarged and painful. Under treatment the gland subsided and the fever disappeared in a week; after that he enjoyed perfect health for nearly two months, when he had a second attack and the same gland again became enlarged and painful. This second attack can be traced to his nursing and almost living in the same house with a plague patient at Matoonga. On this occasion the gland suppurated and was removed by an operation. The patient made a very slow recovery and was finally discharged cured, after living for more than two months in the hospital."

These are all cases of recovery, but Matignon in his account of the bubonic plague in Mongolia records the case of a man who, the previous year, had been attacked with very characteristic plague with buboes and died of plague the following year.

Clot Bey points out that Evagrius, Vallere, Diemerbroech, Chenot, Orréus and Schrauel cite cases of relapses of plague observed by them and refers to Bertrand, who in the Marseilles epidemic mentions some persons who were attacked three times during the same epidemic. Clot.Bey and his colleagues saw in Egypt several patients who died of plague who, on a previous occasion, had recovered from the disease. Russell out of 4400 plague cases met with 28 cases of reinfection[1].

Cases of Plague.

A. B., a Kaffir boy, admitted to hospital, having a swelling in the left groin. His history was that of feeling indisposed three or four days before, having experienced slight shivering, nausea, and loss of appetite, after which a swelling appeared in the groin; next day the malaise disappeared. Examination in hospital showed that the patient had no fever, the temperature being subnormal and registering 97° F. There was a bubo about the size of a pigeon's egg immediately above Poupart's ligament in the left groin; the skin over the bubo was red but mobile. The tongue was coated with a white fur and was red at the tip and edges. The eyes were not congested. There was no lisping nor slurring of the speech, and his intellect was as quick as ordinarily. On examination of the contents of the enlarged glands no bacilli were discoverable, but on

Ambulant variety.

---

[1] *A Treatise of the Plague*, p. 190. By Patrick Russell, M.D., F.R.S., 1791.

culture of the contents, characteristic growths of the plague bacillus were found. A guinea-pig and rabbit inoculated with the culture died in 40 hours from typical plague. The glands had been noticed three days before the patient's visit to hospital. On the third day of his admission the temperature reached normal, he appeared in every way well, and the bubo, instead of suppurating, ultimately disappeared by resolution.

A. B., Malay, 50 years, fell ill on July 9th at 4 a.m. in the Cape Town contact camp, was sent to hospital at 8 a.m., but **Septic and fulminating variety.** died on the way. Thirteen days previously his son died at home after 4 days' illness of plague. A. B. was sent with his family to the contact camp for 12 days' observation and was to have been sent home on the day of the morning on which he fell ill. On the night of the 8th he ate his supper, was apparently well and was seen by the Medical Officer on the latter's evening inspection. Some time after 3 a.m. on the 9th he woke up and remarked to his wife that he did not feel well. At 4 a.m. he suddenly had an attack of shivering and difficulty of breathing and fell almost immediately into a state of collapse, dying at 8 a.m. The patient being a Malay no post-mortem could be obtained at the time, but punctures were made into the spleen, liver and lungs, and the contents drawn off not only gave smear preparations which swarmed with plague bacilli, but also pure cultures of the microbe. No buboes could be detected by careful palpation and examination of the external parts.

C. D., Malay, wife of A. B., fell ill on the 10th July at 9 p.m. and died at 2 a.m. on the 11th. Patient came to the contact camp with her husband. When her husband died on the morning of the 9th July she felt quite well, but on the 10th was depressed, which was attributed to her having lost her son and husband by plague. On the 10th at 9 p.m. Dr McCulloch, the medical officer of the contact camp, made his usual visit and C. D. was found in bed. The daughter states that her mother felt shivery, which she attributed to grief. Professor Levin and Dr McCulloch made a careful examination of her condition. There was no congestion of the face, tongue was normal, temperature 98·3, pulse small, soft and 98 per minute, respiration slightly hurried, rate 28 per minute, lungs and heart sounds normal. Cervical, axillary and inguinal regions carefully examined and no indication of swollen glands or buboes observed. The nurse was instructed to immediately call the medical men if she noticed any change for the worse in the condition of the patient. At 2 a.m. of the 11th the patient suddenly became comatose and died before the arrival of the doctors.

Post-mortem on the 11th. In left axillary region a bubo the size of a pigeon's egg was found. The situation of the bubo was immediately behind the border of the pectoralis muscle and on the dead body was easily discernible, both to sight and touch. Section of the bubo showed a red-violet, granular surface. With pressure there oozed out a red-yellow thick fluid. Nearly all the lymphatic glands in the body were enlarged, congested, and on section showed a red-violet surface. *Pleural cavities* contained about a pint of clear yellow fluid. *Lungs* free, but oedematous. On section a great quantity of reddish-yellow aërated fluid oozed out. *Heart* normal in size, valves and openings free, but the margins of the valves rose-coloured and thickened. *Spleen* much enlarged, pulp dark red colour and friable. *Kidneys* with sub-capsular ecchymoses; section showed cortical substance swollen, picture indistinct, numerous ecchymoses in pelvis, also haemorrhage. *Liver* enlarged, necrotic patches and fatty infiltration on surface. *Stomach* contained coffee-coloured fluid and numerous ecchymoses and haemorrhages on mucous membrane. *Blood* showed leucocytosis.

Bacteriological examination. Smear preparations from bubo, glands, spleen, liver and blood swarming with plague bacilli. Cultures from these organs give pure cultures.

The rapidity of such cases and the absence of buboes or their appearance immediately before death may easily lead to the true nature of the disease being overlooked. In some cases even the most experienced may be left in doubt and it is only by an examination of the blood during life or by a post-mortem examination that an absolute diagnosis can be made.

James Lombard, coloured, 39 years, admitted to hospital on 13th June. *History.* On morning of 10th became suddenly ill with severe shivering and vomiting and severe pain in the joints, especially in the loins. In the afternoon he observed on his face, arms, and chest, patches, which on the following day, the 11th, developed into small bladders which covered the whole body. On the 12th felt pains in axilla and groin. Seen on this day by the Inspecting Medical Officer, who found painful buboes in axillae and groins and a pustular and papular rash on forehead and cheeks. Smears from glands and pustules contained plague bacilli. The pustules were small, irregular in shape, with no umbilication and no surrounding infiltration nor induration of skin.

An atypical case.

Present state[1]. General state grave. Patient is very weak, speech indistinct and stuttering, conjunctivae congested and injected, lips very dry, tongue covered with thick dirty brown and crusty coating. Temperature 100·8° F.; pulse small and soft, 120; respiration hurried, 32 per minute. On the face, arms, legs, on the front side of the body and parts of the back, are numerous pustules from the size of a pin's head to a halfpenny, mostly single but often confluent; some limpid and when pricked a clear fluid oozes out; others opaque and on puncture a dirty yellow thickish fluid oozes out. A number of the pustules dried up, leaving crusts. In the lumbar region on the right side a carbuncle of the size of a halfpenny with dark, raised, undermined, rugged borders; the bottom of the ulcer covered with a thick purulent dirty yellow matter; another carbuncle on the right side on the margin of the lowest rib. In the cervical region buboes of the size of a hazel-nut, two on each side; the skin not red over them but readily mobile; the buboes not painful to pressure but painful when head moved. In each of the axillae a bubo of the size of a pigeon's egg, and of the same character as the cervical buboes. Also on both sides epitrochlear buboes; on the right arm the epitrochlear very swollen and very painful on pressure and movement; the skin very red and not mobile. The whole part very hard and much infiltrated. Femoral buboes on both sides of the size of hazel-nuts, slightly painful on pressure; skin not changed. The first sound of heart indistinct, other sounds normal; lungs normal.

Intravenous injection of 20 c.c. Yersin given. A second dose was given, but when he received 7 c.c. patient began to be restless and the injection was stopped. He became cyanotic and breathed more hurriedly. Ether injection was given subcutaneously and in a few minutes he recovered; 40 c.c. Yersin given subcutaneously.

14th. Patient slept a little during the night and took some nourishment; very weak, pulse small, bad, almost impossible to count. Temperature 100°. 40 c c. Yersin subcutaneously.

15th. General state very bad, patient very restless, incontinence of rectum and bladder, pulse not countable. Temperature 101·8° in morning and 104° in evening.

16th. Coma.

17th. Died.

Post-mortem. On face, arms, legs, and most parts of body encrusted

---

[1] "Bubonpesten i Kap," 1901. *Reseherattelse af Med. Dr Ernest Levin.* Stockholm, 1902.

pustules. Buboes already described. Section of buboes showed a thick, putty-like pus. Both lungs fixed to pleura with easily detached connective tissue. Sub-pleural haemorrhage. Lower part of left lung covered with a thin fibrinous exudation. On section of lower part of left lung, small granular elevated patches of a rosy colour with a distinct slightly depressed centre. In other part of left lung a few similar patches noticed.

Lower lobe of right lung had also a fibrinous covering. Section of right lung showed a grey-red, elevated, granular surface of an hepatic appearance, and on pressure there oozed out a dirty red-yellow fluid devoid of air.

In other parts of lung similar patches as in left. At the base of the heart several sub-pericardial ecchymoses. Heart slightly enlarged; valve openings normal. In the muscular tissue of heart greyish-yellow patches. Spleen not enlarged, dark red; consistence soft and friable. Kidneys with sub-capsular ecchymosis.

Section of kidney. The cortical substance swollen and thickened and not distinct. Liver enlarged with fatty infiltration. Stomach and intestines normal.

Bacteriological examination. Pus from pustules on 14th June exhibited in direct preparation a few typical bacilli. In culture only staphylococci. Axillary bubo, femoral bubo, heart blood and lungs showed no bacilli in either smear preparations or in cultures.

There are two varieties of pneumonic plague. One is primary in its character, and the other is secondary or symptomatic.

Plague pneumonia. Primary plague pneumonia is a type of the disease in which the primary localisation of the plague bacillus takes place in some of the lobules of the lungs instead of in the glands of the groin, arm-pit, or neck or other glands of the lymphatic system.

Secondary pneumonia, on the other hand, develops in the course of other types of plague and is due to a secondary infection which has reached the lungs metastatically through the circulation or lymphatic vessels from some other already infected centre of the body, or has, as in the case of tonsillar plague, been inhaled into the lungs.

The clinical aspects of primary pneumonic plague are not very distinctive, and were it not for the discovery of plague bacilli in the sputum this type of plague may easily be mistaken for broncho-pneumonia. Surgeon-Major Childe's description[1] of the symptoms of

---

[1] Report by Surgeon-Major Lyons, I.M.S., President of the Plague Research Committee.

the illness of Dr Manser of Bombay and of the nurse who attended him, both of whom were attacked with plague, will, with Dr Pöch's description of Dr Mueller's illness, illustrate this type of the disease.

"With regard to the clinical symptoms of these cases, it fell to me to **Dr Manser's** attend on the late Dr Manser, and as he died of this form **illness.** of plague I will mention a few facts about his case. He was in his usual health on January 2nd, and had a sudden rigor in the morning and felt fever coming on. During the day a bad headache developed, he felt nausea and vomited several times, and he had pains and a tired feeling in his limbs; his tongue remained clean and moist, and his skin was slightly moist. At 2 p.m., temperature 103·4, pulse 116, respiration 25, and there were but slight variations during the day. On January 3rd, had passed a bad night and felt worse, and all the symptoms persisted, except the aching in the limbs, and he felt very ill. The temperature remained between 103·5 and 104·5, pulse about 110, and the respirations about 23 throughout the day. During the afternoon he felt some pain at the lower part of the left axilla just underneath the anterior fold, but there was no glandular enlargement or pain in the glands anywhere. On January 4th, had passed a bad night and felt very ill, temperature 104·6, pulse 113, respiration 25, tongue still moist, with a little fur behind, and no sordes about the lips and teeth, other symptoms as before. During the night he began to cough and brought up some watery sero-mucous fluid, slightly blood-tinged, and the pain remained in the same place, only more diffused now, being felt over an area of a square inch. At this part some moist sounds could be heard like early pneumonia, and they could also be heard just below the left clavicle; the rest of the lungs and other organs appeared to be normal, as did the lymphatic glands. Patient considered that he had pneumonia, but the symptoms were not like ordinary pneumonia. For the onset was different, the condition of the mouth and tongue different, there was no dyspnoea or pneumonic disproportion of pulse and respiration, and the sputum was not at all like rusty sputum; for it was loose and free, coming up with the slightest cough, it was watery, looking more like serum than mucus, and it was slightly pink, not rusty yellow at all. Also there was the striking fact that the patient's general condition was far worse than could be explained by the small amount of lung-disease present. So I examined the sputum under the microscope, and found it full of bacilli looking like those of plague, and cultures were made from which a pure growth of the plague bacillus was obtained. During 4th and 5th, patient became steadily worse, his temperature remained about 104, and his expectoration became more profuse; the moist sounds were heard over a larger area, as well as slightly at the bases; the respirations increased to 35, and then to 45, and the pulse to 120 and 135; and he ultimately died early on January 6th.

"There is also the case of the nurse who attended him, who unfortunately died of a similar form of plague. In brief she became ill on the evening of January 7th, and showed symptoms of pneumonia on January 8th. She rapidly became worse and died on the 10th, but her sputum was not nearly so profuse as in the former case, and symptoms of exhaustion came on much earlier. She also had no glandular pain or enlargement whatever and bacteriologically her sputum was exactly as described above. Other cases were met with in which besides plague-pneumonia, there was also general enlargement of the glands,—plague-septicaemia; and clinically it was found that either the pneumonia was primary, and the glandular enlargement secondary, or that the disease first showed itself in the glands and later on in the lungs; and whilst some of the latter recovered, the former were usually rapidly fatal. Also the sputum was not always as has been described above, for in some cases the presence of blood in it was a marked feature, and it was either moderate or abundant in quantity. These pneumonic forms of plague are highly infectious and probably take a large share in the spread of the disease; for in these cases the patient's sputum is practically a virulent pure culture of the plague bacillus, and as there is reason to believe that many of the cases are not recognised as plague at all, precautions are not taken by the patients' friends, and the dangerous nature of the disease is not appreciated."

Dr Pöch[1] begins by referring to the circumstances by which **Dr Mueller's illness.** Dr Mueller contracted the infection. On the 15th Oct. 1898, Franz Barisch, the servant of the pathological institution in Vienna, who had been assigned to the assistance of Albrecht and Ghon to render them service in their investigations on plague, fell ill with the symptoms of a commencing pneumonia. His sputum was examined by Drs Ghon and Albrecht on account of their suspicions being aroused by his previous work, and this examination awakened a suspicion of infection by plague bacilli.

Dr Mueller who was called to examine him clinically had him immediately removed with all precautions to an isolation ward of the

---

[1] *Ueber die Beulenpest in Bombay im Jahre* 1897. Vol. I. Anhang.

Vienna General Hospital. At the same time Dr Ghon personally superintended the disinfection of Barisch's home.

Though Dr Mueller during the first days of the illness could not with certainty confirm a diagnosis of infection with plague bacilli he adopted all precautionary sanitary measures and impressed on the two nurses the greatest caution. He bestowed much attention and care on the patient and did not hesitate to examine him repeatedly and minutely. It was in this service that he contracted plague.

On the 18th of October, on the 4th day of the disease, the servant died of pneumonic plague. This diagnosis was fully confirmed bacteriologically and clinically.

On the 20th of October one of Barisch's nurses, who in the meantime had been strictly isolated, became feverish. On this account both of them were taken to the isolation ward of the Emperor Franz Joseph Hospital, whither Dr Mueller also betook himself, having of his own free will offered himself for the treatment of the sick nurse.

On his arrival in the hospital Dr Mueller was seemingly quite well, but on the same evening he felt continually cold, and walked up and down the room shivering and rubbing his hands, although the room was well heated. He complained of feeling low-spirited and had crural pains. He also coughed, but without expectoration. He attributed this indisposition to fatigue and a chill. The nurse attending on him formed the impression that he was feverish and begged him to take his temperature. This, however, he did not do. He left his supper almost untouched and went to bed at 8 o'clock. He slept quietly and soundly.

On the 21st of October Dr Mueller paid his morning visit to Barisch's two nurses. He looked very pale, felt languid and lay down again at 9 a.m. in order to rest. At this time his pulse was 110, he coughed a great deal but brought nothing up. About midday he got up again, but had to go back to bed shortly after. His temperature was now taken for the first time. It was 38·2 C.

He now began to expectorate; it was a reddish and thin fluid. Dr Kretz who undertook the examination of the sputum confirmed the existence of plague bacilli. Although it was sought to deceive Dr Mueller as to the results of this examination, he himself confirmed the diagnosis of pneumonic plague from his symptoms and held fast to his opinion. The pulse was small, tense, the highest frequency 120. At 2 p.m. his respiration was accelerated to 40 and regular. The fits of coughing became more frequent and copious reddish sputum was

expectorated. The patient did not complain of pain. The fever at
6 p.m. reached its highest point, 40·8° C. Consciousness was maintained.
Digitalis and alcohol were given. He was very thirsty. He decidedly
refused an injection of plague serum.

In the course of the afternoon he had two fluid, not bloody stools.
He had a fairly good night, woke a few times, was delirious a short time:
soon, however, fell asleep again.

On the morning of October 22nd the conjunctivae of the patient were
much reddened. He was unconscious and noisy delirium set in. Speech

Dr MUELLER

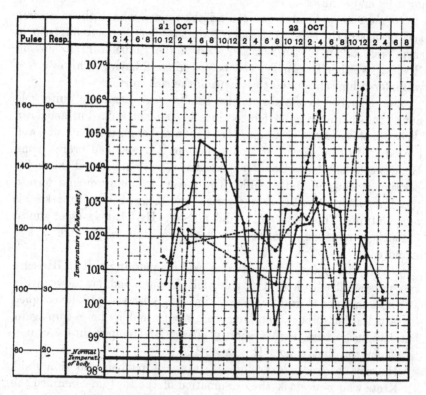

———— Temp.   · · · Pulse.   —·—·— Respiration.

was woolly and indistinct. Large quantities of reddish fluid sputum
were brought up in frequent short fits of coughing. On this day
Dr Mueller took no solid nourishment. He had a second dose of
digitalis and a good quantity of alcohol. In the afternoon he com-

plained of pain in his chest and asked for morphia. He, however, hardly took a third of what was ordered him, the pains having in the meantime diminished. At 6 p.m. the respiration was quickened and very difficult, frequency 59. Cyanosis set in. The fits of coughing became more frequent still and rattling with a quantity of bloody expectoration. There were no skin haemorrhages or glandular swellings. In the afternoon he had 4 thin, not bloody stools, with accompanying pains. Consciousness was dulled. When the thermometer was applied Dr Mueller awoke out of his somnolent condition and began to count pulse and respiration. He made frequent mistakes, and began to count anew until he came to a result. At 10 p.m. the temperature sank to 37·8 and for a short time consciousness was again clearer. Then again great restlessness and delirium set in.

On the 23rd of October at 1 a.m. Dr Mueller stood up and walked up and down the room with help, then he lay down again and went to sleep. Later he woke again and passed urine. There were never involuntary motions or urinating.

At 4 a.m. the temperature was 38°. C., breathing was difficult, cyanosis had increased.

At 4.15 a.m. rattling in the throat began, bloody mucus poured in quantities from the mouth and at 4.30 a.m. death set in.

CHAPTER XV.

DIAGNOSIS AND PROGNOSIS.

In the majority of cases there is no difficulty in the diagnosis of plague. The sudden onset, the severe headache, the giddiness, the high fever of a remittent type, with hot dry skin, the drawn and anxious face, the red and congested eyes without photophobia, the flushed countenance, the stuttering, thick and indistinct speech like that of a drunken man, the coated tongue red at the tip and edges, the staggering gait, the incoordination of the voluntary muscles, the desire to wander about, the quick feeble pulse, the hurried respiration, the rapid development of cerebral symptoms, the heavy drowsy and stupid mental condition, and the formation of a bubo or buboes in the region of the lymphatic glands present such a clear picture of plague that the disease may be readily recognised by a careful observer who is on the alert as to the possible occurrence of plague.

Diagnosis generally not difficult in a typical case of plague.

The bubo which is the most characteristic symptom may at the time of examination not be in evidence. The bubo generally appears within 24 hours but may be delayed till the third, fourth, or fifth day and in some exceptional cases even longer, the other symptoms being well defined. In some cases the affected glands do not form buboes, but are usually recognisable from their exquisite tenderness when touched; in other cases they are deeply situated and it is only by strong pressure over the parts that they are detected. When the clinical symptoms indicate plague, and yet there is no bubo in the groin, arm-pit or neck, a careful examination of the abdomen often reveals a bubo in the iliac or lumbar region.

In milder cases when some of the symptoms are absent, and especially when consciousness and a clear intellect obscure the character of the disease, the pulse is of valuable assistance as a guide to diagnosis.

It is rapid and feeble, and out of all proportion to the condition of the patient.

Before this pandemic the diagnosis of plague had to rest on the clinical symptoms, but now to these is added the bacteriological test.

Bacterio-
logical test.
By puncturing the bubo even at its earliest stage a small quantity of the gelatinous contents can be sucked out with a sterilised glass pipette guarded at the mouth end by sterilised cotton wool. If the contents so obtained are then spread out on a glass slide or cover-glass, gently heated as in the ordinary preparation of a microscopical specimen, coloured with carbol fuchsin or gentian violet, and then examined by a $\frac{1}{12}$ oil immersion lens, the field will be seen to be covered with cocco-bacilli or diplo-bacteria, large numbers of them being more deeply stained at the ends than in the centre. No other disease with swollen lymphatic glands presents microbes such as these. Their presence is sufficient to arouse the greatest suspicion at any time, and the material ought to be taken at once to a laboratory where the bacilli can be cultivated and the confirmatory tests applied. When plague is known to prevail in a country the discovery of bacilli by microscopical examination, combined with the clinical features, is sufficient to make the diagnosis of plague a certainty.

In cases in which the bubo has suppurated the pus only exceptionally contains plague bacilli and the diagnosis must then rest on the clinical features considered as a whole, together with the specific agglutination test of the blood.

The serum test, however, is one not of much practical utility owing

The serum
test.
to the fact that frequently no reaction is given with the blood of patients convalescing from plague, and to the further fact that in an ordinary culture of plague bacilli the microbes are often so massed together that an extra clumping by the agglutinating process of the serum is difficult to recognise. The Indian Plague Commission[1] in summing up their experience on this subject came to the conclusion that "no practical value attaches to the method of serum diagnosis in the case of plague."

On the other hand[2] Cairns in the Glasgow epidemic found by a series of careful experiments that if agar cultures are emulsified with sterile 0·75 % salt solution a homogeneous emulsion of the plague bacillus is obtainable and that the sedimentation test under these

[1] *Report of the Indian Plague Commission*, Vol. v. chap. iii. p. 68.
[2] *Report on certain Cases of Plague in Glasgow in 1900.* By the Medical Officer of Health.

conditions gave good results and that the diagnostic value of the reaction became more apparent during and subsequently to the stage of convalescence when the possibility of a bacteriological diagnosis is more or less remote.

The absence of lymphangitis connected with the bubo serves as
The absence of lymphangitis, a diagnostic point in favour of its being a plague bubo owing to the fact that the microbe of plague very seldom leaves any trace of local reaction at its point of entry. In cases in which a pustule does appear at what may be considered the point of entry, bacteriological examination shows in the case of the plague pustule plague bacilli which at once differentiate it from a malignant pustule or from a septicaemic pustule with lymphangitis, the cultures of which will show streptococci.

The difficulty of clinical diagnosis arises chiefly in recognising the
Chief difficulty arises from the Protean character of plague. several forms and types which the disease assumes, and more particularly is this the case with the ambulant, septicaemic, and pneumonic types without buboes, as well as with the tonsillar form associated with cervical buboes.

If there is no suspicion of plague and no bacteriological examination made, the clinical features and even the post-mortem appearances may be attributed to some other disease. The events which occurred at Paraguay in connection with plague illustrate that which may occur under any circumstances in which plague has never been seen before.

The first case at Asuncion showed a glandular enlargement and some obscure lung affection, death being attributed to disease of the lungs. The second case showed symptoms believed by one medical man to be those of acute gastritis and by another to be those of a general affection, possibly yellow fever. It was because of this latter opinion that several distinguished physicians were sent to attend the post-mortem examination in order to decide the question, as it was of importance that if the disease were yellow fever, precautionary measures to prevent its spread should be immediately adopted. The necropsy revealed general congestion of the internal organs, haemorrhagic swellings in the spleen, an enlarged liver, and an acute gastro-enteritis. The conclusion arrived at was that it was not a case of yellow fever. No one, however, suspected plague, which was unknown in America and which was not known to be nearer than Egypt. The third case, which came off the same ship, was that of a sailor who went to a small village at some distance from Asuncion. He was taken ill there and five months afterwards. on his return to Asuncion he was found on examination to have the signs still on him of buboes characteristic of plague. The three cases are excellent examples of the uncertainty of the diagnosis of plague when no suspicion of plague is in the mind of the medical man. The true significance of these cases in Asuncion was not realised until five months afterwards and then only when a new disease, distinguished by symptoms resembling typhus fever, meningitis, and pneumonia, and frequently accompanied by glandular enlargements in the groin, axilla, or neck, had appeared and prevailed, first of all in a sporadic form in the town for about two months, and later in an epidemic form in the barracks. Only gradually was the suspicion aroused that the disease might be plague, and once that suspicion became general, the discovery, isolation, and culture of the plague bacillus, the classical symptoms of plague which many of the cases presented, and the no less characteristic anatomical features which were observed at the post-mortem examination cleared away every possible doubt. In an investigation which followed this discovery no difficulty was experienced in tracing the new disease back to its commencement; nor was there any difficulty in recognising the symptoms and post-mortem appearances, which had perplexed the medical men six months previously, as belonging to true cases of plague.

The ambulant form is apt to be overlooked from the mildness of the **Ambulant plague.** symptoms. Slight fever, malaise, headache and congested eyes have nothing characteristic about them to indicate such a grave disease as plague, and a glandular swelling may occur under other circumstances, such as syphilis, mumps, and abrasions, wounds, or ulcers with sympathetic glands. It is only possible by a process of careful exclusion combined with a history of the case and a knowledge of plague being in the neighbourhood, that suspicion may be aroused, and it is only by bacteriological methods that a reliable confirmation of the suspicion can be obtained. Microscopical examination is not sufficient, but must be supplemented by cultures of the contents of the bubo and by inoculation of animals. The inoculations are performed in one set of animals with the pure cultures obtained and in another set by the crude contents of the bubo. The latter method, however, is not a reliable one for isolating the plague microbe if mixed with other bacteria. In attempting cultures from the blood the best results are obtained when comparatively large quantities such as 1 c.c. or 2 c.c. are employed. The medical practitioner has seldom the time or the apparatus for a complete bacteriological examination, which in cases of this kind should be delegated to the bacteriologist of the local authority.

The illness is sometimes of a short duration and sometimes of a chronic nature, and some of the symptoms may be absent. Frequently towards the termination of an epidemic diffuse swellings over the cervical and parotid glands with or without fever, together with quick pulse, drawn face and hesitating speech, occur in persons who have been associated with plague persons or plague houses. These cases occurring at the end of an epidemic do not present the same difficulties as ambulant cases at the commencement of an epidemic. Such cases were observed in Bombay and in Cape Town.

In the fulminating, septic and pneumonic types of the disease, in which no buboes may be found, an examination of the blood and sputum for the characteristic bacilli is the chief diagnostic test. In fact in all cases that are clinically obscure bacteriological examination is needed to elucidate them.

In the septic type the bacilli early invade the blood and the patient
Septic type. is prostrated with the intensity and amount of the poison which has penetrated into the system. Besides the common symptoms belonging to all forms of plague this type is characterised by a pallid and apathetic expression and a rapid setting in of extreme nervous prostration, delirium, coma and death, the patient often suffering from haemorrhages from the nose, kidneys, or bowels. In the less rapid septicaemic cases, besides the detection of plague bacilli in the blood, plague bacilli will be found occasionally in the urine, and in the expectoration of those with hypostasis of the lungs and of those with secondary pneumonia. It is a type of disease which is very apt to be overlooked. The absence of buboes, the normal or subnormal temperature in the morning in some cases and the rise of temperature to not more than 100° or 101° are not symptoms which readily raise suspicion as to plague. There are other cases in which a sharp attack of diarrhoea is the most evident symptom. There are other cases again in which the patient is attacked with fever of a remittent type without showing the pulse, tongue, or characteristic appearance of a plague patient, and the bubo if any appears is delayed to the 7th or 8th day. Yet any of these may die suddenly and it is only the sudden death which attracts attention.

Pneumonic plague is specially apt to be overlooked, its physical signs
Pneumonic plague. being often ill-defined. During an epidemic of plague cases of pneumonia should be viewed with suspicion

especially if associated with enlargement of the spleen. In the pneumonic type the bacilli are to be detected in the sputum, the disease localising itself first in the lungs. The symptoms are those of a broncho-pneumonia with much greater prostration. Dyspnoea, cough and expectoration of a watery fluid tinged with blood are the chief clinical features. The absence of any well-marked and special physical signs of serious lung mischief which would account for the gravity and rapidity of development of the general symptoms is a feature that should raise suspicions as to the possibility of primary plague pneumonia. The sputum of all respiratory affections during an epidemic of plague should be examined bacteriologically and tested by inoculation on animals for plague bacilli.

The difficulty connected with the diagnosis of pneumonic plague will be seen from the following case recorded by Dr A. C. F. Halford[1] of Brisbane which was provisionally diagnosed as measles.

" Aged 30, living at South Brisbane, was admitted to the Brisbane General Hospital on the 4th June, 1901. The patient was quite well until the 28th May, 1901, when he complained of headache and feverishness. Next day he complained also of chilliness, headache, feverishness and weakness. He continued in the same condition until the 1st June, when he got up and went for a walk, feeling better. He had on some previous occasions suffered from fever contracted in New Guinea, and put his present illness down to the same cause. He got worse again that night, and remained in bed all the next day. On the 3rd he complained of pains all over his body. On the 4th the pains were more severe and the breathing became rapid and his voice husky. He was seen by a medical man who noticed a rash like that of measles about the body, but more especially marked on the arms. The eyes were injected and the patient had a slight cough. A provisional diagnosis of measles was made, and the patient removed to the General Hospital. On admission his temperature was 103, pulse 140, and respirations 60. No bronchial breathing could be detected, but there were moist sounds from base to apex on both sides. He only lived a few hours in the hospital but he had no serum, and at the post-mortem examination the whole of both lungs were found extensively consolidated. The bronchial glands were enlarged and blackened with haemorrhagic inflammation. No enlarged glands were found anywhere else, nor was there any other macroscopic changes noted in the other organs. Smear preparations

[1] *Report on* 117 *Cases of Plague occurring in Brisbane.* By the Medical Officer to the Metropolitan Joint Board for the Prevention of Epidemic Disease, Brisbane, 1902.

from the affected lungs showed presence of innumerable plague bacilli apparently in pure culture. An infected rat was found at the place of his employment."

In those cases of pneumonic plague in which there is only slight cough and no sputum, it is impossible at an early stage of an epidemic to form more than a suspicion until either the further development of lung symptoms with expectoration gives an opportunity of detecting and isolating the plague bacillus, or the death of the patient allows of a post-mortem examination. During an epidemic it is safer to class all doubtful cases as plague provisionally. If during the epidemic of plague there is also a prevalence of influenza, some of the latter cases

Influenza and plague. may resemble so closely plague cases without buboes, that even the most experienced physician may be unable to differentiate the one from the other, and the diagnosis has to depend on the bacteriological examination of the sputum and the blood. The possibility of the two diseases occurring together in the same patient is not to be overlooked.

The tonsillar variety of plague which is generally associated with

Tonsillus plague. buboes in the neck may be mistaken for diphtheria, as was the case in Bombay. The bacteriological examination of the sputum and of the exudative coating on the tonsils will readily differentiate the diseases. If plague bacilli are not found in these materials, puncture of the enlarged gland or bubo, and examination of its contents will be necessary.

In the pustular variety of the disease plague bacilli are generally found in the pustules, but care has to be taken that the plague microbes are not overlooked as they are sometimes present in these skin eruptions in the atypical or degenerative forms.

Plague has been mistaken for malaria, typhoid, and typhus fever, typhlitis, meningitis, pneumonia, diphtheria, influenza, relapsing fever, syphilis and filariasis with enlarged glands. It has occurred in conjunction with most of these, so that the discovery of the special micro-organism, if any, of these diseases, does not exclude plague unless the microbe of plague has also been searched for and not found.

The prognosis of plague in a particular individual depends on

Prognosis. a number of circumstances, such as the race and age of the person attacked, the period of the epidemic when attacked, the variety of plague, and the degree of reaction which the patient manifests against the disease. In the existing epidemic a white person always has a better chance of recovery than a coloured

person. Taking general averages it may be stated that of white people
attacked two-thirds recover, while of coloured people attacked two-
thirds die. Children between 5 and 10 years of age usually have
the lowest mortality, and persons attacked during the decline of an
epidemic have a greater chance of recovery than those attacked when
the epidemic is on the increase. The variety of plague also makes a
difference. Pneumonic plague is very serious and generally ends fatally.
Septicaemic plague is also of a very grave character and the prognosis
is most unfavourable. In the bubonic type the situation of the buboes
exercises an influence on the gravity of the illness. Axillary buboes
have the highest mortality, femoral and iliac the next, and cervical the
next. The order of the three latter may be reversed. Dr Choksy[1]
analysing 9500 cases treated in Bombay gives the subjoined relative
mortality according to (a) the type of the disease, and (b) the situation
of the bubo in uncomplicated bubonic cases.

(a)

					Mortality
Simple Bubonic Plague	...	...	...	...	77·25 %
Septicaemic Plague ...	...	...	...	...	89·62
Pneumonic Plague ...	...	...	...	...	96·69
Cellulo-cutaneous Plague	...	...	...	...	62·00

(b)

						Mortality
Axillary	...	...	...	...	...	81·29 %
Cervical	...	...	...	...	...	78·87
Inguinal	...	...	...	...	...	77·62
Multiple	...	...	...	...	...	75·87
Femoral	...	...	...	...	...	72·56
Other situations	...	...	...	...	...	71·42
Parotid ...	...	...	...	...	...	70·34

Major W. E. Jennings[2] gives a detailed analysis of 16,132 bubonic
cases and the regional case mortality. They are as follows:—

				Cases	Mortality
Left axillary...	...	...		1712	78·0 %
Right axillary	...	...		1866	77·1
Left femoral	...	...		2429	75·4
Right femoral	...	...		2539	72·3
Left inguinal	...	...		1922	71·7
Right inguinal	...	...		1988	70·1
Cervical	...	...	...	1006	70·5
Multiple	...	...	...	2207	70·0
Parotid	...	..	...	463	68·6

[1] *The Treatment of Plague by Professor Lustig's Serum.* By N. H. Choksy, M.D.
[2] *A Manual of Plague.* By W. E. Jennings, M.B., C.M., Major Indian Medical
Service. 1903.

Of cases admitted into the Parel Hospital, during the Bombay epidemic of 1896–97, Major G. S. Thomson, I.M.S., gives the following details[1]:—

Mortality	Men	Women	Children	Boys	Girls
64·5 %	68·6 %	71 %	52·8 %	42·5 %	64·3 %

Situation of bubo	Total	Percentage	Males	Females	Died	Recovered	Mortality percentage
Right axilla	47	15·5	30	17	34	13	72·4
Left axilla	32	10·5	16	16	24	8	75
Right femoral	59	19·6	45	14	33	26	56
Left femoral	31	10·2	18	13	14	17	45·2
Right inguinal	17	5·6	11	6	10	7	59
Left inguinal	32	10·5	25	7	21	11	65·6
Right cervical	8	2·6	7	1	6	2	75
Left cervical	4	1·3	2	2	2	2	50
Right parotid	7	2·3	3	4	5	2	71·4
Left parotid	1	0·3	1	—	—	1	—
Multiple	24	7·9	15	9	14	10	58·3
No buboes	42	13·8	29	13	33	9	78·6

The utmost circumspection has to be exercised in giving an opinion **Caution as to prognosis.** on the future course of the illness as there is no disease so deceptive and so likely to mislead the physician. Patients, who to all appearances are in a state of convalescence or whose symptoms are mild and augur a speedy recovery, may suddenly die of heart failure with or without some slight exertion in getting out of bed, or they may suddenly develop secondary infection of other glands or organs, or fall into an apathetic or marasmic condition; or patients with the gravest of symptoms whose condition seems hopeless may suddenly and unexpectedly improve and rapidly convalesce. A good pulse not more than 120 or 130 per minute in the acute stage, absence of acute cerebral disturbance, or of dyspnoea, and a rapid development of the bubo without extensive infiltration are collectively favourable signs; so is absence **Favourable signs.** of albumen from the urine and presence of chlorides; also constipation or a few loose motions a day without diarrhoea. Suppuration of the bubo is also favourable, as it indicates that the patient has successfully passed through the first 6 or 7 days, which is the most dangerous period. In Hongkong Wilm showed that 75 % of the deaths occurred within the first 6 days, and this may be taken as the general rule.

---

[1] *A Treatise on Plague.* By Major George S. Thomson and Dr John Thomson, 1901.

Among unfavourable signs are great frequency of the pulse and respiration from the commencement of the illness; high temperature which continues or a sudden fall of temperature with collapse; or a secondary rise which is much higher than the primary; continued insomnia; early and violent delirium; subsidence of the bubo within the first 4 or 5 days, or sudden and extensive infiltration around the bubo; severe vomiting or continuous diarrhoea, tympanitic flatulence, convulsions, haemorrhages from various channels; cyanosis, suppression of urine, the setting in of secondary infections; dicrotic and almost uncountable pulse.

Unfavourable signs.

The discovery of plague bacilli in the blood in large numbers is always a sign of great gravity.

CHAPTER XVI.

TREATMENT.

CURATIVE medicine is powerless to combat the powerful and rapidly disintegrating forces at work in the system in a virulent case of plague. The post-mortem appearances render it too plain that no mode of treatment as yet known to the physician can prevent or neutralise the effects of the plague poison. In the mildest forms at the other end of the scale treatment is seldom required and the patients recover with or without medicine.

Curative treatment powerless in the most virulent forms of plague.

It is between these two extremes that medical treatment may be beneficial, but how much of the cure in successful cases is due to the treatment and how much to nature it is often impossible to estimate.

Many modes of treatment have found favour in plague, and often the most opposite in kind. Their multiplicity throws a certain doubt on their value, especially as the mortality of plague varies much in accordance with the virulence of the virus, the period of the epidemic, and the race and age of the person attacked.

Before considering the modern mode of treatment and its results, it is desirable to glance over the several methods in vogue in the earlier epidemics. It will serve, at least, to prevent them from being resorted to again with exaggerated hopes of success, and it may at the same time prevent an undue estimate of the value of those in use at the present time; for all of them, notwithstanding the energy with which they have been applied and the apparent benefit derived from them at times in some epidemics, have more or less signally failed at other times in the same epidemic, or in others. The general average mortality belonging to the epidemic never seems to have been reduced to any great extent.

Treatment of plague in the past.

Bleeding has been practised since the time of Galen, who appears
to have recovered from the disease after scarifying his
Bleeding. thighs and drawing off a large quantity of blood. Syden-
ham attributes his own success to bleeding, though, as a matter of fact,
he was in London only when the disease was declining and assuming a
milder form. Both Hodges and Boghurst, who practised throughout
the whole epidemic, agree in stating that treatment by bleeding was
most destructive and pernicious, to which Boghurst adds the employment of emetics and purgatives.

Bleeding was employed largely in the epidemic of Egypt of 1834–35
without any satisfactory results, Aubert, alone, reporting favourably
upon it, when combined with other treatment. Leeches have also
been used either alone or with bleeding, to relieve congestions, but
in many cases it was found difficult or impossible to arrest the bleeding
from the wound inflicted by the bite of the leech. Bleeding was also
in some cases combined with emetics, diaphoretics and blisters. Emetics
and quinine were tried in the Moscow epidemic. Evacuants, purgatives,
The evacuant calomel, inunction of mercurial preparations have been
treatment. tried, only in turn to give way to other drugs. Stimulants,
sudorifics, and an occasional bleeding were resorted to in the Marseilles
epidemic.

Stimulants, such as ether, ammonia, camphor, musk, brandy, wine,
The stimulant sarsaparilla, coffee, etc. have been largely used alone or
and tonic combined with tonics. Strychnine has been pushed to
treatment. a dangerous extent with the object of counteracting the
paralysing effect of the plague poison on the nervous system. Often
antiphlogistic, tonic, and stimulant treatment was employed according
to the stage of illness or degree of severity of the case.

Oil frictions enjoyed a great reputation at the end of the 18th and
Oil friction beginning of the 19th century. Assalini referring to this
treatment. mode of treatment says[1]:

"It has been observed that those people who manufacture or carry
oil are never attacked with plague. Hence it has been maintained that
frictions of tepid oil prevent or cure this disease. The result of the
observations made by father Louis of Padua, director of the hospital
for the plague at Smyrna, is the most favourable. He asserts that

---

[1] *Observations on the Disease called the Plague.* By P. Assalini, M.D., one of the Chief
Surgeons of the Consular Guards. Translated from the French by Adam Neale, of the
University of Edinburgh. London, 1804.

during the 27 years he has been in this situation he has seen no means employed against the disease more useful than the friction of oil, and to this day in Smyrna and several lazarettos in the Levant frictions of tepid oil are generally adopted as the best remedy. As soon as a patient attacked with the plague is received into the hospital in Smyrna he is taken into a close chamber, where they light a large pan of coals in which they throw sugar and juniper berries or other perfumes, they then strip off all his clothes and rub his whole body with warm oil until profuse sweats break out. The patient is then put into bed; and whenever the sweating ceases they repeat the friction in the same manner, and so on successively during several days until the disease has spent its violence in consequence of the sweating. One pint of oil is sufficient for each friction, taking care not to commence the second before the sweating occasioned by the first has ceased.

"In the space of 5 years 250 persons infected with plague have been received in the hospital of Smyrna, and I am assured that all those who were thus treated have recovered, and that the number of persons preserved from the plague by frictions of oil is immense."

The buboes and carbuncles have been subjected to many different **Treatment of buboes.** kinds of treatment. They have been incised, blistered, and cauterised with the object of hastening their development on the principle that the sooner they reached maturity the earlier would the virulence of the disease diminish, for it was noticed that with the suppuration of the buboes and the maturation of the carbuncles the patients began to convalesce. A sign of the acute stage of the illness being nearly at an end was evidently mistaken for the cause producing that happy termination. The only occasions on which the knife is found to be useful are when pus has formed in the bubo and when masses of necrosed glands are lying in suppurating buboes.

In contrast to the different kinds of active treatment was that which **Cold water treatment.** confined itself to the giving of the patient cold water, lemonade, acidulated drinks, or rice water. It possessed, at all events, the merits of simplicity and its advocates claimed their successes.

In 1762, on the theory that the pestilential virus was an alkaline **Suggested antiseptic treatment.** ferment exalting and decomposing the humours, it was suggested that after a purge[1] one or two drops of an antiseptic capable of neutralising this alkali and re-

---

[1] Papon. *De la Peste*, 1801, p. 141.

establishing equilibrium should be cautiously injected into the veins of the patient. This suggestion appears never to have been carried out in practice, but it is interesting to recall it, when the hopes of the physician now mainly rest on intravenous injections of serums having for their object the neutralisation of toxines in the blood.

To-day plague, as a disease, is viewed as the manifestation of a struggle between the natural powers of the person attacked and the virulence of the plague microbe. On this basis medicines are administered to maintain the strength of the patient, who is also carefully nursed with the same object in view. Then serotherapy is employed, having for its object the neutralisation of the toxines and the destruction of the plague bacillus; or drugs with disinfecting properties are given to destroy the microbe and prevent its multiplication.

Basis of the present day treatment of plague.

The serum treatment of plague dates only from the discovery of the plague bacillus, and it appears a rational one if the theories on which it is based are correct, the chief of which is that a specific antidote is obtainable from the serum of animals inoculated with the bacillus of the disease.

Attempt at specific treatment.

Serum was prepared by Yersin, Roux, Calmette, and Borrel by the same methods as were employed by Behring in his preparations of antidiphtheritic serum, horses being intravenously injected in order to obtain the antidotal serum.

Observations on the sera prepared by Yersin, Roux, Calmette, and Borrel.

Amoy.

Serum thus prepared was first employed in China by Yersin, in whose hands it gave some marvellous results; the mortality in 26 cases treated, 3 in Canton and 23 at Amoy, being only 7 %. Of the 23 Amoy cases 12 were treated in the first and second day of their illness and all rapidly recovered without their buboes suppurating; 7 were treated on the third and fourth day and they recovered slowly with suppurating buboes; 4 were treated on the fifth day of illness and 2 recovered. There was accordingly no mortality among those treated during the first 4 days, and a mortality of 50 % when the patients did not receive treatment until the fifth day. The dose of serum injected subcutaneously in the last cases was from 60 to 90 c.c.

Bombay.

Yersin was invited to Bombay. Fifty cases were treated by him, but the results were not nearly the same as those obtained at Amoy. The mortality of the cases treated was now 34 %. Analysed, the details are as follows:

17 treated on first { 15 recovered } 12 % mortality.
day of illness { 2 died

17 treated on second { 11 recovered } 35 % mortality.
day of illness { 6 died

12 treated on third { 6 recovered } 50 % mortality.
day of illness { 6 died

3 treated on fourth { 1 recovered } 60 % mortality.
day of illness { 2 died

1 treated on fifth } 1 died.
day of illness

In the same epidemic at Bombay the German Commission treated 26 cases of plague with Yersin's serum with the result that 13 died and 13 recovered, which gave a mortality of 50 %.

11 treated on first { 5 recovered } 54·5 % mortality.
day of illness { 6 died

9 treated on second { 4 recovered } 55 % mortality.
day of illness { 5 died

6 treated on third { 4 recovered } 33·3 % mortality.
day of illness { 2 died

Karad. In Karad Dr Simonds treated 32 cases with serum, of which 21 died, giving a mortality of 65·5 %. Of the 32 cases 27 were bubonic, the details of which are subjoined[1].

2 treated on first { 1 recovered } 50 % mortality.
day of illness { 1 died

17 treated on second { 5 recovered } 70 % mortality.
day of illness { 12 died

5 treated on third { 1 recovered } 80 % mortality.
day of illness { 4 died

3 treated on fourth { 1 recovered } 66·6 % mortality.
day of illness { 2 died

Karachi. In Karachi Dr Simonds treated 51 cases with serum, of which 37 died, giving a mortality of 53 %.

9 treated on first { 5 recovered } 44·4 % mortality.
day of illness { 4 died

28 treated on second { 14 recovered } 50 % mortality.
day of illness { 14 died

[1] *Report of the Indian Plague Commission*, chap. v. p. 303.

19 treated on third day of illness	{ 11 recovered } { 8 died }	42·1 % mortality.
10 treated on fourth day of illness	{ 2 recovered } { 8 died }	80 % mortality.
3 treated on fifth day of illness	{ 1 recovered } { 2 died }	66 % mortality.
1 treated on sixth day of illness	} 1 died.	

In Cutch, Mandvi, Capt. Mason, R.A.M.C., treated 100 cases with serum with a case mortality of 59 %, but it appears that the treatment was applied during the 4 months of a declining epidemic.

The results obtained in the observations made by the Indian Plague Commission showed but a very small balance in favour of the Yersin treatment, and they conclude that on the whole a certain amount of advantage in all probability accrued to the patients injected with Yersin's serum.

.In Oporto Drs Calmette and Salimbeni[1] treated with serum in 1899, from the 3rd of September to the 18th of November, 142 Oporto. cases of plague, 140 in hospital and 2 in the town. Of these 21 died, which is equal to a mortality of 14·78 %. During the same time there occurred in the town 72 cases of plague which were not removed to hospital and not treated with serum. Of these 46 died, which is equal to a mortality of 63·7 %. The details are as follows:

		Cases	Deaths	Mortality
3rd Sept.—30th Sept.	Hospital	28	2	7·14 %
	Town	26	16	61·57
1st Oct.—28th Oct.	Hospital	90	14	15·5
	Town	28	15	53·57
29th Oct.—18th Nov.	Hospital	24	5	20·83
	Town	18	12	66·65

These results more nearly approach those first obtained by Yersin. It is possible that the efficacy of the serum depends largely on its mode of preparation. The serum used at Oporto was obtained by injecting horses first of all with dead cultures and then with living cultures which had been raised in virulence. Greater success was obtained in Oporto when the serum was used in large doses and when employed intravenously. At the beginning of the illness or as soon as the patient

[1] *Annales de l'Institut Pasteur*, tome XIII. Dec. 1899.

came under observation an intravenous injection of 20 cubic centimetres of the serum was given, followed by two subcutaneous injections of 40 cubic centimetres each in the first 24 hours, and subcutaneously of from 10 to 20 cubic centimetres or 40 cubic centimetres on the next and subsequent days until the temperature fell to normal, and even for two days afterwards. Dr Calmette and Dr Salimbeni report that no ill results ensued from these injections further than an occasional erythema and articular pains, which were no more intense after the intravenous than after the subcutaneous injections.

In the few Glasgow cases in which Yersin's serum was tried intra-

Glasgow. venous injections seemed, in most cases, to produce a marked therapeutic effect, except in those cases in which double infection existed from the beginning of the illness[1].

In Cape Town no precise data were kept regarding this mode of

Cape Town. treatment but the results were not so marked as to produce any special impression in its favour.

In Natal 61 cases out of 124 admitted to hospital are recorded as

Natal. having been treated with serum, of whom 33 died, making a mortality of 54 %; while of 63 cases not treated with serum 39 died, giving a mortality of 62 %[2]. It is remarked, however, by the Medical Officer of Health that the administration of the serum was withheld in 10 cases owing to the patients being moribund on admission. Perhaps a more potent factor of the apparent better results of the serum was that this division included all the white patients admitted, numbering 14, of whom 3 died. When these were excluded and the results from its use among natives were compared they are no longer favourable to the serum.

Thus, 47 cases were treated with serum, of whom 30 died, which is equal to a mortality of 63·82 %; while 63 cases were not treated with serum, of whom 39 died, which is equal to a mortality of 62 %.

In Hongkong no favourable results have been observed at any time

Hongkong. from the use of Yersin's treatment. In 1902, 94 cases were treated in the Kennedy Town Hospital with Calmette's serum, with a mortality of 85·1 %. The details are as follows[3]:

---

[1] *Report on certain Cases of Plague occurring in Glasgow in 1900.* By the Medical Officer of Health.

[2] *Report on the Plague in Natal,* 1902–3. By Ernest Hill, M.R.C.S., D.P.H.

[3] *Report on Plague Cases treated in the Kennedy Town Hospital, Hongkong.* By J. C. Thomson, M.D., 1903.

	Cases	Deaths	Mortality
Europeans	3	1	33·3 %
Portuguese	1	1	100
Chinese	80	73	91·3
Other Races	10	5	50·0
	94	80	85·1

In the same hospital the mortality of cases treated in the ordinary way was:

1894	1896	1898	1899	1900	1901
76 %	74 %	81·80 %	81·8 %	77 %	76·5 %

When again the results of the serum treatment are compared with those obtained in the hospital in Hongkong during the first epidemic of 1894 before the plague serum was devised, it will be seen from the subjoined statement that there is not much to choose between the two.

	Affected	Died	Mortality
[1]Europeans	11	2	18·2 %
Japanese	10	6	60
Manila men	1	1	100
Eurasians	3	3	100
Indians	13	10	77
Portuguese	18	12	66
Malays	3	3	100
West Indians	1	1	100
Chinese	2619	2447	93·4

It is thought possible, however, that if the serum were made locally and used fresh better results might be obtained.

On the other hand in Brisbane[2] its efficacy was considered undoubted when given intravenously and in large doses. There were **Brisbane.** no fulminant or septicaemic cases in Brisbane. Its administration in the ordinary bubonic cases was followed by a sudden fall of temperature, a moist skin and profuse perspiration, also by improvement of the mental condition, and of the pulse and respirations.

In 1900 of 56 persons suffering from plague 25 died, yielding a mortality of 44·6 %; no serum was then available. In 1901 of 29 cases treated with serum

$$\left. \begin{array}{l} 20 \text{ recovered} \\ 5 \text{ died} \end{array} \right\} 17\text{·}2 \text{ % mortality.}$$

---

[1] *The Epidemic of Bubonic Plague,* 1894. By James A. Lowson, M.D.
[2] *Report of* 117 *Cases of Plague in sporadic form in Brisbane.* By A. C. F. Halford, M.D., Medical Officer of Health.

In 1902 of 65 cases treated with serum

$$\left\{ \begin{array}{l} 54 \text{ recovered} \\ 9 \text{ died} \end{array} \right\} 13\text{·}8\,\%\ \text{mortality.}$$

It would appear that the benefits derived from the use of Yersin's serum are somewhat uncertain. Sometimes excellent results appear to follow its administration, sometimes only moderately good results are observed, and at other times absolutely no effect seems to be produced. On the whole, for white races in which the disease is comparatively mild the serum treatment is likely to be more efficacious than for coloured people, especially when administered intravenously in large doses. As regards the people of India and of China, in whose countries the disease is now epidemic in a virulent form, serum treatment has not given the brilliant results which were expected.

Lustig's serum, like Yersin's, gave most promising results on its

Observations on Lustig's serum.

first trial. In June and July, 1897, it was administered to six serious cases, all of whom recovered. This was at a time when the epidemic had declined.

Since then it has been tried in some 1500 cases in Bombay, and all that can be claimed for it is that when septicaemic cases, which form over 40 % of the total, are excluded, then it reduces the mortality of the remainder, *i.e.* bubonic cases, to a greater degree than in similar cases under ordinary treatment. The same observation appears to apply equally to the effect of Yersin's serum in Bombay. The virulence of the plague in Bombay, judged of by the case mortality, has increased from 60 % in 1897 to nearly 80 % during the past 4 or 5 years. No evidence is forthcoming as yet that the serum can destroy the plague bacilli in the blood.

The statistical table on page 325 is given by Dr N. H. Choksy, showing the results of the treatment of plague patients with Lustig's serum in some of the municipal hospitals of Bombay from 1898 to 1902.

Dr Choksy, who has had an exceptionally large experience in the treatment of plague in Bombay, is strongly impressed with the value of serotherapy in plague, and expresses his conviction in its efficacy in the following terms: "Should those who are conversant with the application of the serum in plague be entrusted with 100 persons provided the cases are not septicaemic, they would be able to bring round at least 60, if not more, by the use either of Lustig's or Roux's serum of the strength that has been used in Bombay during the last two epidemics." The proviso, it will be noted, is a large one, and accentuates the small assistance to be derived from the most advanced treatment.

Arthur Road Hospital.

Period	System of Treatment	Serum-Treated Patients			Patients under Ordinary Treatment			Difference in favour of the Serum Patients per cent.
		Number	Deaths	Case Mortality per cent.	Number	Deaths	Case Mortality per cent.	
March to Oct. 1898 ...	Selection	257	145	56.4	752	595	79.1	22.7
Jan. to April and June 1899	Do.	189	124	65.60	884	734	83.03	17.4
May 1899 and July 1899 to Aug. 1900	Alternate	484	329	68.00	484	385	79.5	11.5
August 1900 to Feb. 1901 (3 extra cases) ...	Selection	55	36	65.45	184	144	78.26	12.81
March, April and May 1901	Alternate	104	81	77.82	102	81	79.42	1.53

Maratha Hospital.

Period	System of Treatment	Serum-Treated Patients			Patients under Ordinary Treatment			Difference in favour of the Serum Patients per cent.
1898	Selection	28	17	60.71	...	...	80.7	20.0
Nov. 1900 to Jan. 1901	Do.	38	32	84.21	...	...	88.8	4.59
August to Dec. 1901 ...	Do.	44	81	70.45	203	161	79.31	(11.5) 8.86
April and May 1902 ...	Alternate	31	31	100.00	31	29	93.54	*Nil.*

Between November, 1902, and July, 1903, a trial was made in
Observations on Professor Terni's and Bondi's serum. Bombay, under the supervision of the Bombay Laboratory, of serum prepared by Professor Terni and Bondi in Messina[1]. The cases for treatment were taken alternately as they were admitted to hospital. The results were as follows.

111 cases treated with serum $\left\{ \begin{array}{l} \text{21 recovered} \\ \text{90 died} \end{array} \right\}$ 81.08 % mortality.

112 cases treated without serum $\left\{ \begin{array}{l} \text{21 recovered} \\ \text{91 died} \end{array} \right\}$ 81.25 % mortality.

Subsequently, another batch of 16 patients were treated with the same serum in another Bombay hospital, 16 alternate patients being left for comparison. Of the first category 12 died, and of the second, 11. In 1904, a serum prepared by Dr Brazil in San Pavlo, which was reported to give good results in Brazil, was tried by the laboratory. In one hospital the proportion of deaths, among the injected, was 41 out of 50, and among the control cases, 45 out of 50; in another, the

[1] *British Medical Journal*, Sept. 24, 1904.

injected gave a proportion of 17 deaths out of 20, and the control cases
of 15 out of 20. The treatment in all cases consisted in hypodermic
injections, the doses in the latter experiments amounting sometimes to
several hundred cubic centimetres.

Kitasato's serum has been used in Tainan with controls. The odd
Observations on Kitasato's serum. numbers were injected with serum. The even numbers
were not injected, but early extirpation of the glands and
general systemic treatment was adopted. The results
recorded are as follows.

$$56 \text{ cases treated} \left\{ \begin{array}{l} 37 \text{ recovered} \\ 19 \text{ died} \end{array} \right\} 33 \cdot 9\,\% \text{ mortality.}$$

$$56 \text{ cases treated} \left\{ \begin{array}{l} 21 \text{ recovered} \\ 35 \text{ died} \end{array} \right\} 62 \cdot 5\,\% \text{ mortality.}$$

These results are excellent, no doubt, but it is clear from that which
has been observed with the sera prepared by Yersin and Lustig that
the value of a serum for the specific or curative treatment of plague
cannot be determined by one or two series of test experiments, but that
it needs many series of trials under varying circumstances before
anything like an accurate estimate of its efficacy or antidotal powers
can be made.

The serum which shall possess evident and indisputable specific or
antidotal powers against plague during an epidemic has still to be
discovered. To deserve the name of a specific it must do something
more than show good results during the decline of an epidemic or
during the quiescent stage, when only sporadic cases occur. At the
same time the administration of the different sera as employed at the
present time, and more especially if injected intravenously and early,
appears to give the patient a better chance of recovery than any
pharmacopeal drug, which is not appraising their value very highly;
and in some instances the state of the patient after the injection
is so much improved that it can only be attributed to the action of
the serum.

The amount of serum injected intravenously usually varies from
Dosage of serum. 20 to 40 c.c. according to the severity of the case. The
intravenous injection is generally supplemented by a
subcutaneous injection of 20 to 40 c.c. The usual practice is to repeat
the dose every 12 or 24 hours, and continue it for 3 or 5 days after the
general improvement of the patient. A fall in the temperature, less pain
in the bubo, a clearer intellect, and an improvement in the pulse indicate

signs of amelioration.　If the effect of the serum is only slight and the symptoms urgent, intravenous injections may be repeated as frequently and at as short intervals as in the discretion of the medical attendant is advisable.　Larger doses than 40 c.c. have been given intravenously at one time, in some cases amounting to 80, 100, and in one case to 400 c.c., apparently without harmful results.　When subcutaneous injections alone are used it is believed that better results have been noticed in those instances in which the injections have been made in the region which is drained by the affected bubo.　Beyond, possibly, a temporary rise in temperature accompanied by transient rigors, rashes of various kinds, but of an evanescent character, and painful swellings of the joints amenable to doses of salicylate of soda, no other ill-effects have been observed from the administration of plague sera. None of the results from serum treatment have surpassed or even come up to the results obtained at the hospital in Smyrna from the oil friction, and which was used much in the plague at Tangiers in 1809, in the epidemic of Malta in 1813, and again when plague was prevalent in Tunis in 1818–1819.　With a more extended experience, however, it has, like other curative methods, fallen into desuetude.

The internal administration of disinfectants has been tried in Hongkong.　The first experiment was in 1901, when 80 grains a day of carbolic acid were given to each patient: 204 cases were thus treated with a mortality of 76·5%.

Antiseptic treatment. Carbolic acid.

	Cases	Deaths	Mortality
Europeans	24	8	33·3 %
Portuguese	16	12	75·0
Chinese	136	121	89·0
Other Races	28	15	53·6
	204	156	76·5

On the suggestion of Dr Atkinson[1], principal Civil Officer of Hongkong, a fresh trial was made in 1903 with carbolic acid even in larger doses. Accordingly 144 grains of carbolic acid were administered daily, divided into two-hourly doses of 12 grains each in a mixture flavoured with syrup of orange and chloroform water, in some cases over long periods. One patient consumed over 2500 grains of pure carbolic acid before his blood was free from plague bacilli.　Carbolic acid poisoning appears to have been practically unknown.　In a few cases carboluria developed, but the omission of one or two doses was usually sufficient to clear the

[1] *Report on Plague Cases treated in the Kennedy Town Hospital, Hongkong.* By J. C. Thomson, M.D., 1903.

urine and permit resumption of the remedy in full doses. In certain cases dyspeptic symptoms occurred, but in these greater dilution of the mixture with water was all that was required to overcome this obstacle to its consumption. Dr J. C. Thomson, who made the trial in 143 cases, formed the opinion that it was the most hopeful means of treating plague thus far at the disposal of the medical authorities in Hongkong.

Dr Thomson gives the two following tables showing the racial and general mortality before and during the use of carbolic acid.

Before Carbolic Acid was used,

i.e. in the first half of the epidemic.

	Cases	Cured	Convalescent	Deaths	Mortality
Europeans	2	1	...	1	50·0 %
Portuguese	...	...	...	...	...
Chinese	123	15	2	106	86·2
Other Races	14	2	...	12	85·7
	139	18	2	119	85·7

20

Under the use of Carbolic Acid,

i.e. in the second half of the epidemic.

	Cases	Cured	Convalescent	Deaths	Mortality
Europeans	22	17	4	1	4·5 %
Portuguese	1	1	...	...	...
Chinese	80	31	3	46	57·5
Other Races	40	20	15	5	12·5
	143	69	22	52	36·4

91

It is admitted that two circumstances need to be taken into consideration when comparing these figures; the first is that the treatment with carbolic acid was commenced late in the epidemic, at a stage when, as Dr Thomson remarks, there is a greater natural tendency to recovery, the disease being invariably more virulent early in the season; the second is that, owing to the adoption of an improved method of examination of plague blood, a much larger number of very mild cases, many of which would not have been diagnosed as plague in former years, were proved to be plague and sent to Kennedy Town Hospital. These cases swelled the proportion of recoveries.

The internal administration of carbolic acid suggests the possibility Cyllin. of cyllin being useful under similar circumstances. Cyllin has the advantages of being safer, and a more powerful bactericide, but whether it will exercise any curative effect on plague patients is not known.

Notwithstanding the disappointing results of the serum treatment, it has to be confessed that there is no better in the hands of the physician. In falling back on general treatment there is no attempt to deal with the manufactory of poison elaborated in the system. The struggle must be between the attacking force of the microbe and the resisting power of the patient, assisted by the skill of the medical man whose aims are to conserve the strength of the patient, check as much as possible the severity of the symptoms and tide over periods of danger due to exhaustion. Good nursing is a very important factor in preserving the strength of the patient. The nursing is difficult and at times dangerous on account of the delusions of the patient, who may, accordingly, resist being fed and resent being attended, or who may be constantly attempting to get out of bed and escape. Under certain conditions it is absolutely necessary to employ mechanical restraint to keep the patient from inflicting self-injuries or being dangerous. Good nursing combined with early confinement to bed, the maintenance of the recumbent position to prevent syncope, careful feeding and general treatment to maintain the patient's strength and prevent complications if possible, are calculated to give the best results, both with or without serotherapy.

General treatment.

Nursing.

The patient should be placed under the best hygienic conditions. The more abundant the fresh air to which he is exposed, the better are the chances of recovery. In Cape Town at the commencement of the epidemic, when in one ward the accommodation was cramped, the ventilation defective, and the patients overcrowded, it was observed that the cases did badly, and at the same time became dangerously infective. Removal to a large tent, in which the patients were practically treated in the open air, produced a marvellous change in the character of the disease, the symptoms at once ameliorating and becoming milder.

Hygienic conditions.

The treatment is usually commenced by clearing the bowels, calomel followed by a saline or other purgative being administered. Heart failure is perhaps the most important symptom to be contended against. Early signs of it in the course of the disease usually portend a fatal result, and drugs do not appear to be of much value. For sustaining the action of the heart and counteracting the want of tone of the blood vessels the most

Medicines.

successful results have been obtained by the employment of strychnine $\frac{1}{40}$ gr., hypodermically every 4 to 5 hours, or of 5 to 10 minims of the liquor, or a combination of strychnine and strophanthus hypodermically injected. Benefit sometimes follows the administration of digitalis, especially when combined with diffusible stimulants. Digitalis by the mouth and strophanthus by subcutaneous injection have also been found to exercise a particularly good effect. General stimulants, such as carbonate of ammonia and camphor, are indicated at an early stage.

To control the febrile symptoms and check delirium, ice bags to the head, sponging of the body, and the use of hypnotics which are not depressants, are beneficial. Morphine carefully administered, either alone or combined with bromide of potassium or atropine, is generally employed to induce sleep, but many hypnotics may have to be tried before that which suits the patient is found. Antipyrine is not suitable for the reduction of the pyrexia.

Complications are treated on general principles.

The pain and tenderness of buboes are much relieved by ice bags,

Local treatment of buboes. which have also a good effect in circumscribing the infiltrations. Other applications, such as belladonna and poultices, at times prove useful. The bubo is opened when pus forms, but nothing is gained by too early incision. The opened bubo is dressed with antiseptics and drained if required. Gangrenous débris in the suppurating bubo is removed by the knife. Extirpation of the infected gland or glands is sometimes practised, but this mode of treatment is limited in its application, nor can it be applied to buboes within the abdominal wall. It appears not always to have been unaccompanied with risk to the patients. In Bombay injections into the buboes of iodised oil, liquor iodi, carbolic acid, liquor iodi with carbolic acid, creolin, quinine, mercuric chloride, and red iodide of mercury were tried, but without any better results than when the buboes were left alone.

For carbuncles Choksy found that a subcutaneous injection of

Treatment of carbuncles. corrosive sublimate, varying in dose from $\frac{1}{15}$ to $\frac{1}{10}$ or $\frac{1}{5}$ of a grain, had an excellent effect and prevented them from increasing in size.

The treatment of convalescence is mainly directed to restoring the

Treatment during convalescence. general tone and vitality of the system, which, as a rule, have been enfeebled to a remarkable degree by the illness, and treating the anaemia which is associated with the debility. Iron, quinine and tonics are indicated combined with nourishing and easily digested food. During the first week great care requires to be taken to prevent the patient from getting out of or even sitting up in bed owing to the danger of heart failure. In uncomplicated cases the patient is usually well in 5 or 6 weeks. In other cases recovery may be delayed for months, caused by the infection of fresh glands, the formation of abscesses and large sloughing ulcers, and other complications.

The precautions to be taken by the physician to prevent the spread of the disease in the family consists in notifying the case **Prophylactic measures in an infected house.** to the local authorities, on whom rests the responsibility for carrying out the necessary measures, and to prevent extension from the house until the local authorities can take action. If the circumstances of the case do not permit of removal to the hospital, the patient should be strictly isolated in the most secluded and best ventilated room in the house. An acid solution of perchloride of mercury of the strength of 1 in 500 or an alkaline solution of cyllin of the strength of 1 in 200 is recommended as a disinfectant. Sputum, urine and excreta should be received in vessels containing either of these disinfectants. A solution of 1 in 1000 of perchloride of mercury, or 1 in 500 **Use of disinfectants.** of cyllin may be used in vessels for soaking soiled clothes, disinfecting cups, spoons, etc., or washing the hands of the medical attendant and nurse after handling the patient. Nothing from a patient should be discharged down a water-closet or drain without being thoroughly mixed with an abundant quantity of disinfectant, otherwise rats in the sewer may become infected and carry the disease elsewhere. In the event of death a sheet soaked in the strong perchloride solution should be wrapped around the body and carbolised or cyllinised sawdust put into the coffin.

Of prophylactic measures to protect the medical attendant, the **Protective inoculation.** nurse and the relatives who come into close association with the infected, the most important is immediate inoculation with Haffkine's prophylactic or Yersin's plague serum. The dose of Haffkine's prophylactic is usually 2 to 5 c.c. for an adult, and ·5 to 1 c.c. for children, injected subcutaneously into the arm or flank. It causes in a few hours a rise of temperature to 102° F., sometimes to 105° F., headache, nausea, malaise and discomfort, which usually continues for about 48 hours. At the site of the inoculation a painful swelling appears which necessitates rest for a day or two and remains evident for at least a week. Immunity is established in a week's time, but partial immunity much earlier. At no time does it render the inoculated more susceptible to the disease. The protection lasts, it is believed, for at least 6 or 7 months, which is the usual duration of an epidemic.

The dose of Yersin's serum is 10 to 20 c.c., and it is administered hypodermically in the same way as Haffkine's prophylactic. The serum does not cause nearly the same degree of discomfort or local inflammatory action and produces a more immediate immunising effect, but in some persons it may be followed in a week or fortnight's time by symptoms simulating rheumatism, accompanied by swelling of some of the joints, which is successfully treated by the administration of salicylate of soda. The protective effect is also of a very limited duration and is lost in about a fortnight's time. Owing, however, to the small discomfort which it generally produces it can be repeated before the expiration of this period.

Neither Haffkine's prophylactic nor Yersin's serum thus administered afford an absolute protection against a plague attack, but they do protect in a very high degree, and if the person inoculated is afterwards attacked with plague, the chances of recovery are greater than when not inoculated.

Individual prophylaxis will also include scrupulous cleanliness, careful attention to the condition of the skin, especially the hands, regular manner of living, and avoidance of fatigue and of unnecessarily prolonged exposure in a dark, ill-ventilated and infected room, especially at night.

Personal hygiene.

Plague will not spread in a sanitary house if the precautions mentioned are taken. But by a sanitary house is meant, one that is clean, well lighted, well ventilated, and free from rats. If there are any rats measures should be taken at once to destroy them and remove any conditions which are liable to harbour them.

Hygiene of the house.

PART IV.

MEASURES FOR PREVENTION AND SUPPRESSION OF PLAGUE.

CHAPTER XVII.

MEASURES EMPLOYED BEFORE THE DISCOVERY OF THE BACILLUS.

THERE are two periods during which preventive measures against

Two periods to be considered. plague may be considered. The first period embraces the past before the plague bacillus was discovered, and is of historical interest rather than of practical guidance for the measures of to-day. The preventive measures of this period are described because an account of them shows their very slow, chequered, and halting development and the source of many existing practices. The second period deals with the present-day methods employed in combating plague.

Methods of prevention necessarily depend on the views which are

Preventive measures depend on the views which are held concerning the cause of the disease. held concerning the cause of the disease, and as these views change from time to time the measures accordingly vary. When plague was considered to be the scourge of an angered deity or the work of evil spirits, men resorted to penances, sacrifices, and prayers. Thus when the Philistines defeated the Israelites in battle, captured the ark and brought it into their own country, and plague broke out among them causing a deadly destruction in the towns and villages of the victors, the only method of protection adopted appears to have been the

Trespass offerings. making of golden images of their tumours and of the mice that marred the land, and sending them with the ark on a new cart drawn by two milch kine to the Israelites as a trespass offering to the " God of Israel " that He might lighten His hand and take the plague away from them.

Seventeen centuries later another people in possession of Syria entertained the view that plague was caused by the sting of hostile spirits, was a purification from the soil of sin, and that death from it was a martyrdom. These were the Mahommedan Arabs. Holding this doctrine they discountenanced flight from a plague-stricken village, though, at the same time, it was held to be foolish to go to a locality where plague prevailed. Ideas of this kind usually exercised a salutary influence in checking the spread of plague from village to village and in restricting the general dissemination of the disease. But in time of war the protection afforded was lost, for armies moving from place to place carried the disease with them. Omar, in conquering Syria, lost an enormous number of his soldiers from plague. It is estimated that one of the Arabian armies lost 25,000 men. It was only after two com-

Removal from plague-stricken locality. manders-in-chief had succumbed to the disease, that the third commander determined to use preventive measures. He distributed his troops in the mountains and desert, with the result that plague ceased. It is the first record of a successful protective policy being followed with the distinct object of saving a large community from the ravages of plague. From this time, though to remove from a plague-stricken village was still held by many to be a sin, the Caliphs made it a custom to spend a part of the year in the desert to avoid the plague which prevailed at a certain season of the year at their capital, and the measures introduced by Abu Obaidah, the commander, found favour with the majority.

In the more brilliant and cultured period of Arabian history

Fumigation of the dwellings and attention to diet. medical science was largely guided by the teachings of Hippocrates and Galen with reference to epidemics and their causes. The Arabian physicians regarded plague as a disease caused by toxic properties in the air, aggravated by disturbances in the body caused by diet or bad water. Fumigation of the dwellings with musk, camphor, sedge, and sandal wood was advised, with a strict regulation of the diet, certain articles such as onions, vinegar, and pickled fish being recommended, while soup and fruits were forbidden.

With the decline of Arabian culture, the fall of the rule of the first Caliphs, and the rise of the military and uncultured rule of the Ottoman, preventive measures gradually fell into desuetude. The terrible experiences of the epidemics of the 13th and 14th centuries, together with the deep-rooted spirit of fatalism in the Mahommedan faith, appear to have produced in a rude, superstitious, and religious people a blind faith in destiny[1]. But before this was reached, prayers

[1] *Ueber die grossen Seuchen des Orients nach arabischen Quellen.* A. v. Kremer, 1880.

and processions unfamiliar to the earlier Mahommedans as a means of pro-
Prayers and tection against plague, were resorted to. Ibn Batuta[1], the
processions. celebrated Moorish traveller, witnessed a strange procession
in Damascus in 1348, on the occasion of the Black Death. He arrived
at Damascus on a Thursday in the month of July. Argunshah, the
Governor, had proclaimed a public fast of three days. On its completion
the Emirs, Sheikhs, Cadis, Priests, and all classes of the population
assembled by invitation in the principal mosques of the town and passed
the night in prayers and praising God, and in registering vows. On the
Friday morning, having offered up the morning prayer, they left the
mosque and marched barefooted through the town carrying the Koran.
They were joined by the Jews carrying the Bible, and by the Christians
carrying the New Testament. Women and children formed part of the
procession, and all engaged in weeping, supplicating and seeking
protection by means of their books and their prophets. Ibn Batuta
remarks that there was an undoubted alleviation, for the number that
died in Damascus was not greater than 2000 a day, whereas in Cairo and
Old Cairo the mortality reached the appalling number of 24,000 a
day.

To the majority of people, however, as epidemic followed epidemic,
Resignation causing an extraordinary destruction, prayers seemed to be
and fatalism. of no avail, and resignation and fatalism took their place.
To seek safety in flight, or to take any measure against plague, was
held to be useless. The bolt could not miss its aim if God had destined
it to strike. In the 15th and 16th centuries the Turks who held these
views put on the clothes and linen of plague patients even while they
were damp with the death-sweat. They even rubbed their faces with
these clothes, and in doing so would justify the action by saying that if
it be God's will I should die of plague it is unavoidable, and if it be not
His will it cannot hurt me. In Cairo, where the same beliefs prevailed,
the people visited the infected houses and took no precautions, and the
mortality was enormous.

Fortunately for Europe, the fatalism of the East never acquired
Disposal of a strong hold in the West; pilgrimages, processions,
the dead. prayers, and flight continued for a long time to be resorted
to at the time of plague. But the only sanitary measure which pressed
itself as a necessity on all was the disposal of the dead, and, as the
ordinary modes of burial failed to meet the requirement, arrangements
were made by which large numbers of bodies could be buried in trenches
and pits. Later, other measures of protection were tried by individuals

---

[1] *Voyages d'Ibn Batoutah.* Par C. Defremery et le Dr B. R. Sanguinetti, 1853.

under the advice and influence of the more learned physicians. House-

Isolation of the rich.
holds shut themselves up and attempted to avoid contagion by cutting off all communication and intercourse with others. Special attention was paid to diet and cleanliness, and fumigations were practised. It was not, however, until the experiences of the pandemic of 1348 or the Black Death that views regarding the contagious nature of plague, and the infectious condition of the air, became sufficiently general to give rise to any organised attempt to meet

First preventive measures of an organised nature in Venice in 1348.
epidemics of plague by preventive measures other than those open to the individual. At the commencement of this pandemic in Italy efforts were made by some of the towns to save themselves, by refusing admission to the plague-stricken, and by the adoption of other protective measures. The Venetians forbade vessels with plague on board approaching the port, and when plague broke out in Venice the sick were carried into the suburbs to die or recover. The authorities at Milan kept the town free of the epidemic for a long time by shutting up and barricading three houses infected with plague. Boccaccio relates that the plague reached Florence " in spite of all the means that human foresight could suggest, as keeping the city free from filth and excluding all suspected persons, notwithstanding frequent cónsultations what else was to be done, not omitting prayers to God in frequent procession."

The first Governmental measures against infection were organised by

First Governmental measures in 1374.
Count Bernabo in Reggio in January, 1374[1]. The regulations provided that every plague patient was to be taken out of the city into the fields, there to die or recover, that persons who nursed or attended upon a plague patient were to be isolated for 10 days before being free to associate with others, that the priests were to examine the diseased and give notice to the officials, under punishment of confiscation of their goods and of being burnt alive, that persons importing the plague were to forfeit their goods, and that none except those appointed were to attend plague patients under penalty of death and forfeiture of their fortune. In 1383 on plague returning to Lombardy, Count Bernabo rendered his measures still more stringent by forbidding, on pain of death, people from plague-stricken places being admitted to his territories.

Other Governments followed Count Bernabo's example, though perhaps with not the ·same stringency. On plague visiting Italy again

[1] *The Epidemics of the Middle Ages.* By J. F. C. Hecker, M.D. Translated by B. G. Babington, M.D., F.R.S., 1859.

in 1399 measures were introduced to destroy the infection. Infected houses were thoroughly fumigated and ventilated for 8 or 10 days, they were further purified from noxious vapours by fires, and were fumigated by balsams and resins. Straw and rags in infected houses were burnt, and the bedsteads which had been used were set out for 4 days in the rain or sunshine. It was forbidden to use the beds and clothes from an infected house without permission, and without first subjecting them to a thorough cleansing and washing, and then drying them at the fire or in the sun. Thus it is evident that serious efforts were made in some of the Italian states to grapple with the plague, and it is remarkable how closely they resemble those of to-day. Examination of the sick, notification to the authorities, isolation of the patient and of the attendants, and disinfection of the house and household furniture by fumigation and ventilation, burning or washing of certain articles, and exposure to the sun of others were all employed.

In the 15th century a still further advance was made. In 1403[1]

Lazaretto established by the Venetians in 1403.

the Venetians established a lazaretto for the treatment and isolation of plague patients at a distance of about 2 miles from the town. It was situated on an island, and cut off from all communication with the town. In 1467 the Genoese imitated the Venetians and also established a lazaretto. In 1475 there was a plague hospital at Inch Keith in the Firth of Forth. Later, in 1485, the lazaretto system was extended in Venice, to provide not only for the treatment and segregation of plague patients for 40 days, and for the purification of their clothes and effects, but also for an elaborate system of isolation and purification of all persons and passengers coming from countries infected with plague. The merchants of Venice had experienced the injurious effect which the importation and prevalence of plague had exercised on their commerce and prosperity.

In the course of six centuries, from 901 to 1500, the Venetian state had

A council of health and quarantine established in 1485 in Venice.

suffered from 63 epidemics of plague, and they determined to make a strenuous effort to protect themselves as much as possible. With this object in view they established in 1485 a Council of Health, whose duty it was to do everything to meet the invasion of plague. For this purpose they framed certain regulations for the management of the lazarettos, the duration of detention, and the method of purification to be adopted. The places of detention and purification were called the

---

[1] *Essai sur l'Hygiène Internationale.* Par Adrien Proust Paris, 1873.

lazarettos, and the period during which the detention and purification were undergone was called the quarantine, the minimum being 40 days. Gradually the term quarantine was used to embrace the whole system, and will in future be employed in this sense. The quarantine regulations of 1485 are interesting from an historical point of view because they formed the pattern for most quarantine regulations against plague for the past 500 years, and were only materially altered in 1897 at the conference of the European Powers held in Venice, when plague became epidemic in Bombay, and because they indicate the notions of infection that were held in the 15th century, the belief as to the infectious principles being dissipated by exposure to air and sunshine, and the opinion as to the period necessary to cover the development of any latent principle of contagion. It was even then recognised that the infection manifested itself earlier than 40 days in persons, but as it was difficult to separate persons from their belongings, it was determined to require the same length of purification for both. Briefly, the

The Venetian system of quarantine. Venetian system[1] was as follows: Every vessel coming from the Levant was to hoist on the mizen-mast a yellow flag before approaching the port. The vessel was then met by an official who took charge of and anchored it at a particular place. The captain, after all papers and letters were fumigated, accompanied a second official to the Health Office under certain precautions, where he was questioned as to the voyage, the ports he had touched at, and the state of health of those on board. A careful examination was made of his papers with special reference to the number of passengers and crew, the clearness of his bills of health, the kind of merchandise on board, and the ports from which it came. If the ship was from a country that was free of plague, and the Health Office was satisfied, pratique was allowed. If, on the other hand, it came from a suspected place the captain was conducted back to the ship, a list was made of the names of every one on board, and another list of the belongings of each person. Orders were then given for unlading the ship. Goods were distinguished as susceptible and unsusceptible, or receptive and unreceptive, which referred to their powers of retaining infection. The latter did not undergo any purification or retention, and, under certain regulations, were handed at once from the vessel by officials under the control of the Health Office. The former were taken in boats under precautions of the lazaretto for purification. The passengers with their baggage were also taken to the lazaretto, none being allowed to perform quarantine on

[1] *Account of the Office of Health, Venice.* London, 1752.

board for fear that the things worn or wearable should not be sufficiently purified. The lazarettos consisted of a number of buildings in which quarters were arranged for the accommodation of healthy passengers in small groups. Shut off from these by high walls were other buildings consisting of large open and covered sheds designed for the exposure to the air in all weathers of the different kinds of merchandise. Persons falling sick of plague were removed to the old lazaretto, while healthy passengers were housed in the new; and goods and merchandise were taken to the sheds and there opened up. The boxes and trunks of the passengers were also opened and everything in them, whether wearing apparel or merchandise, was hung up and exposed to the air. When these preliminaries were completed the quarantine of 40 days commenced and not before.

The procedure adopted for the goods was to take them out of their bags and cases, or to undo the bales and deposit them in separate heaps about 4 feet high in the sheds. These heaps were then thoroughly aired by being turned over and handled, and then removed from one place to another, the object being that every part in turn should get exposed to the sun and air. There were rules of purification to be adopted for every kind of merchandise. The greatest attention was paid to woollen goods, as these were considered to retain the infection much more tenaciously than other kinds. They were turned over, handled, and removed from place to place daily. Silks, linens, furs, and ribbons were thoroughly aired twice a day, and removed to another place twice a week. Cottons, thread, camel hair, and similar articles which came in bags, were differently dealt with. The bags were unsewn on one side and left for 20 days, the contents each day being stirred up by the naked arms of the workmen appointed to do it. The bags were then turned and unsewn on the other side and the contents similarly treated for 20 days. Wax, sponges, and animals with short hair were purified by being passed through running water. Feathered animals were sprinkled with vinegar. Corn, salt, seeds, minerals, wood, gold-dust, sugars, cheeses, fruits, smoked fish and meat, drugs, liquors, brandies, oils, wines and similar articles were considered non-susceptible, and could be taken away at once. If the period of 40 days were passed in quarantine without sickness of a suspicious nature among the passengers or the workmen who were employed airing the merchandise, the passengers and goods were allowed admission into the town. Should, however, in the course of the 40 days illness of a suspicious character occur, 40 more days were to be passed in quarantine in the lazaretto.

The whole system, it will be seen, was based on the establishment of the lazaretto at a convenient place near the port, and so situated as to be completely isolated from the town, where passengers and merchandise from an infected country could be subjected to a thorough purification which was supposed to take 40 days for its completion. Quarantine in a lazaretto under the Italian system was not simply the retention of passengers and goods in a quarantine station or ship for 40 days, under the impression that the poison of plague would in that time be destroyed, but it was the purification or disinfection of passengers, effects, and merchandise by means of washing and exposure to the air and sun for a certain period, and no goods were considered to be purified unless they were opened up and so arranged that every portion received a thorough airing; the duration of the quarantine depended on the medical opinion of the time, and, though the arbitrary fixing of 40 days seems now with the advance of medical science to be an extraordinary time compared with that which is needed, yet it is impossible not to recognise that with the means of disinfection at their disposal the procedure was admirably adapted for the purposes in view, and the conditions of maritime commerce at that time; and it is equally impossible to withhold our admiration of the completeness of the system adopted by the Venetians, who, from their intimate intercourse with the Levant, necessarily ran the greatest risk from the importation of plague.

The advance made in the mode of disinfection in modern times can effect in less than 40 hours the purification of goods and passengers, effects which were then believed to need 40 days.

The system was adopted slowly by other nations, but with a less appreciation of the underlying principles, so that little remained in common with the Venetian system than the circumstance that both passengers and goods were detained for 40 days. The system of quarantine degenerated often into the mere crowding of people into insanitary buildings in which there was every chance of their becoming ill, and allowing pratique after they had been detained for 40 days, or the keeping of every one on board for that period, not infrequently in an unhealthy anchorage.

Extension of preventive measures against plague to other countries.

Austria and Germany, exposed to plague from Italy and Turkey, early adopted preventive measures in times of plague similar to those employed in the inland states of Italy. These consisted in making large fires in the square and crossways of the towns and villages,

fumigation of the council chambers and private dwellings, prohibition
of the yearly markets, isolation and shutting up of in-
Measures in
Austria and
Germany, in
16th century. fected houses, building of hospitals outside the town, or
using of old leper hospitals, and the closing of the public
bath-houses. The town magistrates were empowered to
enforce these measures in their own districts. But, as this power did
not always prove to be sufficient, the Government of the country, in
order to secure uniformity and a more rigorous administration, issued
general orders. Thus in Austria[1] the Emperor Maximilian, in 1512, issued
a mandate that the gipsies, who were disliked, and looked upon not only
as Turkish spies and thieves, but also as carriers of plague, were not
allowed to stay in Austria, nor to form an encampment, nor even to pass
through the country. As the condition of the air was considered to
materially assist in producing and spreading plague, regulations were
made to keep the streets and lanes clean and to remove heaps of
manure and other refuse from houses under the penalty of a fine:
whoever threw manure or other rubbish into the streams was taken
before the magistrate and fined.

In Vienna the Government printed short and simple directions
written by physicians instructing the inhabitants what
Educational
tracts and
pamphlets in
16th century. to do to protect themselves against plague and what
medicines they should take in case of illness[1]. A general
order was given in 1521 that all people, particularly
heads of households, should be provided with these small publications,
so that, in case of danger, they might exactly know what to do.
In 1522 Dr Johann Saltzman published a pamphlet on the rules by
which protection may be obtained against the pestilence. This was
printed and put up on walls, and on the doors of the churches and the
gates of the city.

In England, the introduction of measures against plague probably
owe their origin to Venetian influence. The first preventive action
recorded is in 1513[2], when two servants of the Venetian envoy died of
Measures in
London in
16th century. plague in London, and their beds, sheets, and other
effects were thrown into the river. It is in this year
that the inhabitants of houses infected with plague
were ordered to keep in their houses and put out wisps to warn
others that the houses were infected. It was in 1516[3], when the
Venetian ambassador removed from London to Putney because of a

---

[1] Peinlich's *Geschichte der Pest*; also *Geschichte der Pest in Steurmark*.
[2] *History of Epidemics in Britain*, Vol. I. p. 288, Creighton.
[3] *Ibid.* p. 290.

death from plague in his house, that the first reference is made to quarantine in England. The ambassador was not allowed to see Wolsey until 40 days elapsed from the case of plague in his house. Again, in 1518, the same Venetian ambassador had plague in his house, and writes to Venice from Lambeth that on the expiration of 40 days, which had nearly come to an end, he would not fail to do his duty as heretofore. It was not, however, until 1543 that any general order on the subject was issued. It is as follows:

"35 Hen. VIII[1]. A precept issued to the aldermen:—That they should cause their beadles to set the sign of the cross on every house which should be afflicted with the plague, and there continue for forty days:

First Government orders issued in London in Henry VIII's reign.

"That no person who was able to live by himself, and should be afflicted with the plague, should go abroad or into any company for one month after his sickness, and that all others who could not live without their daily labour should as much as in them lay refrain from going abroad, and should for forty days after (illegible) and continually carry a white rod in their hand, two foot long:

"That every person whose house had been infected should, after a visitation, carry all the straw and (illegible) in the night privately into the fields and burn; they should also carry clothes of the infected in the fields to be cured:

"That no housekeeper should put any person diseased out of his house into the street or other place unless they provided housing for them in some other house:

"That all persons having any dogs in their houses other than hounds, spaniels or mastiffs, necessary for the custody or safe keeping of their houses, should forthwith convey them out of the city, or cause them to be killed and carried out of the city and buried at the common laystall:

"That such as kept hounds, spaniels or mastiffs should not suffer them to go abroad, but closely confine them:

"That the churchwardens of every parish should employ somebody to keep out all common beggars out of churches on holy days, and to cause them to remain without doors:

"That all the streets, lanes, etc. within the wards should be cleansed:

"That the aldermen should cause this precept to be read in the churches."

---

[1] *History of Epidemics in Britain*, pp. 312, 313, Creighton.

The order about dogs and cats appears to have been a very general one.

Later, in Queen Elizabeth's time, the orders became more stringent, approaching in severity the regulations issued in the 15th century by Count Bernabo. To protect the Court at Windsor a **Orders more severe in the reign of Elizabeth.** gallows was set up in the market-place of Windsor, to hang all such as should come there from London. It was forbidden to bring wares to, through, or by Windsor, or to carry wood or other stuff to or from London on the river by Windsor upon pain of hanging without any judgment, and any people who received wares out of London into Windsor were to be turned out of their houses, and their houses shut up. In London quarantine and sanitation were rigorously insisted on by the Privy Council in orders to the Mayor, while in 1580[1], when the disease was raging in Lisbon, the Lord Mayor was authorised by Lord Treasurer Burghley to take measures in concurrence with the officers of the port, to prevent in regard of arrivals from Lisbon the lodging of merchants or mariners in the city or suburbs, or the discharge of goods from ships until they have had some time for airing and in the meantime to provide proper necessaries on board ships detained.

It was not only in Windsor that severe measures against plague **Severity of measures in Aberdeen.** were carried out. In Aberdeen the orders became gradually more rigorous. As early as 1498 guards were put on the city gates to prevent suspected persons entering during the day, and the gates were locked at night. In 1514 lodges were erected on the links and gallowhill, where the infected or suspected were to remain for 40 days. In 1546 it is recorded that a citizen was burnt on the left hand with a hot iron for not notifying to the authorities that his child was sick of plague. In 1585 three gibbets were erected in different parts of the town, " in case any infected person arrive or repair by sea or land to this burgh, or in case any indweller of this burgh receive, house, or harbour, or give meat or drink to the infectit person or persons, the man be hangit, and the woman drownit[2]."

In Edinburgh the infected families were removed with all their **Enlightened policy in Edinburgh.** goods and furniture to the moor and there lodged in huts hastily erected for their accommodation. They were allowed to be visited by their friends in company with

[1] *English Sanitary Institutions*, p. 94. By Sir John Simon, K.C.B.

[2] *History of Epidemics in Britain*, Vol. I. p. 371. By Charles Creighton, M.A., M.D., 1894.

an officer. Those who concealed the pest in their houses were liable to be punished with death. The clothes were meanwhile purified by boiling in a cauldron erected in the open air, and their houses were cleansed by proper officers. These regulations were under the care of two citizens selected for the purpose; for each of whom, as for the cleansers and bearers of the dead, a gown of grey was made, with a white St Andrew's cross before and behind.

It will be noted that the measures adopted here differed from those practised in London, in which the pest-houses were very few in number, and the plague-stricken were usually shut up in their houses. In fact in every epidemic of ·plague from the time of Henry VIII to that of 1665, which was the last epidemic in England, the practice of shutting up the sick and suspected in the same house became increasingly more rigorous. In the reign of James I an Act was passed for the

First quarantine station for London established in 1664. charitable relief and ordering of persons infected with plague, authority being given to justices of the peace, mayors, baillies, and other head officers to appoint, within their several districts, examiners, searchers, watchmen, keepers, and buriers for the persons and places infected, to give directions for the prevention and avoidance of infection. In 1664[1] the Lord Mayor and Court of Aldermen of London proposed to the Lords of the Council "that after the custom of other countries, vessels coming from infected parts should not be permitted to come nearer than Gravesend or such like distance, where repositories after the manner of lazarettos should be appointed, into which the ships might discharge their cargoes to be aired for 40 days." The proposal was accepted, and the first quarantine station for London was established, the crew and passengers being kept on board while the apparel, goods, household stuff and bedding were aired on shore. Notwithstanding these orders, plague, which had been endemic in London for many years, broke out in the winter of 1664.

In the London plague of 1665 the Lord Mayor, Sir John Lawrence,

Special plague officials appointed in every parish of London. and Aldermen of the City of London issued orders appointing ·in every parish special officials. The examiners were to make a house-to-house inspection, and were to enquire and learn what houses were infected and the number of the sick, and to give orders and see that the infected houses were shut up. The watchmen were to have a special care that no person went in or out of such houses. The searchers, who were women, were to assist the surgeons in examining corpses and

---

[1] *English Sanitary Institutions*, p. 99.   By Sir John Simon, K.C.B., 1890.

to report whether the death was due to plague or not. Nurses were shut up for 28 days after the decease of any person dying of the infection.

Under orders concerning infected houses and persons sick of the plague, certain regulations were framed, and as they define clearly what was the practice in the 17th century I shall transcribe them[1].

Notice to be given of the sickness. The master of every house as soon as anyone in his house complaineth, either of botch or purple or swelling in any part of his body, or falleth otherwise sick without apparent cause of some other disease, shall give knowledge thereof to the examiner of health within two hours after the said sign shall appear.

Sequestration of the sick. As soon as any man shall be found by this examiner, chirurgeon, or searcher, to be sick of the plague, he shall the same night be sequestered in the same house, and in case he be so sequestered then, though he afterwards die not, the house wherein he sickened shall be shut up for a month, after the use of the due preservatives taken by the rest.

Airing the stuff. For sequestration of the goods and stuff of the infected, their bedding, and apparel, and hangings of chambers must be well aired with fire, and such perfumes as are requisite within the infected house, before they be taken again to use; this to be done by the appointment of the examiner.

Shutting up of the house. If any person shall have visited any man known to be infected of the plague, or entered willingly into any known infected house being not allowed, the house wherein he inhabiteth shall be shut up for certain days by the examiner's direction.

None to be removed out of infected houses but etc. Item. That none be removed out of the house where he falleth sick of the infection into any other house of the city (except it be to the pest-house or a tent, or unto some such house which the owner of the said visited house holdeth in his own hands and occupieth by his own servants) and so as security be given to the parish whither such remove be made, that the attendance and charge about the said visited persons shall be observed and charged in all the particularities before expressed, without any cost of that parish to which any such remove shall happen to be made and this remove to be done by night: and it shall be lawful to any person that hath two houses to remove either his sound or his infected people to his spare

---

[1] The author is indebted to Professor Kenwood of University College for a copy of these orders and regulations.

house at his choice, so as, if he send away first his sound he may not after send thither the sick, nor again unto the sick the sound, and that the same which he sendeth be for one week at the least shut up and secluded from company, for fear of some infection at the first not appearing.

Burial of the dead. That the burial of the dead by this visitation be, at most convenient hours, always before sun rising or after sun setting with the privity of the churchwardens or constable, and not otherwise: and that no neighbours or friends be suffered to accompany the corpse to church, or to enter the house visited, upon pain of having his house shut up, or be imprisoned, and that no corpse dying of infection shall be buried or remain in any church in time of common prayer, sermon, or lecture. And that no children be suffered at time of burial of any corpse in any church, churchyard, or burying place to come near the corpse, coffin, or grave, and that all the graves shall be at least six foot deep, and further all public assemblies at other burials are to be forborne during the continuance of this visitation.

No infected stuff to be altered. That no clothes, stuff, bedding, or garment be suffered to be carried or conveyed out of any infected houses, and that the criers and carriers abroad of bedding or old apparel to be sold or pawned be utterly prohibited and restrained, and no brokers of bedding or old apparel be permitted to make any outward show or spread forth on their stalls, shopboards or windows towards any street, lane, common-way, or passage, any old bedding, apparel, or other stuff out of any infected house, within two months after the infection hath been there or his house shall be shut up as infected and so shall continue shut up twenty days at least.

No person to be conveyed out of any infected house. If any person visited do fortune by negligent looking unto, or by any other means, to come, or be conveyed from a place infected, to any other place, the parish from whence such party hath come or been conveyed upon notice thereof given shall at their charge cause the said party so visited and escaped to be carried and brought back again by night, and the parties in this case offending to be punished at the direction of the alderman of the ward; and the house of the receiver of such visited person to be shut up for twenty days.

Every visited house to be marked. That every house visited be marked with a red cross of a foot long, in the middle of the door, evident to be seen and with these usual printed words, that is to say, "Lord, have mercy upon us," to be set close over the same cross, there to continue until lawful opening of the same house.

Every visited house to be watched. That the constables see every house shut up and to be attended with watchmen which may keep them in and minister necessaries unto them at their own charges (if they be able) or at the common charge if they be unable. The shutting up to be for the space of four weeks after all be whole. That precise orders be taken that the searchers, chirurgeons, keepers, and buriers are not to pass the street without holding a red rod or wand of three foot in length in their hands, open and evident to be seen, and are not to go into any other house than into their own or into that whereunto they are directed or sent for; but to forbear and abstain from company, especially when they have been lately used in any such business or attendance.

Inmates. That where several inmates are in one and the same house, and any person in that house happen to be infected, no other person or family of such house shall be suffered to remove him or themselves without a certificate from the examiners of health of that parish, or in default thereof, the house whither they so remove shall be shut up as in case of visitation.

Hackney coaches. That care be taken of hackney coachmen that they may not (as some have been observed to do) after carrying of infected persons to the pest-house and other places be admitted to common use till their coaches be well aired and have stood unemployed by the space of five or six days after such service.

There were also orders issued for the cleansing and keeping of the houses and streets sweet, and the prohibition of the sale of stinking fish, or unwholesome flesh, or musty corn, or other corrupt fruits, or the use of musty and unwholesome casks in breweries and tippling houses. It was further ordered that no hogs, dogs, or cats, or tame pigeons or conies be suffered to be kept within any part of the city.

Plays, public feastings and large assemblies were prohibited, and regulations were made regarding beggars and tippling houses.

Yet as Hodges remarks in his *Loimologia*, or an historical account of the plague in London in 1665, "although both the makers and executors of the laws were very diligent in their duty during the late sickness the contagion notwithstanding spread." He is doubtful whether the shutting up of infected houses proved a serviceable measure, and he is of opinion that many lost their lives by it, the tragical mark on the door driving proper assistance from them. In his chapter on preservation from a pestilence he remarks that "the timely separation also of the infected from the well is absolutely necessary to be done, because the most sure way of spreading it is letting the sick and well

Hodges opposed to the shutting up the sick and the well in the same house.

converse together. Public funerals ought to be forbid, as also all kinds of meetings and frequent intercourse of several persons together; an injunction also of quarantine from infected places according to the custom of trading nations is by any means not to be omitted and carelessly to be executed[1]."

In 1720 these views, which apparently prevailed in Scotland as early

Dr Mead's views in 1720.

as the 16th century, and led to the Scotch system of evacuating infected houses, are more fully developed by Dr Mead on the occasion of the epidemic of plague in Marseilles which gave rise to much alarm in England. In his short discourse concerning pestilential contagion, and the methods to be used

Advocacy of the establishment of hospitals and quarantine stations.

to prevent it, Dr Mead advocates the establishment of lazarettos and quarantine on the Venetian system to prevent the importation of plague by sea, and in the event of the disease breaking out in a locality the abandonment of the shutting up of infected houses, and the substitution of a system by which the houses were evacuated, the sick being removed to special airy buildings and the sound to others, both being three or four miles outside the town. The sound people were to be stripped of their clothes, and washed and shaved before they went into their new

Evacuation of infected houses.

lodgings. After the infected houses were evacuated it was advised that the goods should be buried and if possible the houses demolished or cleansed. In addition to these measures great attention was to be paid to sanitation. If the plague increased to such an extent that the sick were too many to be removed, then he advised the fumigation of the houses with vinegar or smoke of sulphur, and attention to health of the individual, the personal use of issues, smoking, flight, care in burial of the dead, the prohibition of assemblies, and the forbidding of convalescents leaving their houses until a certain time had elapsed. To prevent the plague spreading from town to town he advised a modification of the *cordons sanitaires* that were customary on the Continent. "[2]The best

Passport system for those wishing to leave infected town.

method for which, where it can be done, is to cast up a *line* about the *town infected* at a convenient distance and by placing a *guard* to hinder the people passing from it without due regulation to other towns: but not absolutely to forbid any to withdraw themselves, as

---

[1] *Loimologia, or an Historical Account of the Plague in London in* 1665, p. 106. By Nath. Hodges, M.D. London, 1720.

[2] *A Discourse on the Plague*, p. 142. By Richard Mead, Fellow of the College of Physicians and of the Royal Society. Ninth Edition, 1744.

they have now done in France according to the usual practice abroad, which is an unnecessary severity, not to call it a cruelty. I think it will be enough if all who desire to pass the *line* be permitted to do it, upon condition they first perform quarantine for about 20 days in tents or other more convenient habitation. But the greatest care must be taken that none pass without conforming themselves to this order, both by diligent watch and by punishing with the utmost severity any that shall either have done so or attempt it; and the better to discover such it will be requisite to oblige all, who travel in any part of the country, under the same penalties to carry with them certificates either of their coming from places not infected, or of their passing the line by permission. This I take to be a more effectual method to keep the infection from spreading than the absolute refusing a passage to people upon any terms. For when men are in such imminent danger of their lives where they are, many no doubt if not otherwise allowed to escape will use endeavours to do it secretly let the hazard be ever so great, and it can hardly be but some will succeed in their attempts; as we see fell out in France notwithstanding all their care. But one that gets off thus clandestinely will be more likely to carry the distemper with him than twenty, nay a hundred, that go away under the preceding regulations: especially because the infection of the place he flies from will be by this management rendered much more intense; for confining people and shutting them up in great numbers will make the distemper rage with augmented force, even to the increasing it beyond what can be easily imagined, as appears from the account that the learned Gasendus has given us of a memorable plague which happened at Digno in Provence, where he lived in the year 1619. This was so terrible that in one summer out of 10,000 inhabitants it left but 1500, and of these all but five or six had gone through the disease, and he assigns this as the principal cause of the great destruction, that the citizens were too closely confined and not suffered so much as to go into their country houses."

Dr Mead's recommendations fortunately were never required to be put in practice in England. Some of them were adopted in India during the present epidemic of plague. In England quarantine regulations **First quarantine Act passed in reign of George IV.** were never favourably received, and it was not until the reign of George IV that a quarantine Act was passed by Parliament for Great Britain and Ireland. It was repealed in 1897, and all quarantine was abolished. The countries bordering on the Mediterranean, especially Italy, France, and Spain, always attached much importance to quarantine and the lazaretto system as a protection against plague. Their intimate intercourse with, and comparative proximity to the Levant largely influenced their views, which appear to have been formed not without foundation, for since the epidemic in Marseilles and Provence in 1720, which caused nearly 90,000 deaths, plague has been introduced into

International preventive measures introduced in 1831 and 1838.

the quarantine station at Marseilles before the Chinese epidemic came into being no fewer than nine times, the last being in 1837. In 1838 quarantine stations were formed in the Turkish dominions in order that plague should be dealt with by European measures nearer its

centre. The direction of these sanitary precautions was entrusted to a Superior Council of Health in Constantinople to which the European Powers delegated medical men. Previous to this, at the time of the cholera of 1831, an International Sanitary Council was established at Alexandria for the protection of Europe against moving epidemics from

Disappearance of plague from Turkey and Egypt attributed to these international measures.

the East. It is to the establishment of sanitary stations and an active supervision on the highways of plague, and on the frontiers and gateways of Europe, that the disappearance of plague from Turkey and Egypt is generally attributed, the disease not being truly endemic in these countries, but imported into them from centres in Mesopo-

tamia and Arabia. The retrocession of the plague from Egypt and Turkey was so remarkable an event, and followed so closely on the organisation of protective measures, being not more than 7 years in the one case and 14 years in the other, that it is difficult to dissociate from them the relationship of cause and effect. There is no reason to challenge the beneficial effect which is likely to have been exercised by these sanitary measures, but on the other hand it is possible to

Other causes also at work.

exaggerate their influence. In a previous chapter the great change which took place in the trade routes from the

East is pointed out, and the very great influence which such a change is likely to have exerted in preventing the transportation of the infection of plague from endemic centres is discussed. Plague had been perceptibly receding eastwards for the past 150 years, and not in any known relationship with the introduction of protective measures. Its pandemic area appears to have been contracting considerably both in Europe and the East. In the 17th century plague disappeared from the greater part of Western Europe in ten years, and in every succeeding epidemic the tendency was to recede further eastwards, which is noticeable until the middle of the 19th century, when in the course of five years, from 1839 to 1844, it disappeared entirely from its old haunts in

South-eastern Europe, the Levant, and Egypt. The epidemiological factor is, therefore, not to be forgotten in judging of the value of the restrictive measures, and of the two it would appear that the first was the more influential. Why at one time a disease takes on the character of an invading force with the power of transmissibility, and at other times is possessed of a tendency to remain stationary, or even to contract its area over which it has prevailed, it is impossible with our present knowledge to explain. It is nevertheless a fact, and it is

Failure of measures to prevent spread of strong invading epidemics and the possible cause.
remarkable that whenever a strong invading epidemic has to be dealt with, the organisation of quarantines, cordons sanitaires, and other restrictive measures mostly fail. The failure may be due to the invading epidemic possessing other means of extension than the ordinary, or to the fact that the usual modes of extension of ordinary epidemics are not known, and that the protective measures employed cover only a few of the means of attack, and possibly not the most important. We are still too much in the dark regarding plague, but an illustration of the latter point may be taken from cholera. The discovery that cholera spreads by water and could be introduced into a town by the river from which the inhabitants obtained their drinking water was not antagonistic to the view that cholera was transportable from place to place but it completely demonstrated that, while the cordon sanitaire and quarantine were doing their part in the defence, the disease was capable of entering the town by ways over which these had not the slightest control, and hence they were bound to fail.

In the same way quarantine might be effective in preventing patients suffering from yellow fever being landed from a vessel, and yet yellow fever might not be prevented from gaining access to the port because of infected mosquitoes which would not be dealt with by quarantine.

International conferences of European Powers to consider measures of mutual protection against epidemic disease from the East.
With the disappearance of plague from Egypt and Turkey in the middle of the 19th century, the same urgency for precaution against the spread of plague no longer continued. The lazarettos, quarantines, and cordons sanitaires, which were the weapons employed by each country to safeguard itself against the importation of plague, were now used to meet the invasion of cholera. Failure to prevent importation was attributed to a want of uniformity in the measures adopted, and as the checking of these epidemics was a matter of European interest it was considered advisable that in times of danger representatives of the

European Powers should meet and discuss the means of defence which might be adopted in common for frontier and for seaport. The first of these conferences was held in Paris in 1852, and the second in Constantinople in 1866, but no radical change was effected in the older regulations at either of these meetings. At the third conference,

New basis for maritime preventive measures adopted at the Vienna Conference, 1874. however, held in Vienna in 1874, an important agreement was come to which placed the maritime preventive measures on a different basis than had been the case hitherto. It was decided that the guiding principle for action was not to be the arrival of a ship from an infected country, but the state of health of those on board. Quarantine in its former sense was abolished, and the period of incubation of the sickness on board became the standard or limit of duration of detention. In the conference at Rome in 1885 land quarantines and cordons sanitaires for cholera were declared to be useless. Other conferences, at Venice in 1892, at Dresden in 1893, and at Paris in 1894, were held on the subject of cholera. Plague was not considered. For many years it had appeared to be almost extinct.

There were local outbreaks in Benghazi in 1856, 1858, 1859, and

Quarantine and sanitary cordons brought into requisition in the Russian outbreak of plague in 1879. 1874, and in Mesopotamia in 1867, but it was not until the very fatal outbreak at Vetlianka on the Volga in 1879 that any alarm was caused by the disease. In each of these outbreaks the sanitary cordons and quarantine regulations were brought into requisition. Before these local outbreaks it had been shown by the investigations by Aubert Roche, and the French Commission who enquired into the question in 1843, that notwithstanding some exceptions ordinarily the maximum period of incubation did not exceed eight days. In the Vetlianka outbreak there were special cordons around infected villages, and a general cordon around the district containing the infected villages. Persons who had been in an infected village had to undergo 42 days of quarantine, and persons outside the infected villages, but within the general cordon, wishing to leave had to undergo 10 days' quarantine[1]. Tholozan clearly establishes that neither for the Benghazi nor the Mesopotamian outbreaks did the quarantine or the sanitary cordons exercise the slightest influence in controlling the disease. They were not put into force until the epidemics were nearly at an end. The evidence is not so positive as regards the Vetlianka outbreak on the

[1] *Ninth Annual Report of the Local Government Board.* Levantine Plague, 1879–80.

Volga, though even here the cordons were placed round the village and district only at a late period of the outbreak. Notwithstanding the fatality of the disease in the outbreaks which were investigated in Benghazi, Mesopotamia, Vetlianka and Persia, one fact becomes evident in all, and it is that the disease at that time possessed very slight disposition to spread. On the contrary, each outbreak presented a well-marked tendency to self-limitation and was apparently quite unaffected by the measures tardily introduced for its suppression.

It is the dual character of plague which causes difficulty in estimating the value of the older or even of the newer methods of dealing with an epidemic. At one time the disease possesses most active properties of extension, while at other times it is almost devoid of them. Accordingly in an epidemic wanting in diffusive attributes and strictly self-limited in its character, the measures adopted for its control very readily acquire a reputation for efficacy which they do not deserve, while in an epidemic with strong diffusive powers they may readily be under-estimated from their apparent powerlessness in either altering the course of the epidemic or preventing its spread to other localities. It will only be when more is known of the general laws governing epidemics of plague that a true estimate of such measures can be made.

CHAPTER XVIII.

EXISTING MEASURES AGAINST PLAGUE, AFTER DISCOVERY OF BACILLUS.

Measures to prevent importation of plague.

EXISTING measures against plague may be divided into those taken to prevent the importation of the disease and its spread into other countries and localities, and those for the suppression of the disease in the locality infected. These may be further subdivided into *International* and *Local*.

Two motives have inspired international action against plague; one is a common interest of self-preservation from a disease International which is extremely destructive and the germs of which measures. are transportable from place to place; the other is that there should be some uniformity of action so as not to interfere with commerce more than is absolutely necessary. International measures of prevention as regards Europe are, as has been shown, a product of the early part of the 19th century.

In 1897 an international conference of the European Powers was held at Venice and a convention was signed, in which it was agreed that certain protective measures, having for their object efficiency but at the same time the avoidance of unnecessary restrictions on commerce, should be put into force against the threatened invasion of plague from the East. It was further agreed that any infringement of the convention on the part of any one of the signatories absolved the other Powers from adherence to the agreement with reference to that particular Power and allowed them to adopt towards it, if necessary, more stringent measures.

The regulations framed at the conference were based on the Regulations views entertained at the time that the chief danger of of the Venice the spread of plague was associated with sick persons Convention and their personal effects, and that the period of incu- of 1897. bation was the determining factor in the limitation of detention for observation purposes. The regulations included:

(1) International notification of places infected with plague, so that all being apprised of the fact, each Government has the opportunity of taking in time the necessary precautions for self-protection.

(2) Medical inspection of crew and passengers leaving infected ports, the prevention of the embarkation of any person showing symptoms of plague and the disinfection of infected and suspected articles.

(3) Special precautions with regard to ships coming from infected ports and passing through the Red Sea or Persian Gulf, the gateways of the maritime traffic of the East with Europe.

(4) Special precautions with regard to pilgrims from an infected country.

(5) Measures to be taken at the port of arrival with regard to vessels from an infected port. Such vessels are classified as healthy, suspected, and infected. *Healthy* vessels are those which have left an infected port for 10 days and more and have had no cases of plague on board. *Suspected* vessels are those in which cases of plague have occurred but not within 12 days, and *infected* vessels are those in which plague cases have occurred within 12 days of arrival.

All ships coming from infected ports are subjected to medical inspection and the measures taken depend on the events that have occurred during the voyage. Certain terms are used in this connection. The term "observation" means isolation of the passengers on board a ship or in a lazaretto till they have obtained free pratique, and "surveillance" means that the passengers will not be isolated but on arriving at their destination they will be kept under medical surveillance.

Healthy ships are at once given *free pratique* and the passengers and crew are subjected to "surveillance" for 10 days from the date on which the ship left an infected port. The authorities may also insist on the pumping out of the bilge water and the substitution of good drinking water for the water stored on board.

Suspected ships are treated with more care. The crew and passengers are subjected to "surveillance" for 10 days from the date of arrival of the ship. The soiled linen and personal effects of the crew and passengers are disinfected. The bilge water is pumped out after disinfection and a supply of good drinking water is substituted for that stored on board. All parts of the ship which have been inhabited by plague patients are disinfected and the local authorities have power to order a more thorough disinfection.

Infected ships have their sick landed at once and isolated, and the crew and passengers are, at the discretion of the local authority, subjected to "observation" or "surveillance" for a period varying according to the sanitary condition of the ship and the date of the last case of plague, but which must not exceed 10 days. The other precautions are similar to those laid down for suspected vessels. The soiled linen and personal effects of the crew and passengers suspected of being infected, and all parts of the ship which have been inhabited by plague patients, are disinfected. It is within the power of the local authority to cause a more thorough disinfection. The bilge water after disinfection is pumped out and good drinking water substituted for the water stored on board.

As regards merchandise, cargo, and baggage, the old system of **Merchandise to be prohibited or disinfected if thought necessary but not quarantined.** quarantine has completely given way to either absolute prohibition of the importation of susceptible goods, or to disinfection according to the option of the Governments concerned. The only articles which must be compulsorily disinfected, if admitted, are soiled linen, wearing apparel, clothes, and articles carried as personal baggage, or household goods coming from a local area declared to be infected, and which the local sanitary authority deems contaminated. Disinfection of merchandise is only enforced in the case of merchandise and articles which the local sanitary authority considers contaminated, or whose importation may be prohibited.

The susceptible articles or goods which may be prohibited are:

1. Used linen, clothing, personal effects, and bedding.

2. Rags, including rags compressed by hydraulic force, which are carried as merchandise in bales.

3. Old sacking, carpets, and old embroidery.

4. Raw hides, untanned and fresh skins.

5. Animal refuse, claws, hoofs, horse-hair, hair of animals generally, raw silk, and wool.

6. Human hair.

Quarantine on land frontiers for merchandise is abolished, and letters **Quarantine on land frontiers abolished.** and correspondence, printed matter, books and business documents, except parcels received through post, are subjected to no restriction or disinfection. Quarantine on land frontiers is also abolished for travellers. Medical inspection on the railways, at the custom houses, and at special stations, with the detention of the sick and the surveillance of travellers from an infected area, are the measures on which reliance is placed to screen out the sick from the healthy, and to keep a control over the spread of the disease.

As certain classes of people, such as gipsies and vagabonds, emigrants, and persons travelling or crossing the frontiers in large bodies, are a special danger in conveying disease, the same liberty is not accorded to them, and each Government reserves the right to take special measures against them.

Quarantine not abolished for certain classes and pilgrims.

It is this particular danger attached to crowds moving from one place to another that has necessitated the framing of special and more stringent regulations for the control of the pilgrim traffic to and from the Hedjaz. The Kaabah in Mecca is to the Mahommedan the holiest place on earth, and Medina contains the shrine of their prophet. It is the ardent desire of every Moslem to carry out the injunction of Mahomet to make a pilgrimage to the Holy Land and worship at the Kaabah. They come from India, Persia and the adjoining countries, Java and the Malayan Archipelago, from the Mauritius, Zanzibar and Madagascar, from Africa, from Asia Minor, and from the Turkish and Russian Dominions. All who are able converge to this one centre to be present and to engage in the rites and ceremonies of the Kurban Bairam festival. The fatigues, privations, and insanitary conditions to which the poorer pilgrims are subjected during the voyage to the Hedjaz, the crowding that takes place during the festival, and the misery and filth that follow from the overcrowding, are all conducive to the prevalence of infectious diseases, the seeds of which are apt to be scattered on the track of the pilgrims on their return journey and to be carried back even to their distant homes.

The convention was not signed by Portugal, Turkey, Greece, and Servia.

In 1903 another conference of the Powers was held in Paris for the purpose of codifying the terms agreed to in previous conferences and modifying or adding to them. By this time more was known of plague and it was evident that although the international measures agreed to in 1897 had proved useful and that Europe remained free of epidemic plague, yet since then there had been a small outbreak in Oporto in 1899, in Glasgow in 1900, in Naples in 1901, and in Marseilles in 1903, and in none of these places was the infection traceable to imported cases of plague in human beings. More-

The measures agreed upon at the Venice Convention though useful had not stopped altogether the importation of plague.

over, notwithstanding similar regulations having been put into operation in many of the ports whose Governments were not signatories to the Venice Convention, plague had spread to them and was gradually distributing itself from port to port in different parts of the world. It was obvious that the axiom which applied to cholera and which was adopted in 1874 at the Vienna Conference for that disease and on which protective measures against plague were based, viz. that it is not the arrival of the ship which renders it necessary to treat the same, but the state of health of those on it, had to be modified in the light of experience of plague and shape itself somewhat more in accordance with the older views. Much had been learnt during the six years about the plague bacillus and the disease itself. It was now known that there is a bubonic, septicaemic, pneumonic and pustular form of plague; that only the septicaemic and pneumonic forms are specially infective; that the period of incubation is usually less and rarely more than 10 days; that rats are very susceptible to plague; that there is a connection between rat plague and human plague; that certain animals besides rats may take plague; that plague is transportable by infected human beings, infected animals, especially rats, and by infected clothing and by articles contaminated with infective material, and that Haffkine's prophylactic and Yersin's serum exert a sensible protective effect.

The regulations of the Paris Convention of 1903 confirm those of the Venice Convention except in two important respects.
Regulations of the Paris Conference of 1903. One is that the period of detention of infected ships is reduced from 10 to 5 days, and the second is that in addition to disinfection of an infected vessel all the rats on board must be destroyed. The creation at Paris of an international sanitary office to receive and transmit sanitary information to the countries which adhere to the convention was also agreed to as desirable. The full text of the Paris Convention of 1903 is given in Appendix II of this work.

Local measures to prevent the importation of plague devolves
Local measures. usually on the municipal authorities under the supervision of Government. They mostly consist in providing the machinery to carry out the regulations framed at the Venice and Paris Conventions. Additional protective measures may be taken by the signatories of the convention so long as they do not run counter to the principles and regulations of the convention itself. Arrangements are accordingly made to provide for:

(a)   Medical inspection of all ships coming from infected ports.

(*b*) Hospitals for the isolation of plague cases arriving from an infected country.

(*c*) Observation buildings for persons whom it is thought advisable to place under observation.

(*d*) Medical surveillance.

(*e*) Disinfection of suspected and infected ships, of soiled linen and of luggage.

(*f*) Destruction of rats on board suspected and infected ships, and also on ships from infected ports.

(*g*) Prevention of ships from infected or suspected ports being moored alongside the wharves or quays unless rats have been destroyed.

(*h*) The inspection of forage, fruit crates, grain bags, and other cargo from infected centres to prevent the conveyance of rats in them and the possible importation by rail of some which may be plague-infected.

Next to the prevention of admission of cases of plague and the early isolation of any which may have escaped medical inspection but which were discovered after arrival at their destination during the period of surveillance, the most important measures are the destruction of rats on board ships from infected ports and disinfection of suspected and infected ships. Until recently the destruction of rats on board ship was peculiarly difficult, no method being found to be entirely satisfactory. The generation of carbonic acid gas was tried but it was found to be very expensive, and not very effective; carbonic oxide was also employed but the colourless, odourless and poisonous nature of the gas renders it unsafe and dangerous to use. Only since the introduction of the Clayton process of fumigating with sulphur-polyoxide has a thoroughly satisfactory, efficient and controllable method of destroying rats on board ship with certainty come into use, and it moreover has the advantage of germicidal and insecticidal properties.

Methods employed for the destruction of rats on board ships.

These triple powers, together with the fact that it has no injurious effect on textile fabrics or on grain, render it of the highest value, not only for destroying rats, but also for disinfecting ships, whether empty or full of grain or other cargo except fruit and vegetables. The gas, which analyses show to be a mixture of SO_2 and SO_3 together with some unknown gaseous toxic combination of sulphur and oxygen, is generated by burning rolls of sulphur at an intense heat in a very simply constructed

The Clayton process for the destruction of rats and disinfection of ships.

apparatus, which is usually fixed on a small launch so that the machine may be brought to the side of any ship that requires fumigation. Air is supplied to the burning sulphur by an induced draught, which at the same time draws the heated gases so formed through a cooler attached to the apparatus. This cooler is kept at a low temperature by a continuous passage of water through it. The water can be taken from the dock. From the cooler the gas, reduced in temperature and volume, passes to a blower, which propels it through a hose-pipe to the part of the ship that is to be fumigated. There is a return hose-pipe which draws the air from the chamber that is being fumigated to the furnace. It is this air which first supplies the sulphur in the furnace with oxygen for combustion, but as the percentage of gas in the compartment that is being fumigated rises, the withdrawal of such air to feed the furnace cannot be continued, as 5 % of the gas in air possesses fire-extinguishing properties. Even a smaller percentage would cause the sulphur to burn badly, and tend to put out the fire. Accordingly, whenever the returning air from the compartment registers 3 %, the connection between the return-pipe and the furnace is closed, and a valve is opened near to where the pipe enters, which permits an incurrent of fresh air to the furnace from the outside. When the percentage of gas in the furnace rises to about 18, and there is a tendency to exceed this, in order to prevent any volatilisation and deposit of sulphur along the pipes a second valve is opened, which keeps the percentage of gas formed in the furnace at a regular standard.

The system is first one of propulsion and exhaustion, but when the **Strength and properties of the gas.** air exhausted contains 3 % of gas, the exhaust pipe is shut off, and a high percentage of gas is then continued to be propelled into the chamber until the air in it reaches a saturation of 12 to 15 %. A very simple contrivance indicates the percentage of gas that is being propelled or exhausted through the tubes, and by a similar test the percentage of gas in the compartment that is being fumigated can be ascertained. A percentage of between 10 and 12 is sufficient for all purposes; a large machine is capable of generating 800 cubic feet per minute of 18 % gas. The gas driven into the supply pipe emerges from it into the chamber to be fumigated in the form of a white fuming gas, which is exceedingly irritating to the mucous membrane of the respiratory passages when breathed in small quantities and in a confined space. The presence of the gas is thus readily detected and recognised by the irritating effect it produces on the respiratory passages and by the fact that it is visible. These two qualities are particularly advantageous, because those employed in carrying out the fumigations are able to see the gas when it escapes from the pipes, and they are rendered so uncomfortable by the irritation of the eyes, nostrils, throat and chest as the percentage of gas increases in the room, that it necessitates a speedy retreat from the room to the fresh air outside, and thus there is no chance of the operators being injuriously affected by the gas. This irritating effect on the mucous membrane of the respiratory passages drives rats, insects and other vermin from their holes and hiding-places in search of relief, and they die in the open where their dead bodies can be collected, thus avoiding the great inconvenience of rats dying in their holes from poison or from the use of non-odorous gases such as carbonic oxide and carbonic acid. The gas itself has no effect on the clothes or the person of those exposed to it, provided fresh air is supplied for breathing purposes. In a number of experiments carried out by the writer the engineer who was conducting the operations put on a specially designed diving helmet and several times entered a passage and cabin saturated with 10 to 12 % of the gas, and removed articles which had been exposed.

The readiness with which the gas is detected compares very favourably with carbonic acid and carbonic oxide gases, which are not only odourless but invisible, and if breathed even in small quantities are liable to produce poisonous effects without any warning.

The gases formed by the combustion of sulphur at a high temperature such as is attained in the Clayton furnace, which not infrequently reaches 1800° F., are of a complex and unstable character, consisting of SO_2 and SO_3 and other higher sulphur oxides. When sulphur is burned in the open air the product is almost entirely sulphurous acid (SO_2) with a very minute quantity of sulphuric anhydride (SO_3), but in the Clayton furnace, where the products do not readily escape, besides the production of SO_2 a second reaction takes place and a greater quantity of the sulphurous acid (SO_2) is converted into sulphuric anhydride (SO_3). There are limits to the production of the sulphuric anhydride (SO_3) in the furnace as heat decomposes it into sulphurous acid and oxygen, but analyses show that the amount of sulphuric anhydride sent through the blower is more than 60 times greater than that produced by burning sulphur in the open air under ordinary conditions. Sulphurous acid does not show any signs of cloudiness in the air while sulphuric anhydride is intensely cloudy. It is this smoky character of the gas pumped from the Clayton furnace which distinguishes it from sulphurous acid alone which is colourless, and it is the presence of the sulphuric anhydride and possibly other unstable oxides which endows the gas with its highly toxic properties.

From a series of experiments carried out in the early part of 1903 by Professor R. Tanner Hewlett, Dr H. S. Willson and the writer on board the s.s. *Manora* in the port of London it was ascertained that:

1. The gas generated from the Clayton furnace and saturating the holds of the ship to the extent of 10 and 12% is a toxic gas.

2. That a six hours' and even a four hours' exposure to a 10% or 12% gas is fatal to rats and insects such as cockroaches, bugs, fleas, and grubs, and to mosquitoes and mosquito larvae and pupae. As a matter of fact all of these are destroyed by a much shorter exposure to a gas of 3%.

3. That a similar exposure to a 10 or 12% gas is destructive to the vitality of the bacillus of plague, cholera and typhoid fever, but has no action on the spores of anthrax.

4. That the gas is a preservative of meat when moderately exposed, and is not injurious to food-stuffs except fruit and some kinds of vegetables.

5. That merchandise, such as dyed silks, print stuffs, books, photographs, tea, coffee, etc., if dry, are unaffected by the gas.

6. That upholstering stuffs and machinery sustain no damage from the gas, but that metals are tarnished and afterwards require to be cleaned, when they regain their former appearance.

These observations are in consonance with those observed elsewhere. Dr Calmette, Director of the Pasteur Institute at Lille, found that dry cultures of streptococcus and of typhoid bacillus mixed with or without blood were destroyed by exposure for six hours to an 8% concentration of the gas generated by a Clayton machine, and that cultures of plague and of cholera were destroyed even by a two hours' exposure to an 8% gas.

Steamers with and without cargo, hospitals and other buildings have been fumigated with the gas with destructive effect to every form of vermin, and to cultures of bacilli placed under conditions calculated to test to the utmost the penetrative power of the gas. Large numbers of vessels with cargo of every kind have been fumigated at Dunkerque and elsewhere with success and without any damage to the cargo.

Textile fabrics of the most delicate colours, so long as they are protected by wrappings from the direct action of the gas, are not affected either in texture or colour. In an experiment made with 150 samples of coloured silks, three were slightly changed in tint but not bleached

In merchantable bales they would not be exposed to the direct action of the gas.

Experiments have also been made by Dr Clemow at Liverpool, Drs Savage and Walford at Cardiff, Dr Robertson at Cape Town, in which plague bacilli and rats have been killed in a few hours' exposure to a 10 and 12 % strength. Other experiments made by Dr W. A. Evans of Bradford, by Dr Dzeryhopky of St Petersburg, by Dr Tamayo, who carried on similar experiments in New York on behalf of the Peruvian Government, confirm these observations.

In 1904 the Local Government Board issued a report on the destruction of rats and disinfection on shipboard by J. S. Haldane, M.D., F.R.S., and John Wade, D.Sc., in which from observations on the Clayton process they conclude that:

" For the treatment of a vessel's hold the Clayton method possesses very distinct advantages. In the first place, the process of filling the hold with the gas can be carried out simply by gravitation. The gas must in time find its way to the bottom because it is heavier than air. Any hold can thus be treated, whatever the construction or system of ventilation may be. In the second place the process is perfectly safe. There is not the slightest risk of fire or explosion, and the possibility of asphyxiating any one on board is, with ordinary care, very remote, as the gas is so unpleasant that any one exposed to it would at once become alarmed, and escape long before any dangerous effect was produced; and moreover the gas is visible. A third advantage is that the gas, unlike carbonic oxide, kills insects. A fourth is that, as shown in Dr Wade's report, which on this point confirms and amplifies the results of other observers, the gas produced by the Clayton apparatus is a very efficient disinfectant, provided it penetrates.

" The disadvantages of the process are: (1) That it causes serious damage to various articles of food, such as fruit, flour or meat, and slight damage to metal work, etc. (2) That it is absorbed to a considerable extent by articles of cargo, and therefore penetrates a mass of cargo very slowly. It is thus not nearly so rapid in its action in holds filled with cargo as in empty holds, cabins, etc. Whether it will with certainty kill all rats in a hold after a few hours of continuous treatment is still uncertain."

The damage to metal consists, as stated before, only of slight tarnishing, which cleaning will remove, and as regards the efficiency of the gas in killing rats in a cargo-laden ship there is ample evidence of certainty in the large number of ships that have been successfully treated, provided the gas is retained in the cargo-holds for 12 hours. Cargoes of sugar from the Mauritius are now treated on their arrival at Durban by fumigation with a Clayton machine with excellent results, and with no damage to the cargo.

The objections to fumigation by the ordinary process of burning **Precautions to be taken in carrying out the fumigation.** sulphur are the risk of fire and the bleaching effect which it frequently causes to the goods subjected to the process. Neither of these risks are encountered in fumigating with the Clayton apparatus.

The secret of the success of the method and of no injurious effects being produced either on the texture or colour of the fabrics exposed to the action of the gas, appears to lie in the cooling of the gas before it is forced into the compartment to be fumigated; were it pumped in in a heated condition there would be condensation of moisture and permanent absorption of the gas when it cooled, which would be then liable to damage some of the merchandise. In fumigating, it is important that the compartments already fumigated should not be opened until those adjoining have been filled with gas. This precaution is necessary to prevent the rats escaping into compartments already fumigated. For the same reason it is also necessary to leave no part of

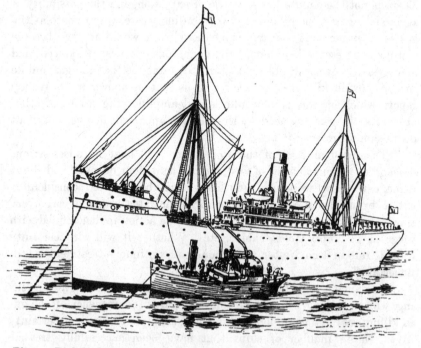

Fig. 1.   Disinfection by Clayton System of laden Steamer infected with Plague.

the ship unfumigated; even the boats should be exposed to the fumes. The duration of the fumigation should be adapted to the size of the ship. For small ships the gas, at a concentrated strength of 10 to 12 %, should be shut into the holds for fully 6 hours, while for the largest vessels and liners it should be for much longer, which need cause no great inconvenience, for if the fumigation is begun in the early morning the cabins which have been disinfected will be fit for occupation at night, while the holds will retain the gas for the whole night. This or similar arrangement will permit of the exposure of the cargo to the action of the gas for 24 hours or longer without inconvenience or much delay. The gas can be used for disinfecting every part of the ship except the decks, which can be washed down with a solution of corrosive sublimate or cyllin. Such a fumigation destroys rats, vermin and plague infection. Fig. 1 shows the Clayton apparatus at work disinfecting a plague-infected ship.

A process which will destroy the rats and insects on ships having commercial relations with plague-infected ports, and will **Uses of the Clayton disinfector on board ship.** at the same time destroy the infection of plague which may be on the ships, and accomplish these without damage to the merchandise and cargo, is a weapon of the utmost value, when properly used in combating the spread of plague. There can be no doubt that the toxic gas generated by the Clayton apparatus is such a weapon, and it is obvious that the general adoption of the Clayton apparatus and its proper use in infected ports, and also in those ports which have commercial relations with infected ports, will secure a greater degree of safety with less inconvenience, delay and expense than has been attained by the existing precautions or by quarantine. Ships, especially mail steamers, carrying a disinfector on board can under the supervision of their medical officer readily be fumigated and have their rats destroyed on the voyage and before arriving in port. Ships carrying emigrants, coolies and soldiers, also cargoes of fodder, forage and grain, would be less liable to transport disease if periodically subjected to the action of the gas.

In the case of transit ports, where only a small amount of cargo is taken on, and it is impossible to clear the hold of the ship of all the rats which have been killed by the fumigation, it is sufficient to fill up the hold with gas and keep it there until the port of arrival is reached, to prevent the rats which have been killed from decomposing.

Baggage on suspected and infected ships is far more expeditiously **Disinfection of baggage.** and conveniently disinfected by the Clayton process than by any other. This can be done before the passengers arrive at port, if a disinfector is carried by the ship, or it can be done by the local authority on arrival of the ship.   If there is no Clayton apparatus, the older processes will have to be adopted, which may be exposure of the baggage and personal effects to the fumes of sulphur, which is useless, or to the fumes of formalin, or boiling of the effects in water, or soaking them in water to which a disinfectant has been added, or subjecting them to steam sterilisation.   The employment of boiling water, disinfectants or steam is inapplicable to feathers, leather, furs, skins, and other goods, as they would be spoiled.

The use of the apparatus is not limited to maritime commerce; it is useful on shore as well.   One of the features of plague in South Africa and elsewhere has been the number of railway stations and stores in which plague rats have been discovered, the infection most probably having been conveyed in the cargo by the trains.   Disinfection of warehouses by the gas, fumigation of cargo at the place of departure and, if need be, at the place of arrival, and disinfection of railway carriages in like manner, are practical measures likely to be most useful in preventing the spread of the disease from infected localities.   Its utility in disinfection of plague-infected houses will be referred to later on.

One of the most conspicuous features in the history of plague epidemics and of the measures taken for their prevention is the constant unpreparedness to combat the disease. In Marseilles in 1720, though there was a quarantine station, there were no arrangements for dealing with plague should it arise.   It was on the 25th of May that the plague ship which is believed to have brought the infection arrived; it was the 9th of July before the first case of plague was recognised among the residents of Marseilles, and it was not until the 3rd of August that it was decided that 150 citizens should be appointed to look after the wants of the poor, and not until the 8th before it was resolved to establish a pest-house.   To combat plague, promptitude, foresight and action on scientific lines are required at every stage.

Necessity to be in a state of preparedness.

The precautionary measures to prevent the importation of plague should be supplemented by others which are of an anticipatory character and which have for their object not only the dealing promptly with a possible outbreak of plague, but also the early discovery of rat plague and the destruction of rats.   The actual organisation for this purpose does not require to be on more than a very moderate scale, but it is necessary that it shall be conceived on a liberal basis, so as to allow of ready adaptation to the circumstances which may arise.

Local measures to be adopted in anticipation of an outbreak.

Preparation should be made beforehand by the health authorities for the rapid and ample provision of temporary hospitals for the sick, and observation wards for doubtful cases; for the selection of reception houses, lazarettos or health camps for contacts, until the infected houses are disinfected; for the burial of the dead; and for a special plague organisation. It is unnecessary to enter minutely into the kind of hospital required for plague cases, which will depend very much on the locality, the resources available, and the people to be treated.

Certain principles should be adopted, whatever the structure of the building. First of all, it is not advisable for the hospital **Certain principles should underlie the erection of plague hospitals.** or hospitals to be erected too far from the infected town, otherwise conveyance from the home to the hospital may be too fatiguing for the patient. There is no danger in a properly constructed plague hospital being erected inside the town so long as it is kept free from rats and is sufficiently isolated from other buildings; secondly, it is of the greatest importance that every ward should have plenty of sunlight and very free ventilation—the more the patients are subjected to the open-air treatment the better is their chance of recovery; thirdly, overcrowding must be avoided at all costs, because crowding together of patients appears to intensify the virulence of infection; fourthly, the cases should as far as possible be classified, mild cases being placed together and not mixed up with the more serious—pneumonic cases appear to do best in tents; and fifthly, accommodation should be provided for different classes. The structure of the hospital should be as simple as possible.

The accommodation in hospital, health camp, observation wards, and their number of staff, medical, nursing, and employees will, in the event of a serious outbreak, require to be increased many times without delay, and arrangements should accordingly be made to meet this contingency.

Attached to the hospital but separate from it within the enclosure of the hospital premises should be receiving rooms, observation wards, administrative block, bacteriological laboratory, mortuary, laundry and disinfecting apparatus, ambulance sheds, destructor for burning excreta, etc., medical officers' quarters, nurses' quarters, and attendants' quarters.

The health camp or observation buildings, in which contacts are lodged until their houses are disinfected, should not be **Health camps.** within the hospital premises, but it is advantageous for them to be near one another. In addition to the necessary accommodation, adequate provision should be made for disinfection and washing the personal effects of those who may be removed. As in the hospitals, so in the health camps or lazarettos, special accommodation is necessary for different classes.

Arrangements require to be made for the proper disposal of the **Arrangements for disposal of the dead.** dead. This has always been a source of difficulty. Burial should not be left to individual and private undertakers without careful supervision, and there should always be in readiness a special organisation to deal with the work, for immediately the mortality rises to any great extent such an organisation only can cope with the pressure of work. Cremation is the most sanitary method of disposal when not objected to.

Nothing ought to be left to the last. A medical service should be **Administrative arrangements.** in readiness for the hospital and health camps and for medical inspection, inoculations, and other medical measures necessary for the town or locality threatened. Similarly, a nursing service has to be provided, and a special plague service under the control of the medical service to carry out the removal of the sick, the transportation of the healthy from infected houses to the reception houses, the cleansing and disinfection of infected houses, the removal of infected articles for destruction or disinfection, the destruction of rats, the inspection of bake-houses, lodging-houses, rag stores, pawnbrokers' shops, warehouses, grain depots, corn and oil chandlers, etc., in the infected locality. Both the special plague service and ordinary sanitary service should be under the direction of the permanent health officer of the town, assisted by a special and adequate medical staff. If there is no medical officer of health then a special officer will be appointed. A dual control is to be avoided if possible. To divorce the ordinary sanitary department from that which is newly constituted for the emergency is to lose the experience of the older department and not to obtain the best work out of the organisation; but to endeavour to deal with plague by the ordinary sanitary department is to court failure, for the routine sanitary work will be neglected and there are measures to be adopted in plague which are not provided for under ordinary circumstances.

The nucleus of a plague department should accordingly be formed capable of rapid extension; provision should also be made for the bacteriological examination of rats, for their regular destruction, and for the general sanitary improvement of the most crowded and insanitary places.

Bacteriological examination of rats should be carried out regularly

in all ports that are in communication with infected ports, and when the ports of a country are infected, then in the inland towns which have commercial relations with these ports. As the docks and the neighbourhood of the docks are the localities in a port in which the rat is likely to become first infected with plague, the health conditions of the rat in these localities should be carefully watched, which can only be efficiently done by systematic and regular bacteriological examination. A bacteriologist should be employed whose duty is to record daily the result of the bacteriological examination of rats brought to him from different parts of the docks. In inland towns the same watch is to be kept over the rats in the markets and their neighbourhood, the railway stations, sheds and store-houses belonging to them, the granaries, warehouses, rag stores, slaughter-houses, workshops, and restaurants. .

The susceptibility of rats and mice to plague, and their powers of

disseminating the disease, render it imperative as . a precautionary measure that these animals should be destroyed in a healthy locality carrying on an extensive traffic with an infected centre. The destruction of the rats and mice removes a dangerous breeding ground for plague. By clearing the healthy port beforehand of its indigenous rats and mice, the locality is, to a certain extent, immunised. The measure is, for plague, as necessary a sanitary precaution as the provision beforehand of an unpolluted supply of water on the occasion of a threatened invasion of cholera. In cholera the water contaminated with the microbe disseminates the disease. In plague rats and mice infected with the plague bacillus disseminate plague. The two agencies may not be of the same importance and rank in their respective spheres. In the case of cholera contaminated water is the chief disseminator and with a protected supply a large epidemic is impossible. It would be rash to assert an equivalent relationship between infected rats and plague epidemics, but there can be little doubt that if there are no rats and mice to infect, plague has a greater difficulty in effecting a lodgement and spreading widely in a locality. The contagion having been transported to a healthy place by sick mice or sick rats or by infected baggage and merchandise, the indigenous rats appear to be, in a number of cases, the link in the chain connecting the new epidemic with the old, and if that link is wanting there is in those cases no serious epidemic.

A systematic destruction of rats should also be carried out both
in ports and in inland towns in those localities which
are apt to be infected.   To accomplish this the co-
operation of the inhabitants should, if possible, be
obtained, who by means of traps and rat poison, such as
arsenic, phosphorus and strychnine mixed with flour, can
destroy large numbers, especially if a small reward is offered for
each rat brought in to the depot.   For the destruction of rats by the
local authorities two processes are useful and can be both used with
advantage.   The first is the fumigation with sulphurous
gas of the sewers, warehouses, depots, stores, markets,
stables, and sheds by Clayton's apparatus; and the second
is by the employment of cultures of Danysz' bacillus for
poisoning rats.   The bacillus of Danysz isolated by him
from field mice suffering from an epizootic which spontaneously broke out in the laboratory is harmless to man and to all
domestic animals, but is pathogenic to mice and rats.   Its power of
causing an epizootic among rats is, however, limited, and it is far from
being able to produce an epizootic either so diffuse or destructive as
plague in these animals.   Even plague which is so destructive to them
does not totally destroy the rat colonies in a town.   The bacilli of
Loeffler and Löser are pathogenic to mice and not to rats.   The Loeffler
bacillus or bacillus typhi murium is pathogenic to ordinary mice (mus
masculus) and field mice (mus agricola); the bacillus of Löser is fatal to
mus agrarius, that of Mereshkowsky to ground squirrels.

A careful watch at the same time has to be kept on the nature of
sickness prevalent and on the causes of death.   The
sputum of lung cases not clearly due to other causes
should be systematically examined and if thought necessary
a thorough bacteriological examination should be made
and the cultures tested on animals.   This watch has to
be specially kept on the sickness prevalent in the poorer
quarters, for plague is essentially a disease of the poor, attaching
itself to the poorest, most crowded, and filthiest localities of a town.
General sanitary measures for the whole of a town or a district
necessarily form a part of the ordinary routine against disease, epidemic
or otherwise, but zeal and expenditure in this direction must not be
allowed to overshadow the special measures that are required against
plague.   The display of exceptional effort and the adoption of extraordinary measures in the general cleaning and disinfecting of the streets

*Methods
available for
the destruc-
tion of rats.
Traps and
poison.*

*Fumigation
with Clay-
ton's appara-
tus.*

*The employ-
ment of
Danysz'
bacillus.*

*A careful
watch on
prevalent
sickness re-
quired,
especially in
the poorer
quarters.*

outside the most susceptible areas may assist in allaying public alarm, but they will not exercise the slightest influence on the progress of an epidemic of plague any more than they will arrest an epidemic of small-pox. It is not general measures that are required but special measures against special localities. Plague, in addition to being disseminated by rats, has been observed to be favoured in its prevalence by darkness and dampness, and is believed to be assisted in its spread by vermin in general. No time should be lost in the application of measures having for their object the removal of these causes, especially in common lodging and tenement houses.

CHAPTER XIX.

MEASURES TO COMBAT AN OUTBREAK OF PLAGUE IN A LOCALITY.

Preliminary observations as to the hindrances to a locality being declared infected with plague.

IN the past all great outbursts of plague have been remarkable for the similarity of their history. The obscurity of the earlier cases, the contradictory opinions of medical men, the apprehension of the merchants as to the injury which plague would inflict on their commerce, and the alarm of the populace at the very name of plague, have always been against the early recognition of the disease and have led to denial of its existence or to great delay in admitting that the disease was plague. Controversy was substituted for immediate action, with the consequence that the necessary precautions which are invaluable at the commencement were not taken until too late. Muriatori, referring to such occurrences in connection with plague, instances the plague at Venice in 1576, at Florence in 1630, at Malta in 1675, and at Venice in 1713. Russell in dealing with the same subject refers to the Marseilles and Messina epidemics of 1720 and 1743. In 1720 Chicoyneau and Verny, sent by the King to study the disease which had prevailed for some time at Marseilles, recognised its true nature three months after the disease first began. Messina is worthy of quotation[1]: "In that plague it appears that after the death of the master and one of the mariners of the ship, which brought the infection from the Morea in the latter end of March, the ship and cargo were destroyed and the remaining crew were put under a rigorous quarantine. That, no other accidents intervening, the first alarm subsiding, the people resumed confidence as if all had been over, and the 15th of May was appointed for a Te Deum in the cathedral. That the ceremony was interrupted after the people were assembled by a physician who declared that he had reason for thinking that the plague

[1] Russell on the Plague, 1791, pp. 513 and 514.

was actually in the place. A declaration which endangered his own life, it being with difficulty he made his escape from the fury of the populace, and though from that period to the end of the month between three and four hundred perished of a distemper which he continued to affirm was the genuine plague, no precautions were taken. He persisted singly in his opinion against the rest of the faculty, who, in spite of unequivocal symptoms, contended it was only an ordinary epidemic distemper. On the 31st of May an assembly of thirty physicians there concurred in a formal attestation of its not being the plague. Lastly, that the funerals soon increased to one hundred daily, Government at length, but too late, took the alarm, and dreadful scenes of unparalleled anarchy followed." The diseases that have been most commonly confounded with plague are typhoid and typhus fever, gastro-enteritis, diphtheria, influenza, pneumonia, different forms of pernicious intermittent fever, parotiditis, scrofula, and syphilis, apoplexy and meningitis.

With the discovery of the plague bacillus one great obstacle in the way of the early adoption of preventive measures against plague has been removed. Still, even with the assistance which is given in the detection of plague cases by bacteriological methods, many difficulties are met with in dealing promptly with plague immediately it appears in a locality. Human nature is still the same and is liable to be swayed in the same way and by the same influences as formerly, and although the diagnosis of plague can with certainty be established with the adoption of accurate methods, yet the different forms that plague assumes, its insidious character, and its likeness often to diseases already prevalent in the locality, are circumstances which surround its early recognition with difficulties, especially when medical men are in-experienced with its symptoms, diagnosis, and Protean forms. Two features are specially characteristic of plague. They are, first, the slow, irregular and gradual manner in which the disease acquires a hold over a locality into which it is imported and which may later on become the scene of an epidemic; and secondly, the obscurity which often surrounds the earlier cases. The first is apt to raise false hopes of the disease dying out, to cause the procrastination of effective measures, and to favour the postponement of careful enquiries into the disease at a stage when its movements and mode of spread are more easily followed than later on. The other gives rise to disputes as to the nature of the disease and consequently to the loss of valuable time.

It is not surprising under these circumstances that the early cases most probably escape detection, and that even when suspicion arises the responsibility which is incurred by the medical man who announces the appearance of plague in a community is shirked while there is the slightest doubt on the subject. That doubt can only be removed by a thorough knowledge of the disease, both from a clinical and bacteriological point of view.

Even when the diagnosis is made, other considerations come into play, tending, if possible, to conceal or minimise the extent of the outbreak. Commercial, political, and social forces nearly always range themselves against the first announcement of plague in a town. Every endeavour is made to show that the medical man is mistaken and that there is some sinister motive underlying his statement. Plague has lost none of its terrors to the general population, to whom it means some ill-defined fear, restriction, or loss, and it is met often by a blind denial of its existence. The same mistake is repeated over and over again. It is forgotten or unrecognised that plague is not influenced by policies however subtle, and that no denial of its presence when in the midst of a community will in the slightest degree affect the course it may take.

Commercial, political, and social forces nearly always range themselves against the first announcement of plague in a town.

No disease has raised so much controversy as to its existence when it first appears in a locality. In Bombay, when Dr Viegas in September, 1896, announced that plague prevailed in the city, ways and means were discovered to throw discredit on his judgment, and valuable time was wasted in controversy. The same controversy happened in 1896 and 1898 in Calcutta, it threatened to recur in Cape Town in 1901, it made itself manifest in San Francisco, and was apparently not absent in 1903 in Johannesburg when the presence of plague might be expected to be particularly dreaded[1].

Controversies in Bombay, Calcutta, Cape Town, and San Francisco.

In connection with Johannesburg, where plague broke out in March, 1904, the following antecedent circumstances in 1903 are instructive because of the difficulties, even with the employment of the bacteriological test, of recognising beyond doubt early cases of plague.

Case No. 1. February 9th, 1903. A Jew (M. L.) living in a crowded tenement house in Becker Street, book-keeper in forage store. Sickened 9th February; high temperature; considerable prostration; when seen on 12th February had large bubo in right groin; no venereal history, but slight abrasion on meatus urinarius afterwards noted. Patient

Reported cases of suspected plague in Johannesburg.

---

[1] Report of the Medical Officer of Health for period from 1st July, 1902, to 30th June, 1903. By Charles Porter, M.D., D.P.H.

removed to venereal ward of lazaretto, where glands were removed. He eventually recovered. *Bacillus pestis* could not be found in the blood and no bacteria of any kind in stained sections of groin glands.

Cases Nos. 2 and 3. March 21st, 1903. Dutch mason and wife in Vrededorp. Man had been suffering from asthma (5 years) and pneumonia (14 days) with some swelling of neck glands, and died suddenly at 8 a.m. from heart failure. Woman who was pregnant miscarried from shock, bled profusely, and died at 9 a.m. Neither in the post-mortem nor bacteriological examination was there the slightest indication of plague, but the organism of pneumonia (pneumococcus) was found in both cases. Before the Medical Officer of Health could get to the house, however, white-helmeted policemen had been posted there and alarm created locally that was most unnecessary.

Case No. 4. March 28th, 1903. Native "John," who died suddenly at 71, Korte Street. Had come from Krugersdorp some three weeks before; large bubo in right arm-pit; right arm and right side of chest swollen and oedematous. Congestion of bases of both lungs. No plague bacillus found, but pneumococcus present.

Case No. 5. April 11th, 1903. Male adult, native, employed at the hospital. Had an ordinary, but very large abscess in right arm-pit. Removed to lazaretto, abscess opened, and boy soon recovered. Neither the organism of plague nor that of pneumonia was found.

Case No. 6. April 19th, 1903. Boy died suddenly in Pritchard Street, and police were informed by medical man who was called in, that death was due to plague. Post-mortem made same day by district surgeon, who returned death due to "scurvy and heart disease," adding that "there was absolutely no sign of plague" and that he thought the practitioner in question should be asked on what he had based his diagnosis and created quite an unjustifiable panic. Nothing suggestive of plague was found bacteriologically.

Case No. 7. April 28th, 1903. Zulu "Pesuana." This boy was removed to hospital from a store in Eloff Street on April 27th; developed a large abscess and brawny swelling in right axilla on April 28th; was removed to the plague camp on the 29th and on admission there presented bloodshot eyes, brown tongue, sordes on lips, and was semi-comatose, dying on April 30th. The medical man who was attending him had no doubt that he was suffering from plague. This belief received confirmation from the naked-eye post-mortem appearances which were typical of that disease, as well as from the boy's statement that he had only arrived in Johannesburg from Natal 16 days before.

This case occasioned grave anxiety and as the boy's pass could not be found some days elapsed before he could be traced at the Pass Office, when, however, it was found that he had been at least four months at Johannesburg. Portions of the affected glands and of the spleen were examined bacteriologically and were both found to contain very virulent pneumococci, but there was no indication of the plague bacillus, and the case was therefore one of severe pneumonia.

Case No. 8. April 28th, 1903. Native boy from Saver Street. Sickened on April 28th. Seen by medical attendant and Medical Officer of Health on April 30th; large bubo and brawny swelling in right groin; bloodshot eyes, extremely prostrate and ill. Removed at once to plague camp and died on May 1st. Had not been out of Johannesburg for ten months. Results of post-mortem and bacteriological examination were almost identical with the preceding case (No. 7) and death was eventually ascribed to pneumonia.

In each of the foregoing cases stringent measures of disinfection were adopted, the names and addresses of contacts were taken, their clothing and persons were purified and they were kept under observation for fourteen days. The only case which caused real anxiety was No. 7, owing largely to the sufferer's statement that he had only just come up from Natal. On May 20th it was reported that four coolies had died very suddenly in the location. They had, however, been attended by a medical man, and he was able to state there was no suspicion of plague.

On December 22nd, 1903, a notice was placarded offering 3*d.* per

Rats.   head for every rat brought in to the Corporation depots, and in every suspicious case the rats were forwarded to the Government bacteriologist for examination but in no instance was the plague bacillus found.

In January, 1903, a notable mortality amongst rats was noticed at Henwood's Arcade and the bodies of several were examined with negative results. In April, 1903, complaint was received of rats dying in large numbers in the Market Buildings, and the bodies of 38 (taken from beneath flooring, etc.) were sent to the Government bacteriologist but were too decomposed for examination by him. Other 15, also decomposed, were afterwards found, and on the strength of this, a local reporter, to whom the true facts of the matter had been carefully explained by the Medical Officer of Health, deliberately published a false and very alarming statement to the effect that the rats in the market were infected, and that 400 rats had been found there.

This statement together with rumours which obtained credence in regard to the Zulu Pesuana (*vide supra*) gave rise to the belief, which was cabled to Europe, that there was plague in Johannesburg, and in consequence the following telegram was sent on May 2nd to the Medical Officer by H.E. the Lieutenant-Governor:—"Suspected cases from Johannesburg not bubonic plague. Five cases have been recently referred to Government Laboratory but none have been plague. All cases have been deaths of natives who died suddenly and three cases presented enlarged glands. Enlargement in all cases was due to bacteria other than plague, namely, bacteria of pneumonia, bacteria to which natives in this country appear to be unusually susceptible. Please publish this information."

In many cases of plague Kitasato's bacillus is the only microbe to be found in the blood and tissues and it has such a resemblance to the diplococcus pneumoniae that it creates hesitation in early cases unless the clinical features of plague are also present. The next that is heard of plague in Johannesburg is on the 21st of March, 1904, when 30 deaths were reported from plague.

For the successful isolation of the plague bacillus when mixed with the pneumococcus care requires to be taken to cultivate the plague bacillus at a low temperature by which the pneumococcus and other bacilli may be eliminated. Dr W. C. Pakes[1] and Dr F. H. Joseph have recently recommended the employment of broth with an acidity of + 25 or + 30, and incubated at 37° C. The acidity inhibits the growth of the pneumococcus but does not affect that of the plague bacillus. The resulting cultivation is then injected into guinea-pigs or rabbits.

There is no disease which creates so much alarm and excitement as plague. When an epidemic has once developed and unless

No disease which creates so much alarm as plague.

care is taken to allay the state of panic that is likely to arise, the feeling of the populace among excitable nations may readily culminate in disturbances or hostile demonstrations. Of course this will largely depend on the nationality affected with plague. In Iquique in Chili the medical authorities were obstructed in their duties; in Calcutta some of the medical men were attacked; in Poona the Commissioner directing plague operations was shot; in Cawnpore the native apothecary engaged on plague duties was

---

[1] "The use of acid media in the isolation of the plague bacillus," *British Medical Journal*, January 21, 1905.

burnt; in Bombay there were riots; in Cape Town the Malays had to be firmly dealt with, as they were inclined to assume a hostile attitude.

The great mortality of plague is apt to produce the impression among the ignorant and turbulent that those taken to hospital are poisoned by the doctors. In past times, when plague patients were not removed to hospital, the great mortality was frequently ascribed to poisoning of the wells by Jews and others, with the result that popular resentment spent its fury on these innocent people.

There are generally two periods of alarm. One is when plague is first announced, the second is when, after a considerable period of slight fluctuations in regard to the daily numbers, there is suddenly a great increase of cases and deaths and the epidemic has fairly set in, rapidly rising to a crisis.

At both periods there is flight of the inhabitants. The first flight is comparatively harmless from the point of view of spreading the disease, because very few of the inhabitants are infected. From this aspect, the flight is likely to be beneficial than otherwise, because it tends to reduce overcrowding, which is an important factor in the spread of plague. The second flight, on the other hand, is dangerous on account of the large numbers of infected persons taking their infected personal effects with them and thus spreading the disease in the healthy localities to which they go

Panic will not be prevented by the authorities concealing the number of cases of plague, for rumour will soon magnify the number of those not reported. A daily report with the actual number of new cases with the locality in which they occur, and the publication in the newspapers and by hand-bills of a few simple rules which may be carried **Firmness and** out by each householder to protect the inmates against **judgment** **required from** plague, will materially assist in restoring confidence, which **the com-** will be strengthened if the authorities act from the com- **mencement.** mencement with firmness and judgment. Vacillation will almost inevitably lead to disturbances, and certainly, later on, to an epidemic.

If there is to be a panic it is better to take place early than late, as flight at the commencement does but comparatively little harm and will at most be short in duration. The risk lies in the possibilities of the authorities relaxing at this stage the active and stringent measures which they have decided on and thus allow the disease to gain ground. When plague has once assumed epidemic proportions no measures that are known will arrest the natural course of the epidemic in the particular locality in which it is raging. They can only act as checks and palliatives and as such require to be used with discretion.

Measures necessary at the commencement not suitable when the epidemic is beyond control. Measures which are imperatively necessary at the commencement, having for their object the arrest or control of the disease, and which entail the removal of every sick person to the hospital, and the isolation of contacts, cannot be fully carried out, unless under exceptional circumstances, at the height of an extensive epidemic. To do so is only to add to the alarm and to increase the desire on the part of the inhabitants to leave the locality, both of which it is most important to allay, first because of the danger of hostile demonstrations, and secondly because of the risk of infection to which the surrounding healthy districts will be exposed. Great activity in the removal of the sick when an extensive epidemic is approaching its height is a waste of energy which might with more profit be expended in other directions. For instance it is better to be directed to the protection of the healthy in the infected districts and to the safeguarding of the surrounding localities in which plague has not yet gained a foothold.

In combating plague an accurate diagnosis is all-important, and **Accurate diagnosis essential, and its difficulties.** unless the most careful examination is made in every instance the difficulties of diagnosis in early cases are manifold, owing often to the masked character of the disease. Plague has been mistaken for influenza, lymphangitis, pneumonia, bronchitis, pleurisy, typhoid fever, typhus fever, malarial fever, relapsing fever, yellow fever, rheumatic fever, septicaemia, pericarditis, endocarditis, peritonitis, appendicitis, dysentery, gastric enteritis, beri-beri, syphilis, venereal bubo, non-venereal bubo, mumps, adenitis, and parotitis. In Bombay some of the earlier cases with swollen cervical glands and throat symptoms were mistaken for diphtheria. In Jedda, where lung symptoms predominated, the earlier cases were taken for influenza. In Calcutta some of the cases were attributed to syphilis, others to non-venereal buboes. Dr Kinyoun[1] relates some instructive cases in this connection.

" In San Francisco a case of illness occurred which, clinically, was that of typhoid fever, passed muster as such until three weeks later the autopsy and bacteriological examination demonstrated plague. Another case was clinically that of diphtheria, but no cultures were made from the throat; antitoxin was administered when the case was

---

[1] "The prophylaxis of Plague," by J. J. Kinyoun, M.D., *The Journal of the American Medical Association*, Vol. XLII. No. 3.

moribund. During his last hours, while in delirium, he coughed and spat in the nurse's face, some of the sputum entering the eye. The nurse was immediately immunised with large doses of diphtheria anti-toxin. Despite this precaution she became ill within less than 30 hours and died of an acute fever four days later. Autopsy revealed an acute septicaemia due to plague. Another gave a typical history of lobar pneumonia and the death certificate was made out accordingly.

" The room in which the patient died was closed for two weeks, when it was occupied by a woman and child. Four or five days after occupancy both became ill, one with bubonic, the other with pneumonic plague. A case was diagnosed as phlegmonous erysipelas and was treated as such for 10 days, but on post-mortem examination plague bacilli were isolated from the phlegmonous tissues, the heart's blood and spleen. Another case occurring soon afterwards certainly did present the evidences of acute myocarditis. The blood, however, showed leucocytes and pest-like bacilli. The autopsy was confirmatory of plague septicaemia. In Hongkong I saw in consultation a case which all of us agreed was one of acute appendicitis requiring immediate surgical interference. The blood showed considerable increase in the number of the white cells and many malarial parasites. The surgeon concluded to wait until quinine had been administered. On the next day the patient was worse, temperature higher, slight effusion into the peritoneum. The operation was deferred and death occurred on the next day. Autopsy revealed a plague infection of the retro-peritoneal glands near the appendix. In a case of a child in Manila presenting all the symptoms of a catarrhal pneumonia, autopsy confirmatory, the bacteriological examination showed the cause to be plague bacillus."

In a country in which beri-beri prevails sudden death from heart failure due to plague would not unlikely at first be assigned to beri-beri. In Japan plague in some instances was mistaken for beri-beri and a similar mistake was made in Manila. It is not improbable that some of the cases were really beri-beri attacked with plague.

The early diagnosis of plague is the first essential to success in dealing with the prevention of the disease in a locality in which it appears. Failure to recognise the nature of the disease allows a start which is not readily overtaken. It requires to be borne in mind that plague may occur without external signs of buboes, and that cases may arise without appearing to have the slightest connection with each other. The diagnosis must rest on the clinical features, on bacteriological examination, and on the history of the case. There are three varieties of the disease which require special attention from the obscurity of their symptoms. These are the siderans, fulminating or septicaemic cases, the pneumonic, and the ambulatory cases. The symptoms of pneumonic plague may be so obscure as to even perplex experts thoroughly acquainted with the disease. This is illustrated by the Vienna outbreak in which Drs Müller and Ghon, members of the Austrian Plague Commission to Bombay, were for several days in doubt as to the true character of the disease from which Barisch, the assistant in the pathological laboratory, was suffering. It is important, therefore, that all lung affections should be bacteriologically examined when plague is threatened. Similarly with ambulant plague or pestis minor, it is not unusual for these cases when occurring at the commencement of an epidemic, to be attributed to some other cause such as malaria, venereal disease, strain, mumps, scrofulous glandular enlargement, and the glandular fever of children. Again, persons with plague may appear to be only slightly indisposed, and yet die suddenly. Accordingly when a district is liable to be threatened with plague, a most careful watch requires to be kept over the character of the prevalent sickness and of the causes of death, and if there occur cases of disease about which uncertainty arises as to whether they are plague or not, or there are cases with anomalous symptoms with sudden or unexpected death, no pains should be spared to arrive at a definite diagnosis by a most careful and thorough examination, and in the event of the slightest doubt the case or cases should be treated as plague and the necessary precautions taken. Over-caution is easily rectified and can do no harm, whereas neglect to deal with a true case of plague because of the doubts which exist as to its exact nature, may be followed by the most unfortunate results: once plague has been recognised in a locality inactivity and procrastination are unpardonable, for it is only at the beginning that preventive measures have a chance of success. It is then that measures which ensure early diagnosis and notification of the disease are of supreme importance.

The diagnosis of plague having been made in an infected locality the machinery previously designed and organised to deal with the plague, and if possible, to stamp it out should be set in motion. The forces to combat plague should, as it were, be mobilised, and operations should be begun at once. The invasion of a locality by the plague bacillus differs from that of a hostile army in that the movements of the former are less discoverable, its resources are greater in that it possesses the power of self-

Plague organisation previously planned to be mobilised.

multiplication, and it is only recognised by its effects. For these reasons its attack is likely to be more serious and destructive than that of any army if not resolutely met at the beginning. No expenditure is considered too great to defeat and get rid of an invading army, but, as a rule, in the case of plague, there is not the same solicitude at the early stage when it is possible, and when the organisation and expenditure are most likely to be effective.

Prompt notification of cases of plague or suspected plague by the medical attendant and householder is one of the means of securing early intelligence of human cases, but it must be supplemented by the search for cases among the very poor by visitation of the houses, by medical officers, and by following up the results obtained by a systematic bacteriological examination of the rats in the different districts into which the infected locality should be divided for the purposes of administration. Special search for cases should always be made in localities in which the rats are found to be infected.

Notification to be supplemented by visitation of houses, and other measures.

Too great reliance is not to be placed on notification by medical men, even in those towns in which notification of infectious disease is a matter of ordinary routine in other epidemic diseases, for the poorer people will very often not call in medical aid in plague cases. The notification is therefore supplemented by house-to-house visitation. The searching out of plague cases is no new system. It was provided for in England in the ordinances of James I. At that time women were employed none of whom had any special knowledge of the disease; most of them were derived from a class that was not very trustworthy. They were assisted, when required, by surgeons. Now the visitors are, or should be, medical men and medical women assisted by sanitary inspectors. In the absence of a trained sanitary service in India, laymen had to direct the operations against plague, and, in a number of instances, soldiers had to be employed for house-to-house inspection. Neither soldiers nor policemen are fitted for this work, and they are more likely than other agencies to cause resentment, panic, and concealment of cases, which are serious obstacles to the proper working of an organisation intended to check the plague. The disease whether in force in a locality or not should be sought out by medical inspectors, and their attention directed not only to sickness among people, but also to sickness and mortality among animals, particularly among rats, mice and cats. Encouragement should be given to all householders, especially in the affected area, to notify to the central or local health officer the occurrence of sudden or suspicious illness in their households. For

Information to house-holders.

this purpose advice to that effect, together with a description of the common symptoms of plague, should be printed on leaflets, distributed in the affected area, and published in the newspapers. Similarly the illness and mortality of rats and mice should be described and the inhabitants urged to report any unusual sickness or mortality they may note among these animals. There is no difficulty in recognising the disease in rats. The rat affected with plague usually leaves its usual hiding-place and comes out into the open. It is seen at once to be very ill, and is generally in a dazed condition; its eyes are watery and bleary, its coat is probably sometimes partially deprived of hair, it hobbles about with difficulty, and it staggers and falls. It has lost its timidity of man in its evident desire for fresh air, and it has no energy to attempt to escape. On account of the disposition of the sick rats to leave their runs when ill of plague, the epizootic among them whether in a house, warehouse, market or street, can hardly fail to attract notice if the attention of the inhabitants is directed to the subject, though in some instances, such as in Cape Town, the mortality of rats was not particularly noticeable until the floors of infected houses were taken up and examined. A daily and systematic inspection by the sanitary staff of houses, especially those that are old and dilapidated, cellars, warehouses, chandlers, corn-chandlers, oil-shops, bakeries, groceries, stables, hay-lofts, and other buildings which are likely to be infested with rats and mice, is necessary to ascertain the presence of sick rats.

The examination of rats which is another means of notification is not

Bacterio-logical ex-amination of rats.

a quick process, and the bacteriologist will seldom be able to examine more than 100 or at most 150 a day, so that to overtake the many that are likely to be brought for examination by the rat-catchers, inspectors, and others, it is essential that a large staff of bacteriologists shall be employed for this work alone. The more rats examined in the infected and other parts of the town, the more exactly can the course of infection be traced, so far as it is disseminated by the rat, the more accurately the non-infected localities be ascertained, and the more precisely preventive measures can be applied. The address or locality at which the rat is found is written on a label and fixed to the animal. If it proves to be an infected animal the information thus recorded permits of preventive measures being taken in the infected house or locality before man may be attacked. All rats after examination should be cremated. At the time of collection from the houses they are taken up with short tongs and dipped in a bucket containing a disinfectant.

It will be unnecessary in a work of this kind to give more than an
Outline of a plague organisation. outline of the organisation required to combat plague. Such an organisation will consist of several sub-departments to carry out specific duties, and the whole will be presided over by a Medical Director with the requisite professional assistance and clerical staff to administer, direct and co-ordinate the necessary operations in the campaign against plague.

The subjoined plan gives an outline of such an organisation.

Outline of Plague Organisation.

Medical Director with Assistants
and clerical Staff.

| Bacterio-logists. | District Medical Officers. | Medical Inoculators. | Hospital and health camp staff, medical and nursing and administrative establishments. | Superintendent and trained Inspectors with establishment. | Medical Inspectors for port and rail-ways. | Committee for scientific investigation of the disease. |

The Plague Department as thus constituted would for executive purposes be associated with the sanitary inspectors. The Chief Sanitary Inspector would probably be appointed as Superintendent of the Plague Department, and under him some of the smartest sanitary inspectors, their places being temporarily filled up for routine sanitary work by new men.

To the bacteriologists would be assigned the duties of (*a*) performing
Duties of the plague organisation. autopsies, (*b*) examining rats and other animals, (*c*) examining suspected cases, (*d*) preparing the virus of Danysz, (*e*) preparing Haffkine's prophylactic.

The same laboratory which would be near the mortuary will suffice for the bacteriological examination of specimens and preparations from suspected cases of plague alive or dead, and of specimens and preparations from the rats brought for examination, but it is advisable to have another laboratory elsewhere for the preparation of Danysz' cultures and Haffkine's prophylactic.

To the district medical officers who should place themselves in close association with the medical practitioners of the district would be allotted the duties of visiting their district to discover, locate, and examine all cases of suspected sickness; of tracing out the history of cases of plague or suspected plague that have been reported; of supervising removal of patients from infected houses, the disinfection of houses, reporting insanitary conditions in houses or buildings visited requiring rectification; and of inspecting the markets in the district.

To the medical inoculators would fall the duties of inoculating as many persons as possible with Haffkine's prophylactic or Yersin's serum.

To the superintendent, trained inspectors, and establishment, which would be divided into convenient corps, would be given the duties to remove plague cases to hospital, and contacts to health camp or reception house, to arrange and carry out the burial of plague cases, to disinfect houses or blocks of houses infected with plague, to disinfect clothes and articles likely to be affected, to distribute Danysz' virus or other rat poison, to destroy rats in sewers, warehouses, etc., by fumigation, to take up floors if necessary and remove dead rats after disinfection, to collect dead rats for bacteriological examination and to cremate them afterwards. As in the course of their duties the inspectors will be sure to come across a number of houses in which there will be a great accumulation of filth there should be an establishment for its removal.

To the medical inspectors and staff for port and railways would be given the duties to examine passengers and crews of vessels leaving port, to fumigate ships before their departure in order to destroy rats on board, to fumigate railway goods vans, or store sheds likely to contain rats, to examine passengers leaving or arriving from an infected place, and to furnish names and addresses to local authorities.

The sanitary inspectors who carry out the ordinary routine duties of their office will redouble their efforts to keep their respective districts in a clean and sanitary condition, and by associating themselves with the district medical officer will be able to serve notices for cleansing or other sanitary requirements which may be thought necessary in houses that have been disinfected. They will also be able to secure the adoption of alterations that may be required to make houses rat-proof.

To the hospital staff would be entrusted the duties of scrutinising the diagnosis of patients brought to hospital and placing them in the observation wards or in the ordinary wards of the hospital; of treating and nursing the patients; and of carrying out the duties appertaining to an infectious isolation hospital.

To the staff of the health camp or reception house would be assigned the duties of receiving, providing for, and discharging contacts in a condition to be free of the danger of infection.

To the Committee for scientific investigation of the disease would be assigned the testing by experiment, observation and enquiry with the object of their solution all those difficult problems, with reference to plague and its methods of extension, which continually arise during a plague epidemic.

The most important suppressive measures employed in a plague-infected locality are isolation of the sick, evacuation of infected houses until they are thoroughly disinfected, disinfection of infected houses, destruction of rats in infected districts, preventive inoculation, and supervision over departures by ship and rail. These are carried out by the special plague organisation with its intelligence department for the early discovery of plague in human beings and in animals, more especially rats.

The most important measures for the suppression of plague.

Isolation of the sick from the healthy is essential in all cases. Plague occurs for the most part in insanitary and over-crowded localities, and under these circumstances the isolation can only be properly effected by removal to hospital. In the early stages of an epidemic, it is safer to remove every case because some even of the bubonic cases may develop secondary pneumonia, and thus becoming highly infectious may give rise to cases of primary pneumonic plague. There are instances, however, in which by reason of the condition of the patient, or the excellence of the surroundings, the disease having been contracted elsewhere, removal to hospital need not be insisted upon, but in these cases special care has to be taken that the nursing be of a skilled kind, which at the same time will ensure isolation and proper disinfection of discharges. For this purpose, then, an organisation against plague is incomplete unless it has skilled nurses, not only for the patients in the plague hospitals, but also for those patients who are permitted to remain at home.

Segregation.

Isolation of the sick in hospital does not remove the infection of the rats and other vermin which probably gave rise to the disease; it only removes one source of danger, which, in the bubonic form, is not an important one but which is more important in the case of the pneumonic and septicaemic types, the sputum and discharges of which are likely to infect whatever articles they come in contact with. An exaggerated opinion of the benefits to be derived from segregation in dealing with plague was entertained at first because of the view that plague spread by human agency only. But now that the main factors in its dissemination appear to be infected clothing, infected animals, and possibly, infected insects, isolation and the results to be obtained by it are likely to be duly estimated at their proper value. At the same time the value of isolation must not be under-estimated because, although the patient is only one source of danger, the infection is of such a character as to produce the others, rats and insects in their turn being liable to be infected by man.

Evacuation of the house until it is free of infection is based on the well-

Evacuation of premises. known fact that plague, once introduced, has a tendency to attack first one and another of the inmates until all or the majority have suffered from plague. To this fact is ascribed in a measure the severity of the epidemics of the 16th and 17th centuries, when the recognised mode of isolating plague patients was to shut them up with the healthy in the infected house and to prevent any egress or ingress by placing a guard or watchman outside the barricaded house. The healthy were thus subjected to the risk of infection from the plague patient as well as from house infection. In every epidemic, even in modern times, there are instances of whole households being destroyed. The infection is remarkably adherent to the house. Not infrequently it has happened that the inhabitants of a house, in which plague has occurred, have been attacked with plague on their return to the house even after a month's absence, and one of the most notable features in cases of annual recrudescences is the persistency with which plague cases occur in the same houses or blocks of houses that were previously infected. The vacating of the infected house until it has been thoroughly disinfected has two objects in view, one of which is to remove healthy persons from a centre of infection; the other is to allow of thorough

Circumstances modifying retention of contacts. disinfection of the house. When the vacating is promptly effected experience has proved that for ordinary bubonic plague the number of contacts falling ill afterwards is comparatively small[1]. If therefore pneumonic cases, and those of the septicaemic variety in which the patient has not been early discovered be excepted, contacts may after two days, which will be generally needed for thorough disinfection of the infected house and household effects, be almost regarded as a negligible factor, and may return to their disinfected houses. They can be kept as well under medical surveillance at their homes as in the health camp or reception house, and can be allowed to go to their work. Inoculation, however, with Haffkine's prophylactic or Yersin's serum should be pressed upon them. This arrangement considerably lessens the number who have to be provided for in the health camp or reception house and at the same

---

[1] Ferrari in 1630, and Cardinal Castaldy in 1657, observed that by evacuation of the infected house less than 5 % of the inmates contracted plague.

time lessens the cost of administration. Before leaving the health camp contacts would require to bathe and put on clean and disinfected clothing. In pneumonic and septicaemic cases it is safer in the early stages of an epidemic to retain the contacts for a period of 8 to 10 days before permitting them to return home. In septicaemic cases much will however depend on the time that has elapsed between the illness of the patient and the notification. If the notification is made soon after illness commences, there is seldom need for a longer period of detention than that necessary to disinfect the house thoroughly. Contacts at home should be visited daily by the medical officer.

When dealing with waifs, strays, migratory people, persons living in lodging-houses, and low-class natives, over whom very little control can be exercised as to their whereabouts at any time, the full period of 10 days in the health camp or reception house should be insisted on. Matters like these would be decided on at the discretion of the medical officer of health or medical director of the plague operations. Evacuation of a whole block of buildings on an infected area, and the transference of the inhabitants to healthy surroundings, is one of the most powerful means of dealing effectually with an epidemic at its commencement. Plague administrators in India are unanimously of opinion that for villages this measure is most effective if it is carried out completely and the villagers are not permitted to visit their infected houses or to reoccupy their houses prematurely. Evacuation on a very large scale is not practicable in towns, but it is found very useful when applied to blocks of buildings or to particular classes of people that may be infected. In Hongkong it was repeatedly found that evacuation of a block of buildings, and housing the people for a time in another block specially provided for them, exercised a very marked influence in controlling the disease in contrast to the result attained when the blocks were not evacuated. The sequence of cases in a block in Hongkong before closing is interesting as it tends to show how plague travels from one house to another in a block or street[1].

No. of House		Date of Case
3	on	April 14th
5	,,	,, 16th
4	,,	,, 18th
7	,,	,, 21st
8	,,	,, 21st
3	,,	,, 23rd
4	,,	,, 24th

[1] Report of the Acting Medical Officer of Health, 1903. Hongkong.

The combined effect of evacuation and inoculation against plague is well illustrated in the occurrences at Cape Town. When plague was found to be spreading rapidly among the natives of Cape Town it was decided to evacuate the plague-infected areas and remove the natives to a location on the outskirts of the town. The accommodation was provided most expeditiously and under great pressure by the Public Works Department. In the course of one afternoon one thousand were removed, and in a short time all the natives in Cape Town, except some that were accommodated by the Harbour Board inside the docks, were removed from the town and placed under sanitary supervision in comfortable huts made of corrugated iron. All except about 12 were inoculated, and with the exception of the first few days of their residence in the location when cases of plague developed among those who already had the disease in their system, there were only four cases afterwards in a community of 7000 persons, and this notwithstanding the fact that the natives went into the town to work at the docks and went into some of the most infected centres of the town. The plague was practically stamped out among the natives but continued among the white and coloured population.

The house having been vacated the next important step is its **Disinfection of** disinfection. For this purpose the practice in vogue in **the house.** towns consists in :

(1) Fumigation of the house by formalin, or by chlorine, or by burning sulphur.

(2) Removal in a closed conveyance of clothes, bedding, and textile articles to a central disinfecting depot to be disinfected by steam.

(3) Stripping of the walls of paper, washing or spraying the walls with a disinfectant, and then scraping them.

(4) Removal of the scrapings and of rags and articles of small value to the yard and burning them.

(5) Washing and scrubbing with disinfectants of the solid furniture, walls, floors, stairs, and other parts of the house.

(6) Disinfection of the drains, yards and premises generally.

(7) The removal of dead rats, if any, from under the floors, and the blocking up of rat runs.

The procedure requires a large staff, first, for the taking of inventories of everything in the house in order that compensation, if claimed, shall be properly adjudged, secondly, for the removal and return of the effects in special conveyances, thirdly, for the disinfection and cleansing of the articles at the central disinfection station, and fourthly for the cleansing and disinfection of the infected house. It, moreover, involves the employment of several methods of disinfection, gaseous, mechanical, chemical, by steam, and by burning, and it is not infrequent after the whole process is completed to find that insects are still alive in the disinfected house, and there is no certainty of having destroyed the rats. With plague increasing rapidly there is difficulty in completing the process in 10 days, and, when completed there are usually many complaints on behalf of the occupiers of infected houses that some of their effects have been spoiled or destroyed by the disinfection, or some are missing and cannot be found. There is nothing which adds so much to the difficulties of dealing with plague as the hostile attitude of the lower classes, who are mainly affected, and much of this hostility is due to the necessity there is under the present methods to remove the healthy from infected houses for periods of 10 days or a fortnight until their houses are disinfected and cleansed, and to the loss or destruction of some of their effects in the procedure. To these may be added the displacement and disturbance of everything in the house.

For these reasons existing methods are cumbersome and far from

Existing methods of disinfection cumbersome and unsatisfactory.
being satisfactory. The formalin is destructive to the microbe in about 3 or 4 hours, but has no penetrative powers and is accordingly insufficient. According to Catterina fumigation with pine wood is more effective, the bacilli being killed in 40 minutes. The sulphur fumigation, although held in high repute in the 16th and 17th centuries, is very uncertain in its action and mostly useless. The burning of sulphur in the open air only gives off a 4 % of sulphurous acid and $\frac{1}{10}$ of a milligramme of sulphuric anhydride in a litre of the gas.

Hankin[1], examining a room after the ordinary sulphur disinfection process carried out by natives in India, found that no disinfection took place. Under better conditions in an experiment carried out by himself, and in which the walls and ceilings were first sprayed with water before the sulphur was burnt in the room, the plague microbe was not killed, and the only effect on agar tubes containing the microbe was that, when transferred to fresh agar, the colonies were not very numerous, suggesting a slightly retarding action.

[1] *The Plague in India*, 1896, 1897. R. Nathan.

The best fumigation with the best results is with the Clayton gas or sulphur-polyoxide. It is a process of disinfection which will take the place of the older methods. In addition to sulphurous acid every litre of the gas contains $6\frac{2}{10}$ milligrammes or over of sulphuric anhydride against $\frac{1}{10}$ of a milligramme contained in a litre of gas by burning sulphur in the open air under ordinary conditions; it contains other unstable compounds of sulphur and oxygen, the exact nature of which has not been determined. The fumigation attains the object in view, viz. the disinfection of the house and the household effects, without having to supplement it with other modes of disinfection, and without having to remove anything from the house. It destroys the infection of plague on clothes, bedding, floor or any

The newest and best method of disinfecting a house infected with plague is fumigating with Clayton's apparatus.

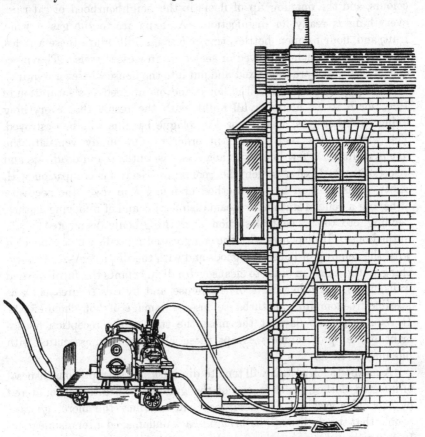

Fig. 2. Portable Clayton Apparatus disinfecting a House.

part of the house that has been contaminated; it destroys the rats, fleas, bugs, or other insects that may be in the house, and if the fumigation is extended to the rat runs and the covered drains, it will destroy any infection that may be in these. Fumigation by a Clayton apparatus brought to the house simplifies the work of disinfection, while at the same time the operation is rendered more certain, more efficient, and safer to the disinfecting establishment. One pound of sulphur is used for every 400 cubic feet of space to be disinfected.

The apparatus having been brought to the front or back of the house and the few preliminaries carried out, such as the sealing of the chimneys and outlets of the house, the opening of the drawers and boxes and cupboards, which can be done by one of the household, the covering over with cloths or paper any stuffs or material of delicate colours, and the opening up of floors in the neighbourhood of rat runs, everything is ready for disinfection. As exposure to the gas of wine, fruit, and flour in open bottles, tins or vessels will injure these articles, they should either be removed or sealed up in close vessels. The pipes and branch pipes are then fixed and put into the house wherever required, and the gas is pumped into the house and maintained at a saturation of 12% for 8 to 12 hours, or all night, with the result that everything living, whether rats, insects, or the plague bacillus will be destroyed. The windows are then opened in order to thoroughly ventilate the rooms, and after a few hours the house can be entered and dead rats and insects removed, after which the rooms are ready for occupation with safety. Disinfection by this method of fumigation saves the necessity of having a central station for steam disinfection and of removing clothes, bedding, etc. to this central station, everything being disinfected *in situ* in the house. It dispenses with the complicated procedure now connected with the removal of household goods and with the displacement of everything in the house in order to cleanse with disinfectants the furniture and walls, floors, and other parts of the house, and by this secures as far as possible freedom from disturbance, loss, or damage of household effects. It reduces to two days at the most the stay in the reception houses or health camp of contacts except those who have been associated with pneumonic cases.

A method such as this will tend to diminish the surreptitious disposal of infected clothes, which is one of the greatest difficulties encountered by the older system. No assurance will convince the more ignorant people that the clothes will be brought back undamaged after disinfection. In a few instances they have had reason to view the assurance with suspicion. Exceptions are always at these times exaggerated into common occurrences.

To prevent the escape of plague-infected rats it is advisable to fill the houses abutting on the infected house with the polyoxide before commencing with the infected house. Once the infected house is filled with the gas, there is no further need of the gas in the adjoining houses, which can be emptied of it at once so that they may be reoccupied. A few hours will suffice for this, which at the same time is a protective measure for the inmates of these houses. The same apparatus by a system of pipes will disinfect several adjacent houses at the same time, a precautionary measure which it is advisable to employ when plague rats are found in more than one house of the block. The underground drains of the house can be disinfected with the gas at the same time and also the sewers of the locality.

In localities in which plague annually recrudesces the systematic
To prevent re- disinfection of houses and destruction of rats in them
crudescences. during the period of quiescence are very important measures
in combating these recrudescences. Occasionally it may not be convenient to disinfect the whole house at one time with the Clayton system. Under these circumstances, with proper arrangements and care, a part of the house can be completed before the other part is commenced. Such an arrangement would prove invaluable for the disinfection of Zenanas, where the women would remove to another portion of the house until their quarters were disinfected. Indian houses with their courtyards are well adapted to such an arrangement, which however would not be suitable for chawls and most tenement houses, which should be disinfected at one operation.

Fumigation has its limits and can only be applied to houses,
buildings, sewers, drains, and other structures that are
Fumigation
has its limits. closed or capable of being enclosed. For surface drains
Employment outside the house, and on the premises, for the yard or
of chemical its contents, which it may be considered advisable to
disinfectants.
disinfect, and for privies and latrines, corrosive sublimate, cyllin, carbolic acid, sulphuric acid, or milk of lime are the most useful disinfectants. Corrosive sublimate 1 in 1000 and 1 in 500 in an acid solution, cyllin 1 in 200 in an alkaline solution, carbolic acid 1 in 20, sulphuric acid 1 in 250 mixed with half the quantity of permanganate of potash, milk of lime 1 in 100, permanganate of potash 1 in 100, are the usual strengths.

In localities where no fumigating apparatus is available recourse must be had to spraying with corrosive sublimate, cyllin, carbolic acid or other efficient disinfectant.

Corrosive sublimate, which has a very powerful destructive action on plague bacilli even in such dilutions as 1 in 5000 and 1 in 10,000 when brought directly in contact with them, in a medium which does not decompose it, possesses certain disadvantages which have to be guarded against; it acts on metals, it is thrown out of solution by alkalis and organic matter, it is precipitated by hard waters, it is decomposed by oxides forming insoluble oxide of mercury, a property which interdicts its use for walls newly lime-washed; it is acted on by the sulphur and sulphuretted hydrogen of decomposing organic matter, and is apt to lose its germicidal effect on discharges, sputum and the like by forming a coating of albuminate of mercury which protects the micro-organism to be destroyed. To prevent liability to decomposition and the formation of inert compounds, there is usually added to the solution of corrosive sublimate, when employed for other purposes than steeping clothes and utensils in the solution or disinfecting the hands, a quantity of hydrochloric acid, which in slight excess adds to the disinfecting power, and some chloride of ammonia or soda, which is conducive to its keeping powers and assists in disintegrating organic matters. The solution commonly employed consists of:

Perchloride of mercury	21 ozs.
Chloride of sodium	15 ,,
Hydrochloric acid	100 ,,
Water	340 ,,
	476 ,,

Five ounces of this solution mixed in a gallon of water gives a strength of 1 in 725, which is a convenient strength for ordinary purposes. By using less water for the standard solution a strength of 1 in 500 may be obtained, which is useful for the interior of houses contaminated with much organic matter. It is useful to add to the solution some aniline dye to give it colour in order to avoid accidents by its being mistaken for water. For steeping clothes and utensils in or for disinfecting the hands a solution of the strength of 1 in 1000 is sufficient. The same strength can be used for washing furniture, which should be first washed down with soft-soap to remove grease; a 3 p.c. solution of soft-soap alone is injurious to the plague bacillus. Under certain circumstances a solution of corrosive sublimate of the strength of 1 in 1000 is not satisfactory for disinfecting purposes. Dr Marsh[1], experimenting in the Plague Research Laboratory of Bombay, found the action of the solution of corrosive sublimate considerably neutralised on floors and walls saturated with organic matter, and especially when dealing with the mud floors of native huts and houses smeared with cow-dung, the properties of the disinfectant being interfered with by the alkalinity of the cow-dung and the compound ammonia bases which it contains. He calculates that 100 square feet of a cow-dung floor require about 8 gallons of the 1 in 725 acid solution to vitally damage any contaminating plague micro-organisms, and that, as the perchloride of mercury solution has only a surface action, its destructive powers would be small if the contaminating material were below the immediate surface, or were the surface protected by leaves, bits of rag, etc.

The Indian Plague Commission as a result of a series of experiments on the material obtained from a paved or cemented floor came to the conclusion that a perchloride solution of the strength of 1 in 500 was efficacious for the interior of houses contaminated with organic matter.

The difficulties in connection with cow-dung floors in native huts would be overcome by the Clayton system of disinfection.

Permanganate of potash possesses an equally powerful destructive effect on plague bacilli as corrosive sublimate, a solution of 1 in 10,000 of the permanganate having been shown by Hankin to destroy the bacillus in 5 minutes. But like the corrosive sublimate it is decomposed when brought into contact with organic matter, which considerably interferes with its action as a disinfectant. A solution of the strength of 1 or 2 p.c. is, however, able to act even in the presence of an excess of organic matter.

In dealing with huts in villages where no means of disinfection exists it is often cheaper and more effective to burn the huts **Burning and exposure to high temperatures.** together with the infected articles in the hut. If this is inadvisable, the hut may be subjected to the desiccating influence of a high temperature by burning cow-dung in a smouldering fashion inside it, and afterwards by unroofing a part and exposing the interior to the direct rays of the sun. The clothes should either be soaked in a disinfectant solution or boiled in a cauldron. **Boiling.** Boiling effectually and rapidly destroys the bacillus of plague, and any clothes in the cauldron in water subjected to a temperature of between 60° C. and 100° C. for half-an-hour will

---

[1] *Minutes of Evidence taken by the Indian Plague Commission*, Vol. III. pp. 68—74; also *Note on Disinfection with Perchloride of Mercury*, by E. L. Marsh.

have been completely sterilised. Where objects such as wool, silk,

Exposure to direct rays of sun for 3 or 4 days. leather, or furs would be injured or destroyed by immersion in boiling water and where no fumigation by formalin is available, they should be spread out in as thin layers as possible and exposed to the direct rays of the sun for 3 or 4 days. Textile fabrics impregnated with plague bacilli have been disinfected experimentally by a 4 hours' exposure to the direct rays of the sun in India and Hongkong. Bedding and clothes that are contaminated should be burnt.

Sanitation. Sunlight, fresh air, good ventilation and dryness are very important factors in the sterilisation of the plague microbe and should always be brought into requisition as sanitary measures both in the prevention and checking of plague. It will be found as a rule that the houses and localities which retain plague the longest are those which are dark, badly ventilated, and damp, and by reason of these conditions are attractive to rats and vermin and are favourable to the prolonged survival and vitality of the plague bacillus, while it is noticeable that even in a badly infected locality houses which possess plenty of light, good ventilation and dryness enjoy a large measure of immunity. The sanitary condition of houses and quarters frequented by tramps, beggars, coolies, emigrants, and pilgrims requires special attention, for they are very liable to become infected and remain centres of infection, being occupied by a migratory class of people who, as a rule, are dirty in their habits and persons and not infrequently covered with vermin.

Destruction of rats. The systematic destruction of rats is a very important measure for combating plague, and with this object in view large quantities of Danysz' virus should be distributed and spread as a poison.

Destruction of rats by the employment of the virus of Danysz. Preparation of the virus of Danysz on a scale which is to be useful requires an adequate staff. Danysz' bacillus is a microorganism of the coli group isolated from field mice suffering from a fatal epizootic, and morphologically identical with the bacillus typhi murium of Loeffler. Danysz was able to set up an illness among grey rats (mus decumanus) by feeding them with cultures of this bacillus. Out of 10 rats there died as a rule two or three, while others fell sick but recovered and others remained quite well. Outside the laboratory the effect of the cultures was tested experimentally in Paris and Hamburg on a small scale with success, but adverse criticism based on unsuccessful results following experiments elsewhere led to its not being applied to any practical use, and it was not until the Cape Town epidemic of plague in 1901 that the destruction of rats by this method was tried on a large scale. The results obtained at first were far from being satisfactory, but those obtained later when new methods were employed were more successful.

It was found after exhaustive tests made by Dr R. W. Dodgson, the Director of the Cape Government Research Laboratory, that **Attenuation and exaltation of virulence of virus.** the cultures sent from the Pasteur Institute had lost their virulence and were either non-pathogenic to the white and grey rat (mus decumanus) and the black rat (mus ratus) or only produced a transient indisposition in the rats after they were fed. Two methods were accordingly adopted to raise the virulence of the microbe. The first was enclosure of the attenuated cultures in collodion capsulés and enclosing them in the peritoneal cavity of a rat for varying periods. The other was the injection of the attenuated cultures into the peritoneal cavity of a rat and allowing the microbe to develop there for a period of 12 to 24 hours. The peritoneal effusion at the expiration of 24 hours was removed and placed in a sterile tube for from 12 to 24 hours for the purpose of aëration. Cultures from this were then made and fresh passages made through rats. After a series of 6 to 8 passages the microbe recovered its virulence, which was easily maintained by an occasional passage in a similar way through rats. The peritoneal fluid was transferred after 12 to 24 hours' aëration to the surface of agar and allowed to grow as a wash culture. This growth was then mixed with bouillon and the resulting emulsion spread evenly over the surface of agar in large flasks or bottles. After 24 hours' incubation the virus was ready for use. The latter method, being much more convenient than the former, was adopted as a matter of routine.

Instead of attempting to set up an epizootic by inoculation of a number of rats and allowing them to escape when ill in **Manner in which cultures of Danysz' bacillus were used in Cape Town.** the hope that their carcases would be eaten by other rats, it was decided to soak pieces of bread in cultures of the virus, and distribute them in the same manner as is done with ordinary rat poison, so that the rats might eat of this infected bread. The virus was made ready for use in the following manner: bouillon was poured into the bottles or flat flasks containing the growth of the bacillus on agar and shaken up until the culture was thoroughly emulsified. It was then poured into dishes, and pieces of stale bread previously dried and of about the size of one cubic inch were dipped into the mixture, care being taken not to soak the bread too long, otherwise it would become pulpy. The agar was also broken up and mixed with the pieces of bread, it being tasty and readily eaten by the rats. When the bread with the virus on it was dry it was packed up in tins and was then ready to be distributed by the rat-catchers or inspectors in the evening. By this method thousands of doses of the virus can be distributed nightly in whatever locality it may be considered to be most required. As the virus does not act on the rats which have eaten the bread for from 8 to 10 days it should be laid nightly for that period in the same places, for experience shows that the rats will continue to eat the bread thus soaked until they fall ill. When, however, illness sets in, the others will disappear from the house, and there is more likelihood of their having eaten some of the bread if the virus is spread nightly. Rats suffering from the disease were found at houses some distance from those in which the virus was laid. The result of the experiment was, on the whole, very satisfactory in Cape Town. Freshly prepared bread will have to be used every night and the media used must always be alkaline. The best alkalinity has been found by experiment to be $N/35\ Na_2Co_3$. All media must be kept alkaline, as the bacillus very rapidly develops acidity, thus inducing an auto-attenuation. The advantage of the virus is that it can be prepared in immense quantities in the laboratory if there is a sufficient staff for that purpose, and that it is harmless to human beings, dogs, cats, fowls, pigs, pigeons, monkeys, and other animals, so that there may be no anxiety in laying down large quantities.

Dr Danysz has recently drawn attention to the tendency of this microbe diminishing in virulence progressively in the course of its passage through the rat and the difficulty of increasing that virulence. There can be no doubt, however, that the virulence was both increased and maintained in Cape Town by the method referred to. Dr Danysz points out that when making experiments on 20 or 30 rats at a time there is certain to be obtained from one or two of these animals a microbe of more virulence than the others, and that in this way the virulence of the culture may be maintained for two or three months. It is in this way that Dr Danysz has been able to maintain a supply of virulent cultures for eight years, and has been able to use them for practical experiments on farms, warehouses, hospitals, workhouses, etc. In 60 % of these operations the rats entirely disappeared, in 15 % the results were entirely negative, and in 25 % complete destruction was not obtained.

In 1902[1] Dr Danysz' bacillus was used to destroy the rats during **Use of Danysz' cultures in the outbreak of plague at Odessa.** the outbreak of plague in Odessa, with the result that the rats completely disappeared. The operation was divided into two parts, one of which was carried out in September, the other in October. In September the proprietors of all houses were ordered to conduct matters themselves, but in October the sanitary authorities enlisted the services of the medical men and medical students of the town. All rats found dead or alive 8 days after the distribution of the virus were examined to ascertain whether they were or were not infected with the microbe. It was found that in those quarters where the instructions were carefully carried out the results of the necropsy of the rats were without exception positive, while in other quarters they only reached 42 to 45 %. Several weeks after the operations it was with the utmost difficulty, even with the offer of a reward, to procure any rats. The Director of the Pasteur Institute of Odessa, who superintended the operations, states that the employment of the virus was far superior to that of other measures used, and that no illness among human beings or domestic animals could be traced to its use.

Other methods may be used for the destruction of rats where the **Other methods employed.** Danysz' virus is not obtainable, and may consist in the employment of professional rat-catchers and the distribution of rat poison in the form of arsenic, phosphorus, and strychnine mixed with other substances; in the event of such poisons being used they should not be distributed without warning in the newspaper, should be laid late at night, and the portions not eaten during the night should be removed early in the morning by the official. These precautions are to avoid accidents to children and the poisoning of other animals.

The following description of the symptoms, post-mortem appearances, and diagnosis of the disease in rats caused by the bacillus of Danysz will be found useful, and is supplied by Dr Dodgson:

The symptoms of the disease usually manifest themselves about **Symptoms in rats suffering from the Danysz' bacillus infection.** 36 hours before death. The rat becomes lethargic, "mopes" with fur erected, and displays an intense thirst. Incoordinate movements are occasionally seen; when they occur the animal will usually be found to be suffering from an acute adhesive (non-suppurative) peritonitis.

---

[1] "A Microbe Pathogenic to Rats," by Dr J. Danysz, *British Medical Journal*, April 23, 1904.

The tail and fur near the anus are usually stained with muco-sanious discharge.

The intestines contain undigested food mixed with glairy mucus or muco-sanious material, and there are usually no formed masses of faeces in the colon or rectum, such as are always found in healthy rats. The intestinal walls are oedematous and translucent, but there is little or no congestion of the blood vessels of either the intestines or the mesentery. Peyer's patches may show infiltration, never ulceration. The spleen is enlarged to from 2 to 10 times its normal size. It is congested, and may show white metastatic growths of the bacillus as large as a pin's head. Lymphatic glands are never enlarged or engorged, except when peritonitis is present, in which case the mesenteric glands may be engorged.

Post-mortem appearances.

The bacillus can readily be isolated from the spleen, blood, peritoneal fluid, etc., by the usual methods. Smears rarely show anything like the number of bacilli as are usually found in those made from the spleen, etc., of rats which have died of plague. The bacilli are actively motile. They are about 2 microm. long by ·75 broad. Nothing characteristic about the growths on ordinary media. In bouillon thread forms soon occur. On acid media coccoid involution forms appear after about 24 hours. Stain readily with aniline dyes. Are decolorised by "gram." In old cultures, and rarely in fresh smears from organs, faint bi-polar staining is met with.

Bacteriological examination.

General biological characters.

Staining.

The bacillus can readily be distinguished from:

Rapid differential tests.

(1) *Bacillus pestis*:

(*a*) Motility.

(*b*) The copious evolution of gas in 2 % glucose agar shake cultures, after about from 6 to 12 hours' incubation at 37°C.

(2) *Bacillus coli communis*:

(*a*) Non-production of gas in 2 % lactose agar shake cultures after 48 hours.

(*b*) Non-coagulation of milk.

Confirmatory tests:

Confirmatory differential tests.

(1) From *B. pestis*:

(*a*) Grows readily in 5 % NaCl bouillon.

(*b*) Causes uniform turbidity in "ghee" bouillon. Never any signs of stalactites.

(2) From *B. coli*:

(*a*) Non-production of gas in gelatine shakes.

(*b*) Non-production of indol. (No smell.)

(*c*) Non-production of HCN in amygdaline bouillon.

Rats eating the carcases of others dead of the disease may die after

Acute toxic cases. 36 hours of acute poisoning (ptomaine?). In these the postmortem appearances are negative, except the condition of the intestines. This closely resembles that described above as occurring in the septicaemic cases. The oedema of the walls of the gut is even more pronounced than in the septicaemic cases, but there may be a few semi-formed faecal masses in the rectum. The bacillus cannot be isolated from the blood or organs in these acute toxic cases, but it is fairly easily isolated from the contents of the intestines by the usual methods. In performing the lactose test, it is necessary to ascertain that the lactose is pure. In ordinary impure lactose, or in lactose that has been kept for some time, especially if damp, a small amount of gas may be evolved in the course of 24 hours.

Large numbers of rats may also be destroyed by fumigating

Destruction of rats in warehouses, etc. buildings with sulphur-polyoxide by Clayton's apparatus. Such fumigation may be applied to warehouses, grain, and rice depots, slaughter-houses and other buildings which harbour rats, also to sewers and drains. For the destruction of rats a 3 or 4 % saturation of the gas in the building for two hours will suffice, and no damage to grain or textile fabrics need be feared.

Plague measures should not cease as soon as the epidemic declines;

Campaigns against plague during the quiescent period. they should continue throughout the period of quiescence with the object of preventing a recrudescence. These measures should consist more particularly in destroying rats generally, in fumigating the houses and blocks of houses that have been infected, along with the neighbouring houses that have remained healthy, together with the drains and rats' runs connected with them, and in bacteriologically examining systematically rats, mice, and sick cats, with the view of ascertaining where active plague is still lurking, and taking measures to eradicate this special source of human plague. Preventive measures should precede and forestall human plague in an infected locality and not wait until a case occurs.

CHAPTER XX.

PREVENTIVE INOCULATION.

THERE is another preventive measure which is of great value. It is preventive inoculation. But unless the danger is urgent few of the poorer classes are likely to resort to it until plague has broken out in a house or in its immediate vicinity. It is advisable to be in possession of an abundant supply of Haffkine's prophylactic in order that those who may be persuaded to be inoculated can be treated.

A preventive prophylactic against plague was discovered in 1896 by **Haffkine's plague prophylactic based on his cholera prophylactic.** Haffkine, his previous experience derived from the results obtained from his cholera prophylactic serving as a guide and leading him to make some material alterations in the mode of preparation of the plague prophylactic. The anti-cholera protective consists of a culture on agar of living comma bacilli fixed at a uniform strength of virulence by passing through an animal. The bacilli when the culture is ready are detached from the agar by suspending them in sterile water, and drawing up the emulsion in a sterile syringe. A small dose of this emulsion injected under the skin produces a certain amount of local inflammatory action accompanied by a temporary rise in temperature and a feeling of malaise lasting from one to two days. The swelling at the seat of the inoculation may last a week and then disappear. The bacteria die in the tissues at the seat of the inoculation; in the process the intracellular toxines become absorbed and immunity is generally established in the course of four days. Sometimes dead cultures preserved in a slightly carbolised solution are used instead of the living cultures. They act in a similar way, the bodies of the bacilli disintegrating with the liberation of the intracellular toxines; but preference is given to the use of living cultures in cholera because the results obtained from them are believed to be better and of longer duration. The immunity varies according to the strength of the prophylactic, the dose, and the length of time that elapses between the inoculations and the infection. With weak vaccines and small doses the immunising effect is more or less transient and rapidly disappears, and even with strong vaccines and ordinary doses the protection does not last longer than two years. In Calcutta a comparison of the inoculated and not inoculated showed an incidence of cholera 22 times greater on the not inoculated than on the inoculated; but this difference only lasted two years, after which the two classes rapidly approached one another in their liability to attack. A remarkable observation was made during the investigation into the effects of the anti-cholera inoculations in India. It was that, though there is always a marked difference between the incidence of the disease on the inoculated and not inoculated, yet the preservative effect of the prophylactic appears to be principally limited to preventing attacks and does not extend to lessening the deaths among those attacked; for when persons are attacked with cholera the inoculation has no effect in reducing the mortality or giving a better chance of recovery. Theoretically this is explained by the serum of the blood of the inoculated containing no antitoxic properties, and consequently being unable to resist or neutralise the effects caused by the pouring in of toxines by microbes which have established themselves in the intestines. Kolle and Pfeiffer, by inoculating a number of students with the anti-choleraic fluid, ascertained by experiment that the serum of those inoculated contains bactericidal products which possess a rapid and destructive effect on comma bacilli to an extent 200 times greater than the serum of those not inoculated. It would appear, therefore, that while the blood of the inoculated against cholera is rich in bactericidal products, it is poor in antitoxins, and that, though it is able by means of its bactericidal products to protect the system against the lodgement and multiplication of the bacillus and so prevent an attack, yet by the absence of antitoxic properties it is unable to prevent the poisonous effects of the toxines should the microbe effecting a lodgement in the intestines overcome the destructive effect of the bactericides and go on multiplying. This is obviously an important defect in the anti-cholera inoculations and one likely to narrow its sphere of usefulness. The experience thus gained proved to be valuable at a time when the question arose as to the possibility of preparing a prophylactic for plague. The defect attaching to the cholera prophylactic had to be remedied if possible, inasmuch as it was not only desirable to provide against the microbe, but also against its toxines. Instead, therefore, of

26—2

preparing the plague prophylactic on similar lines, Haffkine decided to adopt a method which should provide a mixture containing a large quantity of extracellular toxines secreted by the microbes, as well as an abundance of the bodies of the plague bacilli containing in themselves the intracellular toxines. By inoculation with a mixture of this kind it was assumed that both a bactericidal and antitoxic power of resistance would be obtained.

It was impossible to use living plague bacilli for protective purposes, as these grow in the tissues and invade the system; accordingly dead vaccines had to be resorted to, the bacilli, after secreting a sufficiency of toxines, being destroyed before the prophylactic is administered. In the case of employing dead vaccines there is not the same necessity for fixing at a uniform standard the strength of the virulence of the plague microbe as in the case of the cholera microbe, because the plague prophylactic consists of the dead bodies of the bacilli and of their products, and, like the antitoxins of diphtheria, can be measured. A larger measured dose of a mixture prepared from a less virulent microbe will produce the same effect as a smaller dose the product of a more virulent race.

The mode of preparing the prophylactic is simple. To a flask containing nutrient bouillon a very small quantity of melted butter or oil is added; the flask is closed by a cotton plug, placed in the autoclave, sterilised, and then allowed to cool. The fluid is then carefully inoculated through the cotton-wool plug by means of a pipette filled with a culture of the plague bacillus which is obtained first from a plague case or which is maintained in virulence by passing through animals. In India there is no need to place the flask in an incubator; it may be set aside in a shaded place, the growth proceeding at the ordinary temperature of the air. When that temperature falls below 25° C. the air of the room is warmed by lighting some gas-burners. Elsewhere, and out of the tropics, the flask is placed in an incubator with a temperature ranging between 30° C. and 32° C. An alteration in the contents of the flask is soon perceptible; the fluid remains quite clear, but from the particles of fat floating on the surface of the liquid there is seen to be suspended in the depth a series of fine thread-like growths which on the slightest disturbance or oscillation become detached and broken up, falling gradually like fine flakes of snow to the bottom of the flask and which are replaced by a fresh crop in a few days. These growths are the colonies of plague bacilli which have attached themselves to the fat and

Preparation of Haffkine's plague prophylactic.

have grown downwards into the depths of the liquid, giving a peculiar *stalactite* appearance to the growth. The stalactites in the course of 2 or 3 days fill up the upper half or sometimes even the whole volume of the liquid. The flasks are shaken periodically, when the stalactites have been fully grown, to allow the colonies to become detached, and to fall to the bottom in order to permit of fresh growths of a similar kind and so to accumulate at the bottom of the flask a large quantity of the bodies of the bacilli. This is continued for the period of 6 weeks, when by that time the culture contains the bodies of a large mass of plague bacilli and a large quantity of extracellular toxines formed by the microbes in their process of growth. The culture being ripe for use its purity is tested by drawing off a small quantity by a sterilised pipette and transferring it to the surface of an agar tube and noting the physical and microscopical appearances of the growth produced. If the agar is dry and the culture spread evenly over the surface the thin, translucent, colourless growth characteristic of plague will form in 2 or 3 days and any colonies of foreign microbes intermixed with it will be distinctly seen. The test proving to be satisfactory the bacilli are now to be killed. To kill the bacilli the flask containing the prophylactic is placed in a water-bath with another flask containing water and having in it a thermometer which indicates the heat to which both fluids are subjected in the bath. The temperature is raised to 50—55° C. and is then kept at this level for a quarter of an hour. In other laboratories the cultures are usually exposed to a temperature of 60° C. for an hour. This is sufficient to kill the bacilli, after which a small quantity of carbolic acid in the proportion of $\frac{1}{200}$ part of the bulk of the prophylactic is added for preventive purposes. It is not wise to subject the prophylactic to a higher temperature than necessary, though its immunising properties are not wholly destroyed until it has been exposed to a temperature of 100° C.; as a precautionary measure, however, to ensure that all bacilli in the flask are destroyed that portion of the flask which is not submerged in the heated water of the bath should be always heated in the flame of a bunsen burner. The prophylactic consisting of sediment and fluid is now ready for use, and is shaken up so as to make a uniform mixture, which is then decanted into small bottles, and corked with india-rubber stoppers. The standardisation of the prophylactic or the determination of the dose is ascertained by testing the toxic effect of a given quantity on a few individuals, the standard being the smallest quantity which produces an average temperature of 102° F. in a series of cases. For an adult this is as a rule $2\frac{1}{2}$ to 5 cubic centimetres. The test in this instance is

the febrile action produced on man instead of the killing power on
animals. The storage of the prophylactic is important. Bottles with
ordinary corks have frequently failed to keep the vaccine free of
contamination; hermetically sealed tubes or bulbs are undoubtedly the
best and safest method of storage.

A modification of the above method in the preparation of Haffkine's
prophylactic has been employed in the Government laboratory in
Bombay. The flasks of broth are not filled to such a high level as before,
the shallower contents being used in order to secure a more abundant
aëration of the fluid. The cultivation flasks are only slightly vibrated
to dislodge the stalactites and are not shaken up as formerly. When
ready a four days' growth on 300 square centimetres of agar surface is
emulsified in 400 c.cs. of a two-months-old broth cultivation. This
mixture is then sterilised for 15 minutes at 50 to 55° C. and $\frac{1}{2}$% of
carbolic acid added to it. The prophylactic is then tested to ascertain
whether it has been completely sterilised, after which it is decanted into
special laboratory phials which are then stoppered with india-rubber
corks. In Japan and the Pasteur Institute a similar process for preparing
the prophylactic is employed, but more dependence is placed on the
cultures on agar rather than in broth. Kitasato's prophylactic prepared
from agar cultures was used with good results in Formosa.

The method of decanting and storage is open to improvement, and
Dr E. Maynard has devised a storage flask which allows of the cultures
in the flask being decanted without exposure to the air and which admits
of being hermetically sealed instead of being corked. This arrangement
which was much needed reduces the possibility of contamination of the
prophylactic with other microbes.

At the time of inoculation great care has to be taken in securing
Method of complete sterilisation of the syringe and needle. To attain
inoculation. this object the following procedure is recommended if no
portable steriliser is at hand. A Colins syringe, previously boiled to
sterilise it, is filled with a solution of carbolic acid and its needle is
dipped into hot carbolic oil; it is then washed out several times
thoroughly with sterile water, after which it is ready to be filled with
the prophylactic. This is effected by breaking the sealed bulb containing
the prophylactic and drawing it directly up into the syringe. The arm
or loin is generally chosen as the seat of inoculation. This part is first
washed with a swab of cotton-wool soaked in a solution of carbolic acid
of the strength of 1 in 20, the skin is raised by the forefinger and thumb,
the needle of the syringe is plunged into the raised part, $2\frac{1}{2}$ to 5 cubic centi-

metres of the fluid are rapidly injected, the needle is removed and the raised skin allowed to fall back to its old position. The part is once more swabbed with carbolic acid and the operation is over. Before proceeding to inoculate the next person the needle of the syringe is either dipped in hot oil or is rubbed over with cotton-wool soaked in a solution of carbolic acid. This process between every operation secures anti-septicism and avoids any inflammation due to extraneous contamination

Effect of the inoculation. of the wound. The effect of the inoculation is not noticed for the first 3 or 4 hours, then a slight feverishness sets in, and in the course of 12 hours may in some cases reach 102 to 103° F. Occasionally it rises higher, even to 104 and 105° F. At the same time there is a feeling of tenderness at the seat of inoculation, which becomes reddened, swollen and painful, and there may be tenderness and swelling of the nearest glands. Headache, malaise, and general discomfort accompany the local and feverish disturbance, which varies much in different persons, some being but only slightly affected and able to go on with their usual occupation, while others are indisposed for a day or two. The fever disappears in one or two days, and the patient feels well except for the pain at the seat of inoculation, which may last from several days to a week, the swelling not disappearing for a week or two longer.

In the many hundreds of thousands of inoculations that have been performed no injurious result has been known to follow, except in 1902 when a bottle got contaminated with tetanus bacilli, with the result that those who were inoculated died of tetanus. The inoculations, with a prophylactic which has been carefully prepared and stored, are harmless, though the effects for the first few days are far from being pleasant.

The results of the inoculation in plague-stricken districts in India

Results of the inoculations. are summed up by the Indian Plague Commission. 1. Inoculation sensibly diminishes the incidence of plague attacks on the inoculated population, but the protection which is afforded against attacks is not absolute.

2. Inoculation greatly diminishes the plague death-rate among the inoculated population. This is due not only to the fact that the rate of attack is diminished, but also to the fact that the fatality of attacks is diminished.

3. Inoculation does not appear to confer any great degree of protection within the first few days after the operation has been performed.

The Commission were unable to assign a numerical expression to the measure of protection from attack or death which inoculation confers, for it appeared to be subject to considerable variation, dependent on the strength of the virulence of the microbe employed, in the preparation of the prophylactic, the varying length of time to which many of the cultures were subjected, many being much less than 6 weeks, and the difference in the amount of the dose administered. More uniformity in these respects, and improvements in decanting and storage are admittedly required. At the same time there can be little doubt that in a number of the observations recorded after careful investigation, the diminution of mortality among the inoculated as compared with the not inoculated was not less than from 70 to 80 %. The most recent information from India would indicate that the proportion of deaths to attacks in the inoculated was under 25 %, or less than one-half observed in the not inoculated.

It is not to be forgotten that the prophylactic takes 48 hours to act, and in the meantime does not confer protection any more than is afforded by vaccination against small-pox during the first week. In the case, therefore, of nurses or others who have to come into contact at once with plague patients a preliminary inoculation with Yersin's serum, which effects a rapid protection, should be performed.

It is generally advisable to furnish the person inoculated with a short account of the symptoms likely to follow and of the precautions which should be taken to avoid indiscretions. The following hand-bill is useful for this purpose:

INSTRUCTIONS TO PERSONS INOCULATED.

1. Three or four hours after inoculation the patient will experience headache, general malaise, fever, and slight pain at the seat of inoculation. These symptoms will continue for about 48 hours.

2. Patient should rest for 24 hours at least and abstain from all work. The arm should be kept in a sling reaching from the wrist to the elbow in order to ensure perfect rest to the arm.

3. The arm may be bathed with a little hot water or a lotion containing lead and opium, which may be obtained from any druggist.

4. The diet should be light. A purgative on the first day lessens the local reaction.

Another prophylactic has been prepared by Professors A. Lustig and G. Galeotti of Florence. It is a nucleo-proteid prepared from the plague bacillus.

The prophy-
lactic of
Lustig and
Galeotti.

The method of preparation consists in cultivating plague bacilli on agar plates, scraping off the growth and dissolving it in a 1 % sterilised solution of caustic potash[1]. To the mixture is added a very dilute solution of hydrochloric or acetic acid until there is a slight acid reaction and the resulting precipitate is collected on filter-paper, washed, and dried. The precipitate is composed of a nucleo-proteid and is readily soluble in a weak solution of carbonate of soda. The dose for a man is 3 milligrammes, which injected produces in a few hours shivering and general malaise, followed by a rise of temperature to 101° or 102° F. and painful swelling at the seat of inoculation. The general reaction subsides within 36 hours and the local action within 3 or 4 days.

The claims made on behalf of the nucleo-proteid is that its efficacy has been proved on rats, rabbits, guinea-pigs, and monkeys, that it is harmless to man and is devoid of many of the toxic and depressant substances which are contained in liquid cultures of the bacillus. The advantages over Haffkine's prophylactic are set forth as being, first that the substance required for the production of immunity is isolated and used alone and not mixed with extraneous and possibly harmful products; that it is not heated and therefore does not lose any of its immunising properties; that there is no danger of its becoming contaminated, as is the possibility with each separate bottle of Haffkine's prophylactic; that being dry it can be easily preserved; that it can be administered in well-defined doses, which is not the case with Haffkine's; and that it cannot offend the religious susceptibilities of the population of India. There are no data as to the value of this prophylactic in protecting man against plague.

[1] "Preventive Inoculation against Bubonic Plague" by Professors A. Lustig and G. Galeotti. *British Medical Journal*, Feb. 10, 1900.

CHAPTER XXI.

CONCLUSION.

FROM the foregoing it may be gathered that the existing knowledge

More precise information required regarding plague.

of plague is not as precise and exact as it should be to secure unvarying successful control. The little that is known is nevertheless very useful in the prevention of an outbreak in its early stages, especially if it is of the pneumonic type and is limited to human infection. But once an outbreak reaches certain dimensions the lack of exact knowledge regarding many of the modes of dissemination and channels of infection and the conditions which affect the spread of the disease renders the methods of prevention uncertain and ineffective. The extent of an epidemic then depends on those unknown conditions which produce an actively diffusive plague or a self-limited plague.

The discovery of the plague bacillus has given precision to the diagnosis of plague, enabling the disease in man or rats to be recognised at a very early stage of its existence, and this, combined with the notification system and a sanitary organisation which can act at once, robs plague of many of the advantages it possessed in earlier times when attacking a town or district. Preventive measures were seldom introduced in the older epidemics until the outbreak was well-developed, and then, whatever measures were introduced, and however strict they were, they appear to have been of small value in influencing the course of the epidemic. In this respect, therefore, those countries free of plague, and which possess a properly organised sanitary system prepared to act in accordance with the principles which our present knowledge lays down, are in a much better position to prevent the importation and withstand the attacks of the advance-guard of a threatening epidemic of plague than was the case when no such organisation existed.

Still, owing to an imperfect knowledge of the different modes and avenues by which plague attacks, it by no means follows that these measures will always be successful, nor, if the epidemic is small in extent, whether mild or virulent, that the limitation has been due solely to the measures taken. It is impossible to be absolutely certain of either while so much is unknown regarding plague, though at the same time it would be reprehensible not to act vigorously on the guidance given by existing information. The facts known and

The facts known and established regarding plague. established can be easily summarised. They have already been mentioned, but they will bear repetition. They are, that plague is due to a bacillus; that there is a bubonic, septicaemic, pneumonic, and pustular form; that the pneumonic form is very infective; that there is a connection between rat plague and human plague; that rats may disseminate plague as well as man; that the disease both in human beings and in rats is seasonal; that certain animals besides rats take plague; that the disease in man and animals may be of a chronic nature; that Haffkine's prophylactic subcutaneously injected with a syringe has considerable protective effect, but that its mode of administration and the local discomfort produced by it militate against its general use on a large scale; and, lastly, that there is no curative treatment that is effective against virulent plague. It is evident that much more requires to be known if epidemic as distinguished from sporadic plague is to be brought under control, either from a preventive or curative point of view. The suggestion is not that there exists no information on the subjects about to be mentioned as requiring close investigation, but, as will be gathered from a perusal of this volume, the information is not sufficiently exact to ensure absolute safety even in Europe.

The following may be given as examples of questions on which systematic research is needed:

The main lines on which enquiry is needed.   (*a*) The length of time an infected patient or infected animal retains infection. Bacteriological examinations are made for diagnostic purposes but seldom to ascertain period of infection.

(*b*) What proportion of plague cases are traceable to house infection either in dwelling-houses or workshops and what proportion to other causes?

(*c*) In the case of house infection what does it consist of, contaminated food, contaminated floors, or dust, or plague rats, or plague insects, or other agents?

(*d*) The history of plague cases as regards the source of their infection and the conditions under which it took effect.

(*e*) Whether rats or man are the chief disseminators of plague, and in what proportion?

(*f*) Whether other animals are disseminators of plague without being affected themselves, and in what way? It was a common belief when plague used to prevail in Europe that cats and dogs thus conveyed infection. If this is so is it due to insects on these animals?

(*g*) Whether insects such as fleas, bugs, flies, etc., disseminate plague, and if so, the length of time they will retain the infection?

(*h*) What are the species of fleas on the rats, fowls, cats, and dogs in the locality investigated, and which of them attack men?

(*i*) What is the life-history of fleas and other insects in the affected locality in relation to the epidemic and non-epidemic season of plague, and in their relationship to man and the domesticated animals?

(*k*) Whether there are other modes of dissemination besides animals and insects? Are rice stores and granaries, apart from their infected rats, disseminators of plague by the infection of their goods? How long does the bacillus live on fruits and cooked food?

(*l*) How is the infection conveyed from man to man and from animal to animal? except in pneumonic cases the infection does not appear to be direct. What are the indirect agencies and in what way do they act?

(*m*) How is the infection conveyed from man to the rat and in what way from rat to man? Is it by infected food, or by insect carriers? A similar question arises in regard to infection conveyed to and from poultry and other animals. Are vegetable eaters more susceptible to plague than eaters of a mixed diet?

(*n*) Does season affect the bacillus or its carriers and in what way? To what is due the rapid loss of infection of plague after an epidemic has reached its height? Is it climatic and due to the growth of saprophytic organisms destroying the bacillus or rendering it attenuated in virulence, or is it due to some change in the life-history of the carriers such as fleas, etc.?

(*o*) What is the reason of dormancy in non-epidemic seasons, and what are the agents at work producing recrudescence?

(*p*) What are the best agents for destroying the bacillus or its carriers?

(*q*) What modification could be effected in the administration of Haffkine's prophylactic to make its use more general? If it were protected in capsules so as to pass through the stomach into the intestines and escape the digestive and peptonising action of the stomach and upper portion of the small intestine, would it be absorbed in sufficient quantities for prophylactic purposes? What is the action of gastric juice and pancreatic juice on the prophylactic? Do they render it inert? If rendered inert would the intracellular toxines prepared by the liquid air system be also rendered inert or would they more readily pass through the living mucous membrane? If administration by the digestive system should fail in both it might still be well to consider, in any further experimental work upon the preparation of a plague prophylactic, the method employed by Dr Allan Macfadyen for obtaining the fresh cell plasma of pathogenic bacteria for the purpose of vaccination or immunisation and illustrated in his work on typhoid and other organisms.

(*r*) By what means can the antidotal effect of Yersin's serum or of that of others be rendered more powerful and curative against virulent plague? The serum requires to possess properties which shall be not only bactericidal but also powerfully antitoxic in order that it may neutralise the toxines set free by the death of the plague bacillus. Such a combination of properties in the serum is difficult to obtain from the plague bacillus. A serum with bactericidal properties alone is likely to aggravate the disease once the bacteria appear in large quantities in the blood, while if the serum possesses antitoxic properties only it is no protection against the multiplication of the bacteria and the final production of an overwhelming quantity of toxines too great to be neutralised.

The subjects about which more information is needed are by no means exhausted in the list given; much more is required to be known concerning the plague bacillus in nature. But the questions are sufficiently numerous to indicate the amount of uncertainty and ignorance which still exists concerning essentials connected with the epidemiology, prevention, and treatment of plague, and they serve to accentuate the fact that while this state of doubt and ignorance continues no nation is safe against the ravages of plague should the disease, as it threatens to do, present itself in the virulent and diffusive pandemic form.

APPENDIX I.

Reported deaths from Plague in India in 1904, extracted from the official weekly returns.

Province	Bombay Presidency and Sindh	Bengal	Madras	Punjab	United Provinces	Central Provinces	Mysore	Rajputana	Hyderabad	Central India	Other Provinces	Europeans	Grand Total
Week ending													
2nd Jan.	6736	1295	709	1459	2613	1446	662	133	609	828	13		16503
9th ,,	6776	953	740	1394	3291	1574	631	135	972	855	23		17344
16th ,,	5998	2337	875	3080	3567	2388	637	227	1279	862	52		21307
23rd ,,	6996	1752	905	2289	3959	2504	570	(a)	1054	1031	43		21103
30th ,,	6690	2335	908	3251	4914	2589	640	195	644	973	63		23202
6th Feb.	6427	2798	751	2785	5593	2260	533	676	800	1444	137		24204
13th ,,	6461	2787	949	3903	5517	2120	546	496	1259	1352	239		26629
20th ,,	7587	2510	961	4520	5487	1954	479	607	812	1267	352		26537
27th ,,	7609	2986	763	5256	6121	1955	444	487	940	942	352		27858
5th March	7487	3479	674	5550	6910	2040	388	427	813	756	395		28919
12th ,,	8210	4616	525	6431	8504	2290	383	621	577	955	405		33517
19th ,,	8693	5092	385	10174	9427	2804	271	1033	481	1640	526		40526
26th ,,	8422	4580	365	12594	8786	2230	212	(a)	733	1605	540		40075
2nd April	6689	5354	190	19322	8610	1798	223	1385	651	1469	541		46181
9th ,,	7488	4055	208	23775	7641	1386	138	892	1077	1095	4		47759
16th ,,	6128	2442	134	26961	6197	704	134	1005	660	1288	1155(b)		46812
23rd ,,	4535	1879	83	24714	4279	498	162	1072	216	732	579		38748
30th ,,	3706	1332	62	33953	2965	214	145	865	238	512	628		44783
7th May	2873	743	56	34685	2229	133	67	(a)	212	296	313		41607
14th ,,	2041	395	40	30723	1303	62	77	374	68	100	221		35413
21st ,,	1373	349	51	24853	1019	21	66	195	59	109	75		28219
28th ,,	989	290	59	18086	653	8	104	166	8	48	73		20484

1904												Total
4th June	662	199	66	12289	420	2	91	(a)	13	17	81	13770
11th ,,	508	169	71	6491	729	—	165	55	4	21	49	7762
18th ,,	530	159	71	4746	126	—	199	50	8	6	34	5929
25th ,,	495	95	136	1825	40	1	264	(a)	8	2	8	2873
2nd July	746	56	201	1314	17	5	311	6	23	2	7	2688
9th ,,	583	94	197	681	35	1	296	2	28	1	1	1919
16th ,,	1018	116	183	115	39	—	417	14	62	—	1	1995
23rd ,,	1472	114	233	43	58	5	519	7	157	—	—	2608
30th ,,	1706	135	323	58	101	28	629	17	203	7	—	3209
6th August	2973	199	390	24	240	39	605	46	187	90	1	4794
13th ,,	3367	369	413	31	268	58	814	65	266	95	3	5849
20th ,,	3810	338	475	33	361	93	716	134	201	230	7	6398
27th ,,	4900	350	596	99	395	194	794	209	385	388	3	8304
3rd Sept.	6017	375	430	73	634	323	946	385	417	590	10	10199
10th ,,	6579	500	735	102	874	345	807	532	387	929	3	11791
17th ,,	6055	429	365	125	943	379	715	376	284	997	4	10671
24th ,,	7000	305	537	113	628	480	713	446	488	1150	6	11866
1st Oct.	8364	278	597	276	751	677	797	411	440	1138	10	13733
8th ,,	10414	180	540	400	984	661	770	473	494	1548	27	16491
15th ,,	9879	195	426	345	1246	552	852	424	547	1616	27	16111
22nd ,,	8256	190	334	572	1276	485	694	297	570	1170	27	13871
29th ,,	9695	191	475	748	1446	422	663	302	714	798	33	15487
5th Nov.	9570	260	473	1067	1851	514	—	397	1039	755	54	15980
12th ,,	7695	342	398	1357	2476	450	657	500	925	364	32	15197
19th ,,	7180	412	386	1515	2783	478	565	—	474	278	44	14115
26th ,,	6399	421	448	3092	3006	598	589	224	520	208	23	14528
3rd Dec.	6743	735	392	2446	4425	529	1157(e)	292	768	206	30	17728
10th ,,	5913	947	408	2725	5367	458	419	432	609	149	12	17439
17th ,,	5135	1632	402	2989	6186	382	334	409	610	193	12	18284
24th ,,	4325	2023	358	3940	6822	389	319	345	809	132	6	19465
31st ,,	3925	2514	367	4643	9574	379	282	314	516	121	10	22645
Total for the year 1904	281828	68681	21819	354035	163686	41905	24611	18155	26318	33360	7294	1040429

(a) Figures not received.   (b) Figures for two weeks.   (e) Figures for the weeks ending 5th Nov. and 3rd Dec.

Note. There are a few slight discrepancies between several of the weekly grand totals and the sum of the weekly recorded deaths in each province but they are of a very minor and unimportant nature and do not amount in the aggregate to more than a few hundreds.

APPENDIX II.

THE INTERNATIONAL SANITARY CONVENTION OF PARIS, 1903;

WITH APPENDICES,

TRANSLATED BY

THEODORE THOMSON, ESQ., M.D.

PART I.

(Reproduced by kind permission of the Controller of His Majesty's Stationery Office.)

GENERAL PROVISIONS.

CHAPTER I.

PROVISIONS TO BE OBSERVED BY THE COUNTRIES SIGNING THE CONVENTION ON THE APPEARANCE OF PLAGUE OR CHOLERA IN THEIR TERRITORY.

SECTION I.—*Notification and subsequent communications to the other countries.*

Art. 1.—Every Government must immediately notify to the other Governments the first appearance of recognised cases of plague or cholera in its territory.

Art. 2.—Such notification shall be accompanied or very promptly followed by detailed information as to:—
(1) where the disease has appeared;
(2) the date of its appearance, its source, and its type;
(3) the number of known cases and deaths;

(4) in the case of plague, the presence of that disease or of unusual mortality among rats or mice ;

(5) the measures taken immediately on the first appearance of the disease.

Art. 3.—The notification and the information prescribed in Articles 1 and 2 shall be supplied to the diplomatic or consular agencies in the capital of the infected country. In the case of countries not represented there, the notification and the information shall be telegraphed direct to the Governments of these countries.

Art. 4.—The notification and the information prescribed in Articles 1 and 2 shall be followed by subsequent communications furnished regularly and in such fashion as to keep the Governments informed of the course of the epidemic. These communications shall be made at least once a week, shall be as complete as possible, and shall, in particular, indicate the precautions adopted with a view to prevent spread of the disease. They must set out with precision :—

(1) the preventive measures taken in the way of sanitary inspection or of medical investigation, of isolation, and of disinfection ;

(2) the measures adopted in the case of outgoing vessels to prevent exportation of the disease, and, particularly, in the case contemplated in Art. 2 (4), the measures taken against rats.

Art. 5.—It is of primary importance that the foregoing provisions be promptly and scrupulously complied with. Notification is of no real value unless every Government be itself informed, in time, of cases of plague and cholera and also of doubtful cases occurring in its territory. It cannot therefore be too strongly impressed on the several Governments that they should make notification of plague and cholera compulsory, and that they should keep themselves informed as to any unusual mortality among rats or mice, particularly in ports.

Art. 6.—It is to be understood that neighbouring countries reserve to themselves the right to make special arrangements with the object of organising direct exchange of information between the principal administrative officers on their frontiers.

SECTION II.—*The conditions under which a local area may be regarded as infected or as having ceased to be infected.*

Art. 7.—The notification of a first case of plague or cholera shall not lead to the adoption of the measures prescribed in the following Chapter II. against the local area in which the case has occurred. But when several non-imported cases of plague have occurred, or when the cases of cholera constituted a *foyer*[1], the local area shall be declared infected.

Art. 8.—In order that the measures be limited to places which are infected, Governments must apply them to arrivals from infected local areas only. "Local area" means a portion of territory clearly defined in the information that accompanies or follows notification—as, for instance, a province, a "government," a district, a department, a canton, an island, a commune, a town, a quarter in a town, a village, a port, a polder, an agglomeration, etc., whatever may be the extent and population of these portions of territory. But this limitation to the infected local area must be accepted only on the definite condition that the Government of the infected country take the measures necessary (*a*) for preventing the export of the things specified in Art. 12 (1) and (2) derived from the infected local area, unless previously disinfected, and (*b*) for checking the spread of the epidemic.

When a local area is infected no restrictive measure shall be taken against arrivals from that local area, if they have left it not less than five days before the beginning of the epidemic.

Art. 9.—In order that a local area cease to be regarded as infected it must be officially established:—(1) that no death from nor fresh case of plague or cholera has occurred within the five days following either the isolation[2] or the death or recovery of the last case of plague or cholera; (2) that all measures of disinfection have been carried out and that, in the case of plague, measures have been taken against rats.

CHAPTER II.

MEASURES OF DEFENCE, ON THE PART OF THE OTHER COUNTRIES, AGAINST TERRITORIES THAT HAVE BEEN DECLARED INFECTED.

SECTION I.—*Publication of measures prescribed.*

Art. 10.—The Government of each country shall immediately make public the measures which it considers necessary to prescribe with regard

---

[1] *Translator's note. The expression "centre of dissemination" may be taken as a fair equivalent for the word "foyer." It seems desirable, however, to retain the original term in the text, in view of the difficulty of deciding what is to be regarded as constituting a "foyer" of cholera. This question was debated at some length at the Dresden Conference in 1893, and was again raised at the Paris Conference in 1903 by the translator and others. At the Dresden Conference, Professor Brouardel, one of the French delegates, stated that an exact definition of the word "foyer" was a difficult matter. At the Paris Conference in 1903, the word, after some discussion, was retained without definition of its precise significance in relation with cholera.*

[2] "Isolation" means the isolation of the sick person, of those in permanent attendance on him, and the prohibition of visits by any other person.

to arrivals from an infected country or local area. It shall forthwith communicate these measures to the diplomatic or consular agent of the infected country resident in the capital, and also to the International Sanitary Boards. It shall also communicate, through the same channels, the withdrawal of these measures or any modifications of them. In the absence of a diplomatic or consular agency in the capital, the communications shall be made direct to the Government of the country concerned.

SECTION II.—*Merchandise.—Disinfection.—Importation and Transit.—Baggage.*

Art. 11.—No article of merchandise is in itself capable of conveying plague or cholera. Merchandise becomes dangerous only when contaminated by plague or cholera products.

Art. 12.—Only such merchandise and things as the local sanitary authority considers infected may be subjected to disinfection. Provided always that the merchandise or things hereinafter specified may be subjected to disinfection or their importation may even be prohibited, irrespective of any evidence as to whether or not they are infected :—(1) Body-linen, wearing apparel, bedding that has been in use. But when these things are carried as baggage or in consequence of a change of abode (household goods), their importation may not be prohibited but they shall be dealt with as prescribed in Article 19. Soldiers' and sailors' kits, returned to their country after their death, are to be regarded as of the nature of the things specified in the first sentence of (1) of this article. (2) Rags, save, in the case of cholera, rags compressed and carried in bound bales as merchandise in bulk. The importation of the following articles may not be prohibited :—Fresh waste derived directly from spinning, weaving, making up, or bleaching establishments; artificial wools (*Kunstwolle*, shoddy) and new paper clippings.

Art. 13.—The transit of the merchandise and things specified in (1) and (2) of the foregoing article may not be prohibited if they are packed so that they cannot be manipulated on the way. Similarly, when such merchandise and things have been so conveyed that they cannot have come into contact with contaminated articles on the way, their transit through an infected local area must not hinder their importation into the country to which they are consigned.

Art. 14.—Importation of the merchandise and things specified in (1) and (2) of Article 12 shall not be prohibited if it be proved to the authority of the country to which they are consigned that they were despatched not less than five days before the commencement of the epidemic.

Art. 15.—It rests with the authority of the country to which the merchandise and things are consigned to decide in what manner and at what place disinfection shall be carried out, and what shall be the methods adopted to secure destruction of rats. These operations must be performed in such fashion as to injure articles as little as possible. It rests with each State to settle questions of consequent compensation for damage caused by measures of disinfection or of rat-destruction. If, on account of measures taken to secure destruction of rats on board ship, charges are levied by the sanitary authority either directly or indirectly through a company or a private person, the rates of these charges must be in accordance with a tariff made public beforehand, and so drawn up that the State or the sanitary authority shall, on the whole, derive no profit from its application.

Art. 16.—Letters and correspondence, printed matter, books, newspapers, business documents, etc. (not including parcels conveyed by post), shall not be subject to disinfection or to any restriction whatsoever.

Art. 17.—Merchandise, whether it has come by land or by sea, may not be detained at frontiers or at ports ; the only measures that may be taken are those specified in the foregoing Article 12. Provided always that if merchandise, which has come by sea and is either not packed or imperfectly packed, has become infected during the voyage by rats ascertained to have plague, and if such merchandise cannot be disinfected, the destruction of the germs may be secured by storing the merchandise during a period not to exceed two weeks. It is to be understood that the application of this measure shall not in any way delay the ship nor give rise to extra expenses by reason of deficient storage-accommodation in any port.

Art. 18.—When merchandise has undergone disinfection in accordance with the provisions of Art. 12, or has been temporarily stored in virtue of the proviso contained in Art. 17, the proprietor of such merchandise or his representative has the right to exact from the sanitary authority that has ordered the disinfection or the storage a certificate showing the measures that have been taken.

Art. 19.—*Baggage.*—Soiled linen, clothing and articles carried as baggage or as household goods, from a local area declared to be infected, shall undergo disinfection only in those instances where the sanitary authority considers them infected.

SECTION III.—*Measures at ports and land frontiers.*

Art. 20.—*Classification of ships.*—A ship shall be regarded as *infected* if there is plague or cholera on board or if there have been one or more cases of plague or cholera on board within seven days.

A ship shall be regarded as *suspected* if there have been cases of plague or cholera on board at the time of departure or during the voyage but no fresh case within seven days.

A ship shall be regarded as *healthy,* notwithstanding its having come from an infected port, if there has been no death from nor case of plague or cholera on board either before departure or during the voyage or on arrival.

Art. 21.—In the case of *plague, infected* ships shall undergo the following measures :—

(1) medical inspection ;

(2) the sick shall immediately be disembarked and isolated ;

(3) the other persons must also be disembarked if possible, and either be kept under observation[1] during a period which shall not exceed five days and which may or may not be followed by surveillance[2] of not more than five days' duration, or merely be subjected to surveillance during a period which shall not exceed ten days. The period shall date from the arrival of the ship. It rests with the sanitary authority of the port, after taking into consideration the date of the last case, the condition of the ship, and the local possibilities, to take that one of these measures which seems to them preferable ;

(4) such soiled linen, wearing-apparel, and articles belonging to the crew[3] and passengers as are, in the opinion of the sanitary authority, infected shall be disinfected ;

(5) the parts of the ship that have been occupied by persons ill with plague, or that, in the opinion of the sanitary authority, are infected, must be disinfected ;

(6) the rats on board must be destroyed, either before or after discharge of cargo, as quickly as possible and, in any case, within a maximum time of forty-eight hours, and so as to avoid damage to merchandise and to the ship's plating and engines. In the case of ships in ballast, this process must be carried out as soon as possible before taking cargo.

Art. 22.—In the case of *plague, suspected* ships shall undergo the measures specified in (1), (4), and (5) of Article 21.

[1] "Observation" means isolation of travellers either on board a ship or in a sanitary station before they obtain free pratique.

"Surveillance" means that travellers are not isolated ; they receive free pratique immediately, but the authorities of the several places whither they are bound are informed of their coming and they are subjected to medical examination with a view to ascertaining their state of health.

[3] "Crew" means persons forming or having formed part of the crew or staff of the ship and includes stewards, waiters, cafedji, etc. The word must be interpreted in this sense in all instances in which it occurs in this Convention.

In addition, the crew and passengers may be subjected to surveillance, the duration of which, dating from the arrival of the ship, shall not exceed five days. The crew may, during the same period, be prevented from leaving the ship except on duty.

Destruction of rats on board is recommended. This process shall be carried out, either before or after discharge of cargo, as quickly as possible and, in any case, within a maximum time of forty-eight hours, and so as to avoid damage to merchandise and to the ship's plating and engines. In the case of ships in ballast, this process, if there be occasion for it, shall be carried out as soon as possible and, in any case, before taking cargo.

Art. 23.—In the case of *plague, healthy* ships shall be given free pratique immediately, whatever their bill of health may be. The only measures which the authority of the port of arrival may take as regards these ships are the following :—

(1) medical inspection ;

(2) disinfection of soiled linen, wearing apparel and other articles belonging to the crew and passengers, but only in exceptional instances, when the sanitary authority has special reasons for regarding them as infected ;

(3) the sanitary authority may subject ships from an infected port to a process intended to secure destruction of rats on board, either before or after discharge of cargo, although this measure must not be resorted to as a general rule. This process must be carried out as soon as possible and, in any case, must not take longer than twenty-four hours, and so as to avoid damage to merchandise and to the ship's plating and engines, and also so as not to interfere with the coming and going of passengers and crew between ship and shore. In the case of ships in ballast, the process, if there be occasion for it, shall be carried out as soon as possible and, in any case, before taking cargo.

If a ship from an infected port has been subjected to measures of rat destruction, these cannot be repeated unless the ship has called at an infected port and has there brought up to the quay, or unless sick or dead rats are found on board.

The crew and passengers may be subjected to surveillance during a period which shall not exceed five days reckoned from the date on which the ship left the infected port. The crew may, during the same period, be prevented from leaving the ship except on duty.

The competent authority at the port of arrival may, in all cases, exact a certificate, given on oath, from the doctor of the ship, or, in his default, from the captain, testifying that there has not been a case of plague on board since departure and that unusual mortality among rats has not been observed.

Art. 24.—When rats on a *healthy* ship have been shown by bacteriological examination to have plague, or when unusual mortality among these rodents has been observed, the measures to adopt are as follows :—

I.   Ships with rats having plague :—

(*a*) medical inspection ;

(*b*) the rats must be destroyed, either before or after discharge of cargo, as quickly as possible and, in any case, within a maximum time of forty-eight hours, and so as to avoid damage to merchandise and to the ship's plating and engines. Ships in ballast shall undergo this process as soon as possible and, in any case, before taking cargo ;

(*c*) such parts of the ship and such articles as the local sanitary authority regards as infected shall be disinfected ;

(*d*) the passengers and crew may be subjected to surveillance during a period which must not exceed five days reckoned from the date of arrival, save in exceptional instances in which the sanitary authority may prolong the surveillance up to not more than ten days.

II.   Ships on which unusual mortality among rats has been observed :—

(*a*) medical inspection ;

(*b*) the rats shall be examined for plague as far and as quickly as possible ;

(*c*) if it be considered necessary to destroy the rats, such destruction shall take place subject to the conditions specified above as regards ships with rats having plague ;

(*d*) until all suspicion shall have been removed, the passengers and crew may be subjected to surveillance for a period which shall not exceed five days reckoned from the date of arrival, save in exceptional instances in which the sanitary authority may prolong the surveillance up to not more than ten days.

Art. 25.—The sanitary authority of the port shall, whenever requested, furnish the captain, the ship-owner, or the ship-owner's agent, with a certificate stating that measures of rat-destruction have been carried out, and giving the reasons why they were resorted to.

Art. 26.—In the case of *cholera, infected* ships shall undergo the following measures :—

(1) medical inspection ;

(2) the sick shall be immediately disembarked and isolated ;

(3) the other persons must also be disembarked, if possible, and either be kept under observation or subjected to surveillance during a period which shall vary with the health conditions of the ship and the date of the last case, but which shall not exceed five days reckoned from the arrival of the ship ;

(4) such soiled linen, wearing apparel, and articles belonging to the

crew and passengers as are, in the opinion of the sanitary authority of the port, infected shall be disinfected;

(5) the parts of the ship that have been occupied by persons ill with cholera, or that the sanitary authority regard as infected, shall be disinfected;

(6) the bilge-water shall be disinfected and pumped out.

The sanitary authority may order that a supply of wholesome drinking-water be substituted for that stored on board.

Casting human excreta, or allowing them to pass, without preliminary disinfection, into the waters of the port may be prohibited.

Art. 27.—In the case of *cholera, suspected* ships shall undergo the measures prescribed in (1), (4), (5), and (6) of Article 26.

The crew and passengers may be subjected to surveillance during a period which must not exceed five days reckoned from the arrival of the ship. It is recommended that the crew be prevented, during the same period, from leaving the ship except on duty.

Art. 28.—In the case of *cholera, healthy* ships shall be given free pratique immediately, whatever their bill of health may be.

The only measures that the authority of the port of arrival may prescribe as regards these ships are those specified in (1), (4), and (6) of Article 26.

The crew and passengers may be subjected to surveillance, in respect of their state of health, during a period which must not exceed five days reckoned from the date on which the ship left the infected port. It is recommended that the crew be prevented, during the same period, from leaving the ship except on duty.

The competent authority at the port of arrival may, in all cases, exact a certificate, given on oath, from the doctor of the ship or, in his default, from the captain, testifying that there has not been a case of cholera on board since departure.

Art. 29.—In applying the measures specified in Articles 21–28, the fact of a ship of any of the three classes before-mentioned carrying a doctor and disinfecting apparatus (disinfecting chambers) shall receive due consideration on the part of the competent authority. In the case of plague, like consideration shall be given when the ship is provided with apparatus for the destruction of rats.

The sanitary authorities of States that find it convenient to come to an agreement on the matter, may dispense with medical inspection and other measures in the case of healthy ships carrying a doctor specially commissioned by their country.

Art. 30.—Special measures may be prescribed as regards ships that are overcrowded, and more especially as regards emigrant ships, or any other ship in an unsanitary condition.

Art. 31.—Ships refusing to submit to measures prescribed by a port authority, in virtue of the provisions of this Convention, shall be at liberty to put out to sea. Such ships may be permitted to land goods after the following necessary precautions have been taken, viz. :—

(1) isolation of the ship, crew, and passengers ;

(2) in the case of plague, request for information as to whether there has been any unusual mortality among rats on board ;

(3) in the case of cholera, disinfection and evacuation of the bilge-water and the substitution of wholesome drinking-water for that stored on board.

Such ships may also be authorised to disembark passengers at their request, on the condition that such passengers submit to the measures prescribed by the local authority.

Art. 32.—Ships from an infected place, that have been disinfected and have undergone adequate sanitary measures, shall not, on their arrival in another port, be subjected to these measures a second time, if no case has occurred since the disinfection was performed and if they have not called at an infected port. A ship which has merely disembarked passengers and their baggage, or mails, without having been in communication with the shore, shall not be regarded as having called at the port.

Art. 33.—Passengers arriving by an infected ship are entitled to exact from the sanitary authority of the port a certificate showing the date of their arrival and the measures taken as regards themselves and their baggage.

Art. 34.—Coasting traffic shall be dealt with by special regulations to be agreed upon by the countries concerned.

Art. 35.—Without prejudice to the right of Governments to agree to establish sanitary stations in common, every country must provide at least one port on each of its seaboards with an organisation and an equipment sufficient for the reception of a ship, whatever its health conditions may be.

It is recommended that, when a healthy ship from an infected port arrives in a large sea-port, such ship should not be sent away to another port with a view to the carrying out of the sanitary measures prescribed.

In every country, the ports open to arrivals from ports infected with plague or cholera must be so equipped that healthy ships can there undergo the prescribed measures upon their arrival and be not sent to another port for the purpose. Governments shall make known what ports in their country are open to arrivals from ports infected with plague or cholera.

Art. 36.—It is recommended that there be provided in large sea-ports :—

(*a*) a properly-organised port medical service and permanent medical supervision of the health-conditions of crews and of the population of the port ;

(*b*) suitable accommodation for the isolation of the sick and for keeping suspected persons under observation.

(*c*) bacteriological laboratories and the buildings and plant necessary for efficient disinfection;

(*d*) a supply of drinking-water of quality above suspicion at the disposal of the port, and a system of scavenging that offers every possible guarantee for the removal of excrement and refuse.

SECTION IV.—*Measures at land frontiers.—Travellers.—Railways. —Frontier tracts.—River-ways.*

Art. 37.—Land quarantine must no longer be resorted to. Only such persons as show symptoms of plague or of cholera may be detained at frontiers.

This principle does not deprive a State of the right to close a portion of its frontiers in case of need.

Art. 38.—It is important that the railway staff keep watch over the state of health of travellers.

Art. 39.—Medical intervention shall be limited to inspection of travellers and care of the sick. When this inspection is resorted to, it shall, as far as possible, be combined with the Customs' examination in order that travellers may suffer as little delay as possible. Only those persons who are visibly ailing shall be subjected to a thorough medical examination.

Art. 40.—It is a measure of the greatest value to subject travellers that have come from an infected place, on their arrival at their destination, to surveillance for a period which should not exceed ten or five days, reckoned from the date of their departure, in the case of plague or cholera respectively.

Art. 41.—Governments have the right reserved to them of taking special measures in regard of certain classes of persons, notably gipsies, vagrants, emigrants, and persons travelling or crossing the frontier in bands.

Art. 42.—Railway-carriages for passengers, mails, or luggage may not be detained at a frontier. If one of these carriages be infected or shall have been occupied by a person suffering from plague or from cholera, it shall be detached from the train for disinfection at the earliest possible moment. The same procedure shall apply in the case of goods trucks.

Art. 43.—Measures in relation with the crossing of frontiers by railway and postal staff come within the scope of the administrations concerned. They shall be arranged so as not to hamper the service.

Art. 44. —The regulation of frontier traffic and questions connected therewith, as also the adoption of exceptional measures of surveillance, must be left as matters for special arrangement between adjoining States.

Art. 45.—The sanitary control of river-ways is a matter for special arrangement by the Governments of States abutting thereon.

PART II.

SPECIAL PROVISIONS REGARDING COUNTRIES OUTSIDE EUROPE.

CHAPTER I.

ARRIVALS BY SEA.

SECTION I.—*Measures at infected ports on the departure of vessels.*

Art. 46.—The competent authority shall take effectual measures to prevent the embarkation of persons showing symptoms of plague or of cholera.

Every person taking passage by a ship must be individually examined at the time of embarkation, by day and on shore, during such time as may be necessary, by a doctor appointed by the public authority. The consular authority of the country to which the ship belongs may be represented at this examination.

In exception of this provision, the medical examination may, at Alexandria and Port Said, take place on board whenever the local sanitary authority consider this course to be of service; subject, however, to the reservation that third-class passengers shall not afterwards be authorised to leave the ship. The medical examination may be conducted by night in the case of first-class and second-class passengers, but not in the case of third-class passengers.

Art. 47.—The competent authority shall take effectual measures:

(1) to prevent the exportation of such merchandise or articles of any sort as it may regard as infected and which have not previously been disinfected on shore under the supervision of a doctor appointed by the public authority;

(2) in the case of plague, to prevent rats gaining access to ships;

(3) in the case of cholera, to see that drinking-water taken on board is wholesome.

SECTION II.—*Measures regarding ordinary ships from infected northern ports, on their arrival at the entrance to the Suez Canal or at Egyptian ports.*

Art. 48.—Ordinary *healthy* ships from a port, infected with plague or with cholera, in Europe or in the Mediterranean basin, proposing to pass through the Suez Canal, shall be granted passage in quarantine and shall continue their voyage under five days' observation.

Art. 49.—Ordinary *healthy* ships, wishing to touch at Egypt, may put in at Alexandria or Port Said, where their passengers shall complete the period of five days' observation, either on board, or in a sanitary station, as the local sanitary authority may decide.

Art. 50.—The measures to be taken as regards *infected* and *suspected* ships from an European or Mediterranean port infected with plague or with cholera, wishing to touch at an Egyptian port or to pass through the Suez Canal, shall be settled by the Egyptian Sanitary Board in conformity with the provisions of this Convention. The regulations embodying these measures must, to become effective, be accepted by the several Powers represented on the Board : they shall establish the measures to which ships, passengers, and merchandise are to be subjected, and must be submitted with the least possible delay.

Section III.—*Measures in the Red Sea.*

A.—*Measures regarding ordinary ships from the South, touching at Red Sea ports or bound for the Mediterranean.*

Art. 51.—In addition to the general provisions comprised in Part I, Chapter II, Section III, concerning the classification of ships as infected, suspected, or healthy, and the measures regarding them, the special provisions, embodied in the following articles, shall apply to ordinary ships entering the Red Sea from the south.

Art. 52.—*Healthy* ships must have completed or must complete five full days' observation reckoned from the time of their departure from the last infected port touched at.

They shall be entitled to pass through the Suez Canal in quarantine and shall enter the Mediterranean continuing the above-mentioned five days' observation. Ships with a doctor and a disinfecting chamber shall not undergo disinfection prior to the passage in quarantine.

Art. 53.—*Suspected* ships shall be treated in a manner which shall differ according as to whether they have or have not a doctor and a disinfecting apparatus (disinfecting chamber).

(*a*) Those that have a doctor and a disinfecting apparatus (disinfecting chamber) that fulfils the requisite conditions shall be allowed to pass through the Suez Canal in quarantine subject to the regulations prescribed for the passage.

(*b*) Those that have neither doctor nor disinfecting apparatus (disinfecting chamber) shall, before being allowed to pass through the Canal in quarantine, be detained at Suez or at Moses' Wells for such time as may be necessary for the performance of the disinfection prescribed and for assurance that the health conditions on board are satisfactory.

Passage in quarantine shall be granted to mail-boats or packets specially devoted to passenger traffic that have a doctor but no disinfecting apparatus (disinfecting chamber), if it be officially established to the satisfaction of the local authority that cleansing and disinfection have been properly carried out at the place of departure or during the voyage.

Free pratique may be granted at Suez, on the termination of the procedure prescribed by the regulations, to mail-boats or packets specially devoted to passenger traffic that have a doctor but no disinfecting apparatus (disinfecting chamber) if the last case of plague or cholera occurred more than seven days before and if the health conditions of the ship are satisfactory.

In the case of a vessel that has had a healthy voyage of less than seven days' duration, passengers for Egypt shall be landed at an establishment appointed by the Alexandria Board and isolated for such time as may be necessary for the completion of five days' observation. Their soiled linen and their wearing apparel shall be disinfected. They shall then be granted free pratique.

Ships that have had a healthy voyage of less than seven days' duration and that wish to have free pratique for Egypt shall be detained at an establishment, appointed by the Alexandria Board, during such time as may be necessary for the completion of five days' observation; they shall undergo the measures prescribed by the regulations for suspected vessels.

When plague or cholera has occurred among the crew only, no soiled linen shall be disinfected save that of the crew, the whole of which, however, shall undergo disinfection; the crew's quarters shall also be disinfected.

Art. 54.—*Infected* ships shall be divided into two classes, ships with a doctor and a disinfecting apparatus (disinfecting chamber), and ships without a doctor and without a disinfecting apparatus (disinfecting chamber).

(*a*) Ships without a doctor and without a disinfecting apparatus (disinfecting chamber) shall be detained at Moses' Wells[1]; persons that show symptoms of plague or cholera shall be disembarked and isolated in a hospital. Disinfection shall be thoroughly carried out. The other persons shall be disembarked and isolated in as small groups as possible so that, if plague or cholera break out in one group, the whole party will not be affected. The soiled linen and the clothing of passengers and crew, and other articles used by them, shall be disinfected, as also shall the ship.

It is to be understood that there is no question of discharging merchandise, but only of disinfecting the infected part of the ship.

The passengers shall remain five days at an establishment appointed by the Egyptian Sanitary Maritime and Quarantine Board. When cases of

---

[1] The sick shall, as far as possible, be landed at Moses' Wells; the other persons may be kept under observation at a sanitary station appointed by the Egyptian Sanitary Maritime and Quarantine Board (pilots' lazaret).

plague and cholera have not occurred for several days the term o isolation shall be shortened. Its duration shall vary according to the date of recovery, death, or isolation of the last case. Thus, if six days have elapsed since the recovery, death, or isolation of the last case, the period of observation shall be one day; if only five days have elapsed, the period shall be two days; if only four days have elapsed, the period shall be three days; if only three days have elapsed, the period shall be four days; if only two days or one day have elapsed, the period shall be five days.

(*b*) Ships with a doctor and a disinfecting apparatus (disinfecting chamber) shall be detained at Moses' Wells. The ship's doctor must state, on oath, which persons on board have symptoms of plague or of cholera. These persons shall be disembarked and isolated.

After these persons have been disembarked, such of the soiled linen of the other passengers as the sanitary authority regards as dangerous and that of the crew shall be disinfected on board. When plague or cholera has occurred only among the crew, the disinfection of linen shall be carried out only as regards the soiled linen of the crew and the linen of the crew's quarters.

The ship's doctor must also declare, on oath, which part or compartment of the ship was occupied by the sick and to which section of the hospital they were removed. He must also declare, on oath, which persons have been in relation with the plague or cholera patient since the first appearance of the disease, either by direct contact or by contact with objects that may have been infected. Only these persons shall be regarded as suspected.

The part or compartment of the ship, and the section of the hospital, that have been occupied by the sick, shall be thoroughly disinfected. "Part of the ship" shall mean the cabin of the sick person, the adjoining cabins, the passage to these cabins, the deck, the parts of the deck where the sick person or persons have remained for some time. If it be impossible to disinfect the part or compartment of the ship that has been occupied by plague or cholera sick without disembarking the persons declared to be suspected, these persons shall either be transferred to another ship specially reserved for the purpose, or be landed and accommodated in the sanitary station without being brought into contact with the sick, who must be kept in the hospital. This stay on board ship or on shore, for purposes of disinfection, shall be as short as possible and shall not exceed twenty-four hours.

The suspected persons shall be kept under observation, either on their own ship or on the ship reserved for that purpose, for a period which shall vary according to the circumstances and in the manner set out in the third paragraph of sub-section (*a*) of this article.

The time occupied in carrying out the measures prescribed by the regulations shall be included in the observation period.

Passage in quarantine may, if deemed possible by the sanitary authority, be allowed before expiry of the periods of detention indicated above. It shall in any case be granted on the completion of disinfection if the ship leaves behind, in addition to its sick, the persons classed above as "suspected."

A barge fitted with a disinfecting chamber may be brought alongside the ship with a view to hastening the process of disinfection.

Infected vessels seeking free pratique in Egypt shall be detained five days at Moses' Wells; they shall, in addition, undergo the same measures as are taken in the case of infected ships arriving in Europe.

B.—*Measures regarding ordinary ships from infected ports in the Hedjaz during the pilgrimage season.*

Art. 55.—If, during the Mecca pilgrimage, plague or cholera is prevalent in the Hedjaz, ships from the Hedjaz or from any other part of the Arabian coast of the Red Sea, that have not there taken on board any pilgrims or like collections of persons and on which there has been no suspicious incident during the voyage, shall be classed as ordinary suspected ships and shall be subjected to the preventive measures and the treatment prescribed for such ships.

If they are bound for Egypt they shall undergo, at a sanitary station appointed by the Sanitary Maritime and Quarantine Board, five days' observation, reckoned from the date of their departure, whether it be cholera or plague that is in question. They shall, moreover, be subjected to all the measures prescribed for suspected ships (disinfection, etc.), and shall not be granted free pratique until after favourable medical inspection.

It is to be understood that, if there have been suspicious incidents on board during the voyage, the period of observation shall be undergone at Moses' Wells and shall be five days whether it be cholera or plague that is in question.

Section IV.—*The organisation for securing surveillance and disinfection at Suez and at Moses' Wells.*

Art. 56.—Every ship arriving at Suez shall undergo the medical inspection prescribed by the regulations. This inspection shall be conducted by one or more of the doctors attached to the station, and shall, in the case of ships from a port infected with plague or with cholera, be made by day. It may, however, in the case of ships wishing to pass through the Canal, take place by night when the ship is lighted by electricity, and in all cases in which the local sanitary authority is satisfied that the ship is sufficiently well lighted.

Art. 57.—There shall be at least seven doctors at the Suez station,—a principal medical officer and six medical officers. They must hold a recognised diploma and, in their selection, preference is to be given to medical men who have made a special study of practical epidemiology and practical bacteriology. They shall be appointed by the Minister of the Interior on the recommendation of the Sanitary Maritime and Quarantine Board of Egypt. The salary of the medical officers shall commence at 8000 francs and rise by progressive increments to 12,000 francs; that of the principal medical officer shall commence at 12,000 francs and rise to 15,000 francs.

Should this medical staff prove insufficient, naval doctors of the several States may be employed, under the orders of the Principal Medical Officer of the sanitary station.

Art. 58.—The supervision and performance of the Suez Canal prophylactic measures at the Moses' Wells and Tor stations, shall be entrusted to a staff of sanitary guards.

Art. 59.—This staff shall consist of ten guards. They shall. be selected from retired non-commissioned officers, of higher than corporal's rank, of the armies and navies of Europe and Egypt. These guards are elected, after the Board is satisfied as to their fitness, according to the procedure laid down in Article 14 of the Khedivial Decree of 19th June, 1893.

Art. 60.—There shall be two classes of guards; four of the first class, six of the second class.

Art. 61.—The yearly pay of these guards shall be £160 Egyptian, rising by progressive increments to a maximum of £200 Egyptian, for the first class; and £120 Egyptian, rising by progressive increments to a maximum of £168 Egyptian, for the second class.

Art. 62.—These guards shall have the status of police officers, with the right to invoke aid in cases where the sanitary regulations are infringed. They shall be under the immediate control of the administrator-in-chief of the establishment at Suez or Tor. They must have practical knowledge of all the methods of disinfection in use, and must know how to manipulate disinfecting materials and apparatus.

Art. 63.—The disinfecting and isolation station at Moses' Wells shall be under the control of the principal medical officer at Suez. If sick persons are landed at the Moses' Wells Station, two of the Suez medical officers shall be kept in residence there, one to attend to cases of plague or cholera, the other to attend to persons not suffering from these diseases. If there should be cases of plague, of cholera, and of other diseases at the same time, three medical officers shall be kept in residence; one for plague cases, one for cholera cases, and the third for persons suffering from other diseases.

Art. 64.—The disinfecting and isolation station at Moses' Wells must be provided with :—

(1) at least three disinfecting chambers, of which one shall be on a barge, and the plant required for rat-destruction ;

(2) two isolation hospitals, each with twelve beds, one for cases of plague and persons suspected of having plague, the other for cases of cholera and persons suspected of having cholera. These hospitals must be so arranged that, in each of them, the sick, the suspected, and men and women can be segregated from one another ;

(3) buildings, hospital-tents, and ordinary tents, for the accommodation of persons landed ;

(4) a sufficient number of baths and shower-baths ;

(5) the necessary buildings for general staff, doctors, guards, etc. ; a store, and a laundry ;

(6) a reservoir for the water-supply ;

(7) the several buildings must be so arranged that the sick, or infected or suspected articles, cannot be brought into contact with other persons.

Art. 65.—The disinfecting chambers at Moses' Wells shall be entrusted to the special care of a skilled mechanic.

SECTION V.—*The passage of the Suez Canal in quarantine.*

Art. 66.—Permission to pass the Suez Canal in quarantine shall be granted by the Suez sanitary authority ; the Board shall be immediately informed when such permission is given. In doubtful cases, the decision shall rest with the Board.

Art. 67.—When the permission provided for in the preceding article has been given, a telegram shall at once be sent to the authority appointed by each Power. The telegram shall be sent at the expense of the ship.

Art. 68.—Each Power shall issue an edict subjecting to penalties those vessels which depart from the course declared by the captain and enter without license one of the ports of that Power. Exception shall be made in the case of circumstances beyond control and when a break in the voyage cannot be avoided.

Art. 69.—When the health-visit takes place, the captain must declare if he has on board gangs of native stokers, or hired servants, of any description, not included in the roll of the crew, or the register kept for the purpose. The following questions, in particular, shall be put to the captains of all ships arriving at Suez from the south and shall be answered by them on oath :—

Have you any supernumeraries : stokers, or other hands not included in the ship's roll or in the special register ?

What is their nationality ?

Where did you embark them ?

The medical officers must satisfy themselves as to the presence of these supernumeraries, and if they find that any of their number are missing, they must enquire carefully into the cause of their absence.

Art. 70.—A sanitary officer and two sanitary guards shall go on board. They must accompany the ship as far as Port Said ; their duty is to prevent communication, and to see to the execution of the measures prescribed for the passage of the Canal.

Art. 71.—All embarkation and disembarkation, and all transhipment of passengers or goods, are forbidden during the passage of the Canal from Suez to Port Said.

Provided always that travellers may embark at Port Said in quarantine.

Art. 72.—Ships passing through the Canal in quarantine must make the journey from Suez to Port Said without lying up.

In case of the vessel running aground, or being compelled to lie up, the necessary operations shall be carried out by the staff of the ship, all communication with the staff of the Suez Canal Company being avoided.

Art. 73.—Infected or suspected transports passing through the Canal in quarantine with troops must do so only by day. If they are compelled to pass the night in the Canal, they shall anchor in Lake Timsah or in the Great Lake.

Art. 74.—Ships that pass through the Canal in quarantine are forbidden to stop at Port Said except as provided for by the second paragraph of Article 71 and by Article 75. Revictualling must be effected by the means at the disposal of the ship. All stevedores and others who have gone on board shall be isolated on the quarantine barge, where their clothing shall be disinfected as prescribed by the regulations.

Art. 75.—When it is absolutely necessary for ships passing in quarantine to coal at Port Said, they must do so at a place to be fixed by the Sanitary Board, where the necessary isolation and sanitary supervision can be secured. The coaling may be done by the labourers of the port in cases where effective supervision of this operation is possible, and when all contact with the crew can be avoided. At night, the coaling-place must be lighted by electricity.

Art. 76.—Pilots, electricians, agents of the Company, and sanitary guards shall be disembarked at Port Said outside the port, between the jetties, and shall be taken thence direct to the quarantine barge, where their clothing shall be disinfected if necessary.

Art. 77.—As regards the passage of the Suez Canal, the following advantages shall be accorded to ships of war as hereinafter specified.

The quarantine authority shall accept them as healthy on their presenting a certificate signed by the ship-surgeons, countersigned by the captain, and stating on oath :—

(*a*) that there has not been, either at the time of departure or during the voyage, a case of plague or of cholera on board ;

(*b*) that a careful examination of everyone on board, without exception, has been made within 12 hours of arrival at the Egyptian port, and that no case of either of these diseases has been detected.

These ships shall not undergo medical inspection, and shall be given free pratique at once subject to their having completed five clear days since leaving the last infected port at which they called. Such of these ships as have not completed the requisite period may pass through the Canal in quarantine without medical inspection provided they produce the certificate above mentioned to the quarantine authority.

Notwithstanding the foregoing provisions, the quarantine authority shall have the right of medically inspecting, by its officers, ships of war in all instances in which it considers this procedure necessary.

Infected or suspected ships of war shall be subject to the regulations in force.

Only fighting-units shall be regarded as ships of war. Transports and hospital-ships shall be classed as ordinary ships.

Art. 78.—The Egyptian Maritime and Quarantine Board may arrange the conveyance, by rail, over Egyptian territory, of mails and ordinary passengers from infected countries in quarantine trains, under the conditions specified in Appendix No. 1.

SECTION VI.—*Measures in the Persian Gulf.*

Art. 79.—Ships shall undergo the health-visit at the Island of Ormuz sanitary station before they enter the Persian Gulf. They shall undergo the measures specified in Section III, Chapter II, Part I, that their health conditions and the place whence they have come render applicable. Ships, however, that have to proceed up the Shatt-el-Arab shall be permitted, if the period of observation has not been completed, to continue their voyage, on condition that they traverse the Persian Gulf and the Shatt-el-Arab in quarantine. A chief guard and two sanitary guards, taken on board at Ormuz, shall keep the ship under supervision as far as Bassorah, where a second medical inspection shall be made and the necessary measures of disinfection carried out. Pending the organisation of the Ormuz sanitary station, the sanitary guards shall be taken on at the temporary station provided in accordance with paragraph 2 of Article 82 hereinafter, and these guards shall accompany ships proceeding in quarantine up the Shatt-el-Arab to the station provided in the neighbourhood of Bassorah.

Ships that have to call at Persian ports to disembark passengers or goods may do so at Bender-Bushire.

It is to be clearly understood that a ship which continues healthy after five days, reckoned from her date of departure from the last port infected by plague or cholera at which she has touched, shall be granted free pratique at Persian Gulf ports, provided she is ascertained to be healthy on arrival.

Art. 80.—In so far as the classification of ships and the measures they are to undergo are concerned, Articles 20 to 28 of this Convention apply in the Persian Gulf, subject to the three following modifications :—

(1) observation, for the same period, shall always be substituted for surveillance of passengers and crew ;

(2) healthy ships cannot be granted free pratique unless they have completed five full days since leaving the last infected port at which they have touched ;

(3) in the case of suspected ships the period of five days' observation of passengers and crew shall be reckoned from the time at which there ceased to be a case of plague or of cholera on board.

Section VII.—*Persian Gulf Sanitary Stations.*

Art. 81.—Sanitary stations must be provided, under the direction and at the expense of the Constantinople Board of Health, one at the Island of Ormuz, the other at a spot to be selected in the neighbourhood of Bassorah.

At the Ormuz sanitary station there shall be at least two doctors, sanitary officers, sanitary guards, and a complete plant for disinfection and for destruction of rats. A small hospital shall be erected.

At the station near Bassorah there shall be provided a large lazaret with a staff of several doctors, and buildings and plant for the disinfection of goods.

Art. 82.—The Constantinople Superior Board of Health, which has the control of the Bassorah sanitary station, shall have the same power as regards the Ormuz station.

Pending the construction of the Ormuz sanitary station, a sanitary post shall be provided there by the Constantinople Superior Board of Health.

CHAPTER II.

ARRIVALS BY LAND.

SECTION I.—*General provisions.*

Art. 83.—The measures taken in respect of arrivals by land from districts infected with plague or with cholera must be in conformity with the sanitary principles laid down in this Convention.

Modern methods of disinfection must be substituted for land quarantine. With this object, disinfecting chambers and other disinfecting plant shall be established at properly selected points on the roads frequented by travellers. The same methods shall be adopted on railways, whether now in existence or constructed hereafter. Merchandise shall be disinfected in accordance with the principles of this Convention.

Art. 84.—Every Government is at liberty, in case of need, to close a portion of its frontiers to passengers and merchandise in localities where there is difficulty in organising sanitary supervision.

SECTION II.—*Turkish land frontiers.*

Art. 85.—The Constantinople Superior Board of Health must organise without delay the sanitary stations of Hanikin and Kizil-Dizié, near Bayazid, on the Turko-Persian and Turko-Russian frontiers.

PART III.

SPECIAL PROVISIONS REGARDING PILGRIMAGES.

CHAPTER I.

GENERAL PROVISIONS.

Art. 86.—The provisions of Articles 46 and 47, Part II, are applicable to persons and things that have to be taken on board a pilgrim-ship leaving a port in the Indian Ocean or Oceania, even when the port is not infected with plague or with cholera.

Art. 87.—When there are cases of plague or of cholera in the port, embarkation on pilgrim-ships shall not take place until the persons, collected in groups, shall have been subjected to observation sufficient to ensure that none of them are suffering from plague or cholera. It is to be understood that, as regards the adoption of this measure, every Government may take local circumstances and possibilities into account.

Art. 88.—If local circumstances permit, pilgrims must prove that they possess the means absolutely necessary for the accomplishment of the pilgrimage, and, in particular, that they have a return-ticket.

Art. 89.—Only steamships shall be permitted to carry pilgrims on long voyages. The carriage of pilgrims by other ships on such voyages shall be prohibited.

Art. 90.—Pilgrim-ships that are coasters intended for short passages known as "coasting voyages" shall be subject to the provisions of the special regulations for the Hedjaz pilgrimage, which shall be published by the Constantinople Board of Health, in conformity with the principles laid down in this Convention.

Art. 91.—A ship which, in addition to ordinary passengers, among whom pilgrims of the upper classes may be included, carries pilgrims of the lowest class in less proportion than one pilgrim per 100 tons gross, shall not be considered a pilgrim-ship.

Art. 92.—Every pilgrim-ship, on entering the Red Sea or the Persian Gulf, must observe the provisions of the special regulations for the Hedjaz pilgrimage, which shall be published by the Constantinople Board of Health, in conformity with the principles laid down in this Convention.

Art. 93.—The captain must pay all sanitary imposts leviable on pilgrims. These imposts must be covered by the price of the ticket.

Art. 94.—As far as practicable, pilgrims who embark or disembark at sanitary stations must have no contact with one another at the landing-places.

Ships that have disembarked their pilgrims must change their anchorage before commencing re-embarkation.

Pilgrims who have been disembarked must be distributed in camp in as small groups as possible. It is necessary that they be supplied with wholesome drinking-water, obtained either from local sources or by distillation.

Art. 95.—When there is plague or cholera in the Hedjaz, provisions brought by pilgrims shall be destroyed if the sanitary authority consider it necessary.

CHAPTER II.

PILGRIM-SHIPS.—SANITARY STATIONS.

Section I.—*General conditions applying to ships.*

Art. 96.—The ship must be capable of accommodating the pilgrims in the between decks.

Over and above the space required for the crew, the ship must provide for each person, irrespective of age, an area of 1·50 square metres, equivalent to 16 English square feet, and a height between decks of about 1·80 metres. In coasting vessels, each pilgrim must be allowed a space at least 2 metres wide along the gunwales.

Art. 97.—On each side of the ship, on deck, a place must be set apart, screened from view and furnished with a hand-pump, for the supply of sea-water for the needs of the pilgrims. One such place must be reserved exclusively for women.

Art. 98.—The ship must be provided, in addition to closets for the crew, with latrines, fitted with a flushing apparatus or with a water tap, in a minimum proportion of one latrine per hundred passengers. Some of these latrines shall be reserved exclusively for women.

There must be no closets between decks or in the hold.

Art. 99.—The ship must have two places for cooking set apart for the use of the pilgrims. Pilgrims shall be forbidden to light fires elsewhere, especially on deck.

Art. 100.—A properly fitted hospital, constructed with due attention to safety and health, must be reserved for the accommodation of the sick. It must be capable of accommodating, at the rate of three square metres per patient, not less than five per cent. of the pilgrims taken on board.

Art. 101.—The ship must be provided with the means of segregating persons showing symptoms of plague or of cholera.

Art. 102.—Every ship must carry such medical remedies, disinfectants, and things as are necessary for the treatment of the sick. The regulations framed for this class of ship by each Government must specify the nature and the quantity of these remedies[1]. Medicine and attendance shall be provided for the pilgrims free of charge.

Art. 103.—Every ship taking pilgrims must carry a duly qualified doctor, commissioned by the Government of the country to which the ship belongs or by the Government of the port where the pilgrims are embarked. A second doctor must be carried when the number of pilgrims on board exceeds 1000.

Art. 104.—The captain must cause notices, in the languages chiefly spoken in the countries inhabited by the pilgrims he is taking, to be posted up on the ship in a conspicuous place, accessible to all concerned, showing :—

    (1) the destination of the ship ;
    (2) the price of tickets ;
    (3) the daily ration of food and water allowed to each pilgrim ;

---

[1] It is to be desired that every ship be provided with the chief immunising agents (anti-plague serum, Haffkine's prophylactic, etc.).

(4) the price of articles, not included in the daily ration, which may be procured on extra payment.

Art. 105.—The heavy baggage of pilgrims shall be registered, numbered, and put in the hold. Pilgrims may keep with them only such things as are absolutely necessary. The nature, amount, and dimensions of these things shall be decided by regulations framed by each Government for its own ships.

Art. 106.—The provisions of Chapter I, of Sections I, II, and III of Chapter II, and of Chapter III, of Part III of this Convention shall be posted up, in the form of regulations, in the language of the country to which the ship belongs, and also in the languages chiefly spoken in the countries inhabited by the pilgrims to be embarked, in a conspicuous and accessible place on every deck and between-decks of every ship carrying pilgrims.

SECTION II.—*Measures before departure.*

Art. 107.—The captain or, in his default, the owner or agent of every pilgrim-ship must, not less than three days before departure, declare to the competent authority of the port of departure his intention to embark pilgrims. At ports of call, the captain or, in his default, the owner or agent of every pilgrim-ship must make the same declaration twelve hours before the departure of the ship. This declaration must specify the proposed date of departure and the destination of the ship.

Art. 108.—On receipt of the declaration provided for by the preceding article the competent authority shall proceed, at the expense of the captain, to inspect and measure the ship. The consular authority of the country to which the ship belongs may be present at this inspection. Inspection alone shall take place if the captain already has a certificate of measurement furnished by the competent authority of his country, unless it be suspected that the certificate no longer represents correctly the real condition of the ship[1].

Art. 109.—The competent authority shall not permit the departure of a pilgrim-ship until satisfied :—

(a) that the ship has been thoroughly cleaned and, if necessary, disinfected ;

(b) that the ship is in a condition to undertake the voyage without danger, that she is properly manned, equipped and ventilated, and provided

---

[1] At present the competent authority is : in British India, an officer appointed for the purpose by the Local Government (Native Passengers' Ships Act, 1877, Article 7) ; in the Dutch Indies, the master of the port ; in Turkey, the sanitary authority ; in Austro-Hungary, the port authority ; in Italy, the captain of the port ; in France, Tunis, and Spain, the sanitary authority ; in Egypt, the sanitary quarantine authority.

with a sufficient number of boats ; that there is on board nothing that is, or may become, injurious to the health or safety of the passengers, and that the deck is of wood or of iron sheathed in wood ;

(*c*) that there is on board, properly stowed away, over and above the rations for the crew, sufficient food and fuel of good quality for all the pilgrims, during the declared duration of the voyage ;

(*d*) that the drinking-water is of good quality and from a source free from risk of contamination ; that it is in sufficient quantity ; that the tanks for drinking-water are safe from all contamination and so closed that the water can be supplied only by means of taps or pumps. The water-supply fittings known as "suçoirs" shall be absolutely prohibited ;

(*e*) that the vessel carries a condenser, capable of distilling a minimum quantity of five litres of water per diem for every person on board, including crew ;

(*f*) that the ship possesses a disinfecting chamber, ascertained by the sanitary authority of the port where the pilgrims embarked to be safe and efficacious ;

(*g*) that, in accordance with Articles 102 and 103, the vessel carries a duly qualified doctor commissioned[1] either by the Government of the country to which she belongs or by the Government of the port where the pilgrims embark, and that she carries medical stores ;

(*h*) that the deck is free from merchandise and all encumbrances ;

(*i*) that the arrangements on board are such as to allow of the measures prescribed in the following Section III being carried out.

Art. 110.—The captain may not start without having in his possession :—

(1) a list, countersigned by the competent authority, showing the name, sex, and total number of pilgrims he is authorised to carry ;

(2) a bill-of-health, giving the name, nationality, and tonnage of the ship, the name of the captain and of the doctor, the exact number of persons embarked—crew, pilgrims and other passengers—the nature of the cargo and the place of departure.

The competent authority shall note on the bill-of-health whether the number of pilgrims permissible under the regulations has been embarked or not, and, in the latter case, the additional number of passengers the vessel is authorised to embark at subsequent ports of call.

SECTION III.—*Measures during the voyage.*

Art. 111.—During the voyage the deck must be kept free from encumbrances ; it must be reserved, night and day, for the passengers, and placed at their disposal without charge.

---

[1] Exception is made in the case of Governments without commissioned doctors.

Art. 112.—The between-decks must be carefully cleansed and rubbed with dry sand, mixed with disinfectants, every day while the pilgrims are on deck.

Art. 113.—The latrines allotted to the passengers, as well as those for the crew, must be kept clean, and must be cleansed and disinfected three times a day.

Art. 114.—The excretions and dejecta of persons showing symptoms of plague or of cholera must be received in vessels containing a disinfecting solution. These vessels shall be emptied into the latrines, which must be thoroughly disinfected every time this is done.

Art. 115.—All bedding, carpets, and clothing that have been in contact with the sick persons referred to in the preceding article must be immediately disinfected. The observance of this rule is specially enjoined in respect of the clothes of persons who have been near the sick, and which may have been contaminated. Such of the above-mentioned articles as are of no value must be either thrown overboard, if the ship is not in harbour or in a canal, or else burnt. Other articles must be carried to the disinfecting chamber in impermeable bags washed in a disinfecting solution.

Art. 116.—The quarters occupied by the sick, referred to in Article 100, must be thoroughly disinfected.

Art. 117.—It is compulsory on pilgrim-ships to undergo such measures of disinfection as are in accordance with the regulations on this subject that are, for the time being, in force in the country under whose flag they sail.

Art. 118.—Not less than five litres of drinking-water must each day be put at the disposal of every pilgrim, irrespective of age, free of charge.

Art. 119.—If there be any doubt as to the quality of the drinking-water or any reason to suspect that it may possibly have become contaminated, either at its source or during the voyage, it must be boiled or otherwise sterilised, and the captain shall be responsible for seeing that it is thrown overboard at the first port of call at which he can procure a purer supply.

Art. 120.—The doctor shall visit the pilgrims, tend the sick, and see that the principles of hygiene are observed on board.

He must in particular :—

(1) satisfy himself that the rations issued to the pilgrims are of good quality, that their quantity is in accordance with contract, and that they are properly prepared ;

(2) satisfy himself that the provisions of Article 118, regarding the distribution of water, are observed ;

(3) if there be any doubt as to the quality of the drinking-water, call the attention of the captain, in writing, to the provisions of Article 119 ;

(4) satisfy himself that the ship is always kept clean, and particularly that the latrines are cleansed in accordance with the provisions of Article 113;

(5) satisfy himself that the pilgrims' quarters are kept wholesome, and, in case of the occurrence of infectious disease, that disinfection is carried out in accordance with Articles 116 and 117;

(6) keep a diary of all occurrences related to health during the voyage, and submit this diary to the competent authority at the port of arrival.

Art. 121.—Only the persons charged with the care of plague or cholera patients shall have access to them, and these persons must not come in contact with the other persons that have been embarked.

Art. 122.—In the event of a death occurring during the voyage, the captain must enter the fact opposite the name of the deceased, on the list countersigned by the authority of the port of departure, and must also enter in the log the name of the deceased, his age, the place from which he came, the supposed cause of death according to the medical certificate, and the date of death.

In the event of a death from infectious disease, the corpse, wrapped in a shroud impregnated with a disinfecting solution, must be committed to the deep.

Art. 123.—The captain must see that all preventive measures taken during the voyage are entered in the log. The log shall be submitted by him to the competent authority at the port of arrival.

At each port of call the captain must cause the list drawn up in accordance with Article 110 to be countersigned by the competent authority.

In the event of a pilgrim disembarking during the voyage, the captain must note the fact on the list, opposite the pilgrim's name.

In the event of persons embarking, their names must be entered on the list in accordance with the foregoing Article 110. This must be done before the competent authority, as in duty bound, again countersigns the list.

Art. 124.—The bill-of-health given at the port of departure must not be changed during the voyage.

It shall be countersigned at each port of call by the sanitary authority, who shall enter :—

(1) the number of passengers disembarked or embarked at the port;

(2) anything that has happened at sea affecting the life or health of the persons embarked;

(3) the health conditions of the port of call.

Section IV.—*Measures on arrival of pilgrims in the Red Sea.*

A. *Sanitary control of ships from an infected port, going from the south to the Hedjaz with Mohammedan pilgrims.*

Art. 125.—Pilgrim-ships from the south, bound for the Hedjaz, must, in the first instance, put in at the Kamaran sanitary station, and shall be dealt with as provided by Articles 126–128.

Art. 126.—Ships found, on medical inspection, to be *healthy* shall be given free pratique on completion of the following procedure :—

The pilgrims shall be disembarked ; they shall take a shower-bath or bathe in the sea ; their soiled linen and any portion of their personal effects or their baggage, open, in the opinion of the sanitary authority, to suspicion, shall be disinfected. The duration of these operations, including disembarkation and embarkation, must not exceed forty-eight hours.

If no recognised or suspected case of plague or of cholera be discovered during these operations, the pilgrims shall immediately be re-embarked and the ship shall proceed to the Hedjaz.

In the case of plague, the provisions of Articles 23 and 24 regarding rats shall apply in the event of there being any of these vermin on board.

Art. 127.—*Suspected* ships, which have had cases of plague or of cholera on board at the time of departure, but no fresh case of plague or of cholera within seven days, shall be dealt with as follows :—

The pilgrims shall be disembarked ; they shall take a shower-bath or bathe in the sea ; their soiled linen and any portion of their personal effects or their baggage, open, in the opinion of the sanitary authority, to suspicion, shall be disinfected. In time of cholera, the bilge-water shall be pumped out. The parts of the ship occupied by the sick shall be disinfected. The duration of these operations, including disembarkation and embarkation, must not exceed forty-eight hours.

If no case or suspected case of plague or of cholera be discovered during these operations, the pilgrims shall immediately be re-embarked and the ship shall proceed to Jeddah, where a second medical inspection shall take place on board. If the result be favourable and if the ship's doctor certifies in writing and on oath that there has been no case of plague or of cholera during the passage, the pilgrims shall be landed forthwith. If, however, one or more recognised or suspected cases of plague or of cholera prove to have occurred during the voyage or on arrival, the ship shall be sent back to Kamaran where she shall again be dealt with as infected.

In the case of plague, the provisions of the third paragraph of Article 22 shall apply in the event of there being rats on board.

Art. 128.—*Infected* ships, that is to say, ships with cases of plague or of cholera on board, or that have had cases of plague or of cholera on board within seven days, shall be dealt with as follows :—

Persons suffering from plague or from cholera shall be disembarked and isolated in hospital. The other passengers shall be disembarked and isolated in as small groups as possible, in order that, if plague or cholera break out in one group, the whole party may not be affected.

The soiled linen, clothing and personal effects of the crew and the passengers shall be disinfected, as also shall the ship. The disinfection shall be carried out thoroughly. Provided always that the local sanitary authority may decide that heavy baggage and merchandise need not be unloaded, and that only part of the ship need be disinfected.

The passengers shall remain at the Kamaran station seven or five days, according as to whether plague or cholera is in question. When no cases of plague or of cholera have occurred for several days the period of isolation may be shortened, and may vary according to the date of occurrence of the last case and the decision of the sanitary authority.

The ship shall then proceed to Jeddah, where everyone on board shall undergo a thorough medical examination. If the result be favourable the ship shall be given free pratique. If, however, recognised cases of plague or of cholera have occurred on board during the voyage or on arrival, the ship shall be sent back to Kamaran, where she shall again be dealt with as infected.

In the case of plague, the measures specified in Article 21 regarding rats shall be adopted in the event of there being any of these vermin on board.

1.   *The Kamaran Station.*

Art. 129.—At the Kamaran station the following conditions must be fulfilled :—

Complete evacuation of the island by its inhabitants.

For the safety and convenience of shipping in the bay of Kamaran Island, provision of :—

(1) a sufficient number of buoys and beacons ;

(2) a main pier or quay for the landing of passengers and baggage ;

(3) a separate stage for the embarkation of the pilgrims in each encampment ;

(4) a steam-tug and sufficient barges for the disembarkation and embarkation of pilgrims.

Art. 130.—The disembarkation of pilgrims from infected ships shall be effected by the ship's own resources. If these be inadequate, the persons and the barges that assist in the disembarkation shall undergo the same measures as the pilgrims and the infected ship.

Art. 131.—The equipment of the sanitary station shall comprise the following :—

(1) A railway-system connecting the landing places with the administrative buildings, the disinfecting stations, the various staff premises, and the encampments ;

(2) administrative buildings and premises for the sanitary and other staff ;

(3) buildings for the disinfection and washing of wearing apparel and other articles ;

(4) buildings where the pilgrims are to have shower-baths or sea baths while their clothes are being disinfected ;

(5) separate and completely isolated hospitals for both sexes :—

   (*a*) for the observation of suspected persons,
   (*b*) for plague patients,
   (*c*) for cholera patients,
   (*d*) for patients suffering from other contagious diseases,
   (*e*) for ordinary patients ;

(6) encampments completely separated from each other, the distance between them to be as great as possible ; pilgrims' quarters constructed on the most approved sanitary principles, and not to contain more than 25 persons each ;

(7) a well-situated cemetery, distant from all dwellings, free from sub-soil water, and drained to the depth of half a-metre below the level of the graves ;

(8) steam disinfectors in sufficient number, and fulfilling all the conditions of safety, efficacy and rapidity ; apparatus for destroying rats ;

(9) spray-producers, disinfecting chambers and the necessary appliances for chemical disinfection ;

(10) water-distilling machines ; apparatus for the sterilisation of water by heat ; ice machines. A system of pipes and covered reservoirs, impervious, and from which water can be taken only by means of taps or pumps, for the distribution of drinking-water.

(11) a bacteriological laboratory with the necessary staff ;

(12) provision of portable receptacles for the reception of faecal matters after disinfection, and a system of disposal of these matters on one of the parts of the island farthest from the encampments, due regard being had to the conditions necessary for the proper working, from a sanitary point of view, of the land used for this purpose ;

(13) a system of removal of slop and waste waters from the encampments, which shall prevent their stagnation or use for drinking purposes. The slop and waste waters of the hospitals must be disinfected.

Art. 132.—The sanitary authority shall provide, in each encampment, a store for food and a store for fuel.

The tariff of prices fixed by the competent authority shall be posted up in several places in the encampment, in the languages commonly spoken in the countries inhabited by the pilgrims.

The doctor of the encampment shall be responsible for the daily control of the quality and quantity of the provisions.

Water shall be provided free of charge.

2. *The stations at Abu-Ali, Abu-Said, Jeddah, Vasta, and Yambo.*

Art. 133.—At the sanitary stations of Abu-Ali, Abu-Said, Vasta, as well as those of Jeddah and Yambo, the following conditions must be fulfilled :—

(1) the construction of four hospitals at Abu-Ali, two for cases of plague, male and female, two for cases of cholera, male and female ;

(2) the construction of a hospital for ordinary cases, at Vasta ;

(3) the provision, at Abu-Said and at Vasta, of stone buildings capable of accommodating fifty persons each ;

(4) the provision of three disinfecting chambers at Abu-Ali, Abu-Said, and Vasta, with laundries, accessories, and apparatus for destroying rats ;

(5) the provision of shower-baths at Abu-Said and Vasta ;

(6) on each of the islands of Abu-Said and Vasta, provision of distilling machines capable together of yielding 15 tons of water per day ;

(7) the disposal of faecal matters and slop and waste waters on the lines accepted in the case of Kamaran ;

(8) the provision of a cemetery on one of the islands ;

(9) the provision, at Jeddah and Yambo, of the buildings and plant for sanitary purposes referred to in Article 150, particularly disinfecting chambers, and other means of securing disinfection for the pilgrims returning from the Hedjaz.

Art. 134.—The rules laid down regarding food and water at Kamaran shall apply to the encampments of Abu-Ali, Abu-Said, and Vasta.

B. *Sanitary control of ships from the north going to the Hedjaz with Mohammedan pilgrims.*

Art. 135.—If it be not established that there is plague or cholera at the port of departure or in its neighbourhood, and if no case of plague or of cholera has occurred during the voyage, the ship shall be granted free pratique forthwith.

Art. 136.—If it be established that there is plague or cholera at the port of departure or in its neighbourhood, or if a case of plague or of cholera has occurred during the voyage, the ship shall be dealt with, at El-Tor, in the manner prescribed for ships coming from the south and stopping at Kamaran. The ships shall thereafter be granted free pratique.

SECTION V.—*Measures for pilgrims returning home.*

A. *Homeward-bound pilgrim-ships, going north.*

Art. 137.—Every ship from a port in the Hedjaz or from any other port on the Arabian coast of the Red Sea, carrying pilgrims or any like collection of persons, and bound for Suez or a Mediterranean port, must proceed to El-Tor, there to undergo the observation and the sanitary measures specified in Articles 141–143.

Art. 138.—Ships bringing back Mohammedan pilgrims to the Mediterranean shall not pass through the Canal save in quarantine.

Art. 139.—Agents of shipping lines and captains of ships are warned that, on completion of their period of observation at El-Tor sanitary station, only Egyptian pilgrims will be permitted to leave the ship definitively, in order to return to their homes. Only pilgrims with a certificate of residence, issued by an Egyptian authority and made out in the form prescribed, shall be recognised as Egyptians or inhabitants of Egypt. Specimens of this certificate shall be deposited with the consular and sanitary authorities at Jeddah and Yambo, where they may be seen by shipping agents and ship captains.

Non-Egyptian pilgrims, such as Turks, Russians, Persians, Tunisians, Algerians, inhabitants of Morocco, etc., may not, after leaving El-Tor, be disembarked at an Egyptian port. Agents of shipping lines and ship captains are therefore warned that the transhipment of non-Egyptian pilgrims at Tor, Suez, Port Said, or Alexandria, is prohibited.

Vessels carrying pilgrims belonging to the nationalities mentioned in the preceding paragraph shall be treated according to the rules for such pilgrims, and shall not be permitted to enter any Egyptian port in the Mediterranean.

Art. 140.—Egyptian pilgrims shall undergo at El-Tor, Suakim, or any other station appointed by the Egyptian Sanitary Board, observation for a period of three days and medical inspection, before being given free pratique.

Art. 141.—If it be established that there is plague or cholera in the Hedjaz or at the port whence the ship has come, or that either of these diseases has occurred in the Hedjaz during the pilgrimage, the ship shall be dealt with, at El-Tor, in the manner prescribed for infected ships at Kamaran.

Persons suffering from plague or cholera shall be landed and isolated in hospital. The other passengers shall be landed and isolated in as small groups as possible in order that, if plague or cholera break out in one group, the whole party may not be affected.

The soiled linen, clothing and personal effects of the crew and the passengers, and such baggage and merchandise as are suspected of being infected, shall be landed for purposes of disinfection. These articles, and also the ship, shall be thoroughly disinfected. Provided always that the local sanitary authority may decide that heavy baggage and merchandise need not be unloaded and that only part of the ship need be disinfected.

The provisions of Articles 21 and 24 regarding rats shall apply in the event of there being any of these vermin on board.

Whether it be plague or cholera that is in question, all the pilgrims shall be kept under observation for seven clear days, reckoned from the day on which the measures of disinfection were completed. If a case of plague or of cholera occur in a section, the period of seven days for that section shall be reckoned from the day on which the last case occurred.

Art. 142.—In the circumstances provided for by the foregoing article, Egyptian pilgrims shall, in addition, be kept under observation for a further period of three days.

Art. 143.—If it be not established that there is plague or cholera in the Hedjaz or at the port whence the ship has come, or that either of these diseases has occurred in the Hedjaz during the pilgrimage, the ship shall be dealt with, at El-Tor, in the manner prescribed for healthy ships at Kamaran.

The pilgrims shall be landed; they shall take a shower-bath or bathe in the sea; their soiled linen and any portion of their personal effects or their baggage, open, in the opinion of the sanitary authority, to suspicion, shall be disinfected. The duration of these operations, including disembarkation and embarkation, must not exceed 72 hours.

Provided always that a pilgrim-ship, belonging to a country that has given its adhesion to the provisions of this Convention and of previous Conventions, if she has had no case of plague or of cholera during the voyage from Jeddah to Yambo and El-Tor, and if it be established by medical examination, conducted at El-Tor after disembarkation, of every one on board, that she has no such case, may be permitted by the Egyptian Sanitary Board to pass through the Suez Canal in quarantine, even by night, subject to the fulfilment of the four following conditions :—

    (1) that, in order to secure medical attendance of persons on board,

the ship carries one or more doctors, commissioned by the Government of the country to which she belongs ;

(2) that the ship is provided with disinfecting chambers, and it is established that the soiled linen has been disinfected during the voyage ;

(3) that it is proved that the number of pilgrims is not in excess of that permitted by the pilgrimage regulations ;

(4) that the captain undertakes to sail direct to a port in the country to which the ship belongs.

The medical examination, after disembarkation at El-Tor, must be made with as little delay as possible.

The sanitary tax, payable to the Quarantine Administration, shall be the same as the pilgrims would have had to pay if they had remained in quarantine for three days.

Art. 144.—In the event of a suspicious case occurring on board during the voyage from El-Tor to Suez, the ship shall be sent back to El-Tor.

Art. 145.—Transhipment of pilgrims at Egyptian ports is strictly prohibited.

Art. 146.—Ships from the Hedjaz, carrying pilgrims bound for the African coast of the Red Sea, shall be permitted to proceed direct to Suakim or such other place as the Alexandria Sanitary Board shall appoint, there to undergo the same quarantine measures as those at El-Tor.

Art. 147.—Ships from the Hedjaz, or from a port on the Arabian coast of the Red Sea, with a clean bill-of-health, not carrying pilgrims or like collections of persons, and without suspicious incident during the voyage, shall, on favourable medical inspection, be given free pratique at Suez.

Art. 148.—When it is established that there is plague or cholera in the Hedjaz :—

(1) caravans of Egyptian pilgrims must, before proceeding to Egypt, undergo strict quarantine at El-Tor for seven days, whether it be plague or cholera that is in question ; they must thereafter be kept under observation at El-Tor for three days, after which they shall not be granted free pratique until after favourable medical inspection and disinfection of effects ;

(2) caravans of pilgrims from other countries, returning home by land, shall undergo the same measures as Egyptian caravans, and must be accompanied by sanitary guards to the borders of the desert.

Art. 149.—When plague or cholera has not been reported to have occurred in the Hedjaz, caravans of pilgrims coming from the Hedjaz by way of Akaba or Moila shall, on their arrival at the canal or at Nakhel, undergo medical inspection and disinfection of soiled linen and personal effects.

B.—*Homeward-bound pilgrims, going south.*

Art. 150.—The ports of embarkation in the Hedjaz shall be provided with buildings and plant for sanitary purposes sufficient to permit, in the case of pilgrims homeward-bound to the south, the taking of the measures rendered compulsory by the provisions of Articles 46 and 47, on the departure of these pilgrims from ports beyond the Strait of Bab-el-Mandeb. These measures shall be optional; that is to say, they shall not be carried out unless the consular authority of the country to which the pilgrims belong, or the doctor of the ship by which they propose to go, considers them necessary.

CHAPTER III.

PENALTIES.

Art. 151.—Any captain convicted of a breach of his contract for the supply of water, food, or fuel, shall be liable to a fine of 2 pounds Turkish[1]. This fine shall be paid to the pilgrim who has suffered from the breach of contract on proof that he demanded its fulfilment without effect.

Art. 152.—Any infringement of Article 104 shall be punished by a fine of 30 pounds Turkish.

Art. 153.—Any captain, who commits, or knowingly allows to be committed, any fraud with respect to the list of pilgrims, or of the bill-of-health provided for by Article 110, shall be liable to a fine of 50 pounds Turkish.

Art. 154.—Any ship-captain arriving without a bill-of-health from the port of departure, or without its having been countersigned at the ports of call, or unprovided with the prescribed list, duly kept in accordance with Articles 110, 123, and 124, shall be liable, in each instance, to a fine of 12 pounds Turkish.

Art. 155.—Any captain convicted of having or of having had on board more than 100 pilgrims, without a commissioned doctor, in accordance with the provisions of Article 103, shall be liable to a fine of 300 pounds Turkish.

Art. 156.—Any captain convicted of having or of having had on board more pilgrims than he is permitted, by the provisions of Article 110, to carry, shall be liable to a fine of five pounds Turkish for each pilgrim in excess of the proper number.

The pilgrims in excess of the proper number shall be disembarked at the first station where there is a competent authority, and the captain is bound

---

[1] A Turkish pound is of the value of 22½ francs.

to provide the pilgrims so disembarked with sufficient money to enable them to reach their destination.

Art. 157.—Any captain convicted of having disembarked pilgrims at a place other than their destination, unless with their consent, or from unavoidable cause, shall be liable to a fine of 20 pounds Turkish for each pilgrim wrongfully disembarked.

Art. 158.—Any other infringement of the provisions relating to pilgrim-ships shall be punished by a fine of from 10 to 100 pounds Turkish.

Art. 159.—Any known infringement during the voyage shall be entered in the bill-of-health, and in the list of pilgrims. The competent authority shall prepare a statement of the case and submit it in the proper quarter.

Art. 160.—In Turkish ports, infringements of the provisions relating to pilgrim-ships shall be tried before, and the fine imposed by, the competent authority, in accordance with the provisions of Articles 173 and 174.

Art. 161.—All agents required to assist in carrying out the provisions of this Convention regarding pilgrim-ships shall be liable to punishment, agreeably to the laws of their respective countries, for any failure on their part in carrying out the aforesaid provisions.

PART IV.

ADMINISTRATION AND CONTROL.

I.—*The Egyptian Sanitary, Maritime, and Quarantine Board.*

Art. 162.—The provisions of Appendix III of the Venice Sanitary Convention of January 30th, 1892, regarding the composition, the functions, and the manner of discharge of the functions of the Egyptian Sanitary, Maritime and Quarantine Board, as provided by the Decrees of His Highness the Khedive under the dates of June 19th, 1893, and December 25th, 1894, and also by the Ministerial Order of June 19th, 1894, are confirmed.

The said Decrees and Order are appended to this Convention.

Art. 163.—The ordinary expenses arising out of the provisions of this Convention, and in particular those due to increase of the staff employed by the Egyptian Sanitary, Maritime and Quarantine Board, shall be defrayed by an additional yearly contribution by the Egyptian Government of a sum of four thousand pounds Egyptian, which may be paid out of the surplus of the lighthouse dues remaining at the disposal of that Government. Provided always that from this sum shall be deducted the amount produced by an additional quarantine charge of 10 P. T. (piastre tariff) on each pilgrim, to be levied at El-Tor.

In the event of the Egyptian Government finding difficulty in bearing this proportion of the expenses, it would be for the Powers represented on the Sanitary Board to approach the Khedivial Government with a view to securing part of these expenses being borne by the latter.

Art. 164.—It devolves upon the Egyptian Sanitary, Maritime and Quarantine Board to bring into harmony with the provisions of this Convention the regulations it now applies to plague, cholera, and yellow fever, and also the regulations regarding arrivals from Arabian ports in the Red Sea during the pilgrimage season. If necessary, it shall revise, to the same end, the general sanitary, maritime, and quarantine police regulations now in force.

To become effective, these regulations must be approved by the several Powers represented on the Board.

II.—*The Constantinople Superior Board of Health.*

Art. 165.—The framing of the measures to be taken with a view to preventing the introduction into the Turkish Empire and the transmission to other countries of epidemic disease, devolves upon the Constantinople Superior Board of Health.

Art. 166.—The number of Turkish delegates on the Superior Board of Health, having the right to vote, shall be four, namely:—

the President of the Board, or, in his absence, the Acting President of the meeting. They shall have a casting vote only;

the Inspector-General of the sanitary service;

the Assistant-Inspector;

the Delegate acting as intermediary between the Board and the Sublime Porte, known as *Mouhassébedgi.*

Art. 167.—The appointment of the Inspector-General, the Assistant-Inspector, and the Delegate before-mentioned, nominated by the Board, shall be ratified by the Turkish Government.

Art. 168.—The High Contracting Parties recognise the right of Roumania, as a maritime Power, to representation by a delegate on the Board.

Art. 169.—The delegates of the several States must be duly qualified doctors, holding the diploma of a European faculty of medicine, and belonging to the nation they represent, or consular officials of rank not lower than Vice-Consul or of equivalent rank. The delegates must be in no way connected with the local authority or with a shipping company.

These provisions shall not apply to the delegates now in office.

Art. 170.—The decisions of the Superior Board of Health, carried by a majority of its members, shall come into force, without appeal.

The Governments signing this Convention agree that their representatives at Constantinople shall be instructed to inform the Turkish Government of this Convention and to approach that Government with a view to securing its accession thereto.

Art. 171.—The enforcement and the control of the provisions of this Convention regarding the pilgrimages and of measures against the introduction and the spread of plague and of cholera, shall be entrusted, within the scope of the Constantinople Superior Board of Health's jurisdiction, to a Committee selected from among members of that Board exclusively, and composed of representatives of the several Powers adhering to this Convention. The representatives of Turkey on this Committee shall be three in number; one of them shall be the President of the Committee. When the votes are equally divided, the President shall have a casting vote.

Art. 172.—There shall be a staff of qualified doctors, well-trained disinfecters and mechanics, and also sanitary guards selected from persons who have been officers or non-commissioned officers of higher than corporal's rank in the military service, whose duty it shall be to secure, within the jurisdiction of the Constantinople Superior Board of Health, the proper working of the several sanitary establishments enumerated in and prescribed by this Convention.

Art. 173.—The sanitary authority of a Turkish port of call or of arrival, which has convicted anyone of an infringement of the regulations, shall prepare a statement of the case, to which the captain is entitled to add comments in writing. A certified copy of this statement shall be sent, at the port of call or of arrival, to the consular authority of the country under whose flag the ship sails. The amount of the fine imposed shall be deposited with the consular authority or, if there be no consul, with the sanitary authority. The fine shall not be definitely handed over to the Constantinople Superior Board of Health until the consular Commission, described in the article next following, shall have given judgment as to whether such fine be valid.

Another certified copy of the statement must be forwarded by the convicting sanitary authority to the President of the Constantinople Board of Health, who shall bring the document to the notice of the consular Commission.

The nature of the infringement and the deposit of the fine shall be noted upon the bill-of-health by the sanitary or the consular authority.

Art. 174.—A consular Commission shall be established at Constantinople to decide between contradictory statements made by sanitary agents and incriminated captains. It shall be appointed yearly by the consular authority. The Sanitary Administration may be represented by a person discharging the duties of public prosecutor. The consul of the country concerned shall always be invited to attend; he shall be entitled to vote.

Art. 175.—The cost of providing, within the jurisdiction of the Constantinople Superior Board of Health, the sanitary posts, both permanent and temporary, prescribed by this Convention, shall be, in so far as construction of buildings is concerned, debited to the Turkish Government. The Constantinople Superior Board of Health is authorised, if necessary and in case of emergency, to advance from the reserve fund the necessary money, which shall, upon demand, be furnished by the "Mixed Commission entrusted with the revision of sanitary charges." In this event, the Board must see to the construction of these establishments.

The Constantinople Superior Board of Health must organise, without delay, the sanitary stations of Hanikin and Kizil-Dizié, near Bayazid, on the Turko-Persian and Turko-Russian frontiers, out of the moneys now placed at its disposal.

The other expenses arising, within the jurisdiction of the said Board, from the measures prescribed by this Convention, shall be mutually borne by the Turkish Government and the Constantinople Superior Board of Health, as agreed upon by the Government and the Powers represented on the Board.

III.—*The Tangier International Board of Health.*

Art. 176.—In the interests of the public health, the High Contracting Parties agree that their representatives in Morocco shall again direct the attention of the Tangier International Board of Health to the necessity of carrying out the provisions of the sanitary Conventions.

IV.—*Miscellaneous provisions.*

Art. 177.—Each Government shall decide as to the means it shall employ to secure disinfection and the destruction of rats[1].

[1] The following methods of disinfection are given by way of guide :—

Wearing apparel, old rags, infected dressings, papers and other articles of no value should be burnt.

Personal effects, bedding, mattresses infected with plague can be efficiently disinfected either by means of a high-pressure steam disinfecting chamber or a current-steam disinfecting chamber at a temperature of 100° Centigrade, or by exposure to formol vapours.

Articles, such as coverlets and bed-linen, that can be steeped in antiseptic solutions without damage, can be disinfected by 1 per 1000 solutions of perchloride of mercury, 3 per 100 solutions of carbolic acid, 3 per 100 solutions of lysol or commercial cresyl, 1 per 100 solutions of formol (one part of the commercial solution of formaldehyde at 40 per 100), or 1 per 100 solutions of the alkaline hypochlorides (sodium or potassium), that is to say, 1 part of the ordinary solution of commercial hypochlorite. The period of contact

Art. 178.—·The sums realised by sanitary charges and fines may not, in any instance whatever, be used for any purposes other than those under the control of the Boards of Health.

Art. 179.—The High Contracting Parties undertake that their Public Health Departments shall frame a set of instructions intended to enable ship-captains, particularly when there is no doctor on board, to carry out the provisions of this Convention regarding plague and cholera, and also to carry out the regulations regarding yellow fever.

V.—*The Persian Gulf.*

Art. 180.—·The cost of construction and upkeep of the sanitary station to be provided, in accordance with Article 81 of this Convention, on the Island of Ormuz, shall be debited to the Constantinople Superior Board of Health. The said Board's Mixed Commission of revision shall meet at the earliest date possible in order to furnish, on the Board's request, the necessary moneys to be derived from the available reserve funds.

VI.—*International Health Office.*

Art. 181.—The Conference having taken note of the resolutions, hereto appended, passed by its Commission of Ways and Means regarding the creation of an International Health Office in Paris, the French Government shall, at such time as it may think fit, submit, by diplomatic channels, proposals on this subject to the States represented at the Conference.

must obviously be long enough to allow dried germs to be well penetrated by the antiseptic solution: four to six hours will suffice.

To secure destruction of rats, three processes are now made use of :—

(1) Sulphurous acid mixed with a small quantity of sulphuric anhydride, driven under pressure into holds and mixed with the air. This destroys rats and insects and will, it is stated, destroy the plague bacillus also if the proportion of sulphuro-sulphuric anhydride be sufficiently great.

(2) An incombustible mixture of carbon monoxide and carbon dioxide, passed into holds.

(3) Carbonic acid so employed as to constitute 30 per cent. of the air in the ship.

The last two methods kill rodents but it is not claimed that they destroy insects or the plague bacillus.

The Technical Commission of the Paris (1903) Sanitary Conference specified the three following processes—a mixture of sulphuro-sulphuric anhydrides, a mixture of carbonic oxide and carbonic acid, and carbonic acid—as being among those to which Governments might resort, and expressed the opinion that the sanitary authority should, in every instance where it did not itself do the work, superintend its performance and make sure that the rats had been killed.

PART V.

YELLOW FEVER.

Art. 182.—The countries concerned are recommended to modify their sanitary regulations in such fashion as to bring them into harmony with the present scientific data as to the manner in which yellow fever is transmitted, and, in particular, as to the part played by mosquitoes in carrying the germs of the disease.

PART VI.

ADHESION AND RATIFICATION.

Art. 183.—The Governments that have not signed this Convention are allowed to become parties thereto at their request. Such adhesion shall be notified, by diplomatic channels, to the Government of the French Republic, and by that Government to the other Governments that have signed the Convention.

Art. 184.—This Convention shall be ratified, and the ratifications thereof shall be deposited at Paris as soon as may be practicable.

It shall be put in force as soon as it shall have been made public in such manner as is in accordance with the laws of the States that sign it. As regards the relations between the Powers that ratify or become parties to it, it shall replace the International Sanitary Conventions signed on January 30th, 1892, April 15th, 1893, April 3rd, 1894, and March 19th, 1897.

The previous Conventions, above cited, shall continue in force in the case of Powers which, having signed or become parties to them, do not ratify or become parties to this Convention.

APPENDIX I. (*See Art.* 78.)

REGULATIONS

REGARDING THE CONVEYANCE OF PASSENGERS AND MAILS FROM INFECTED COUNTRIES THROUGH EGYPT BY QUARANTINE TRAIN.

Art. 1.—The Egyptian Railway Executive that wishes to run a quarantine train in connection with ships arriving from infected ports, must give notice thereof to the local quarantine authority not less than two hours before the time of departure of such train.

Art. 2.—The passengers shall land at a place appointed by the quarantine authority with the consent of the Railway Executive and the Egyptian Government,

29—5

and shall proceed, without any communication, direct from the ship to the train, under the supervision of a transit-officer and of two or more sanitary guards.

Art. 3.—The passengers' personal belongings, baggage, etc., shall be conveyed in quarantine, by the means at the disposal of the ship.

Art. 4.—In so far as quarantine measures are concerned, the railway staff shall obey the orders of the transit-officer.

Art. 5.—The carriages employed in this service shall be corridor-carriages. In each carriage there shall be a sanitary guard, whose duty it shall be to keep watch over the passengers. The railway staff shall not hold any communication with the passengers.

A doctor on the quarantine staff shall go with the train.

Art. 6.—The passengers' heavy baggage shall be put in a special van which the transit-officer shall seal before the train starts. Upon arrival the seals shall be removed by the transit-officer.

Transference of passengers to another train or taking passengers during the journey is prohibited.

Art. 7.—The closets shall be furnished with pails, containing a certain amount of antiseptic, for the reception of the passengers' dejecta.

Art. 8.—No one, except the staff absolutely necessary, shall be allowed on railway platforms at which the train may have to stop.

Art. 9.—Every train may have a restaurant-car. The remnants of meals shall be destroyed. The staff of the restaurant-car and such other railway servants as have come in contact, from any cause, with passengers, shall undergo the same measures as the pilots and electricians at Port Said or Suez, or such measures as the Board may consider necessary.

Art. 10.—Passengers are absolutely prohibited from throwing anything whatever out of the windows, doors, etc.

Art. 11.—In every train a hospital compartment shall be kept empty so as to secure isolation of the sick therein, should such contingency arise. This compartment shall be fitted up in accordance with the direction of the Quarantine Board.

If plague or cholera appear among the passengers, the sick person shall immediately be isolated in the special compartment, and shall, on the arrival of the train, be removed forthwith to the quarantine lazaret. The other passengers shall proceed on their journey in quarantine.

Art. 12.—If a case of plague or of cholera occur during the journey, the train will be disinfected by the quarantine authority.

In all instances the vans carrying baggage and mails shall be disinfected immediately after the arrival of the train.

Art. 13.—The transference of passengers, baggage, etc., from train to ship shall be effected in the same way as on arrival. The ship that takes the passengers shall immediately be put in quarantine, and any incident that may have occurred during the journey shall be noted on the bill-of-health, with specific mention of any persons that may have been in contact with the sick.

Art. 14.—The expenses incurred by the quarantine administrative body shall be debited to whoever requisitioned the quarantine train.

Art. 15.—The President of the Board, or his substitute, shall have the right to exercise supervision over the train during the whole of its journey. The President may, moreover, entrust the duty of such supervision to a high official (above and beyond the transit-officer and the sanitary guards). This official shall have access to the train on his showing an order signed by the President.

APPENDIX II. (*See Art.* 162.)

[*This Appendix, consisting of the Khedivial Decrees of* 19*th June*, 1893, *and* 25*th December*, 1894, *and of the Ministerial Order of* 19*th June*, 1893, *is not here reproduced.*]

APPENDIX III. (*See Art.* 181.)

RESOLUTIONS

PASSED BY THE COMMISSION OF WAYS AND MEANS OF THE SANITARY CONFERENCE OF PARIS REGARDING AN INTERNATIONAL HEALTH OFFICE.

I.—An International Health Office shall be established on the lines followed in the institution and conduct of the International Office of Weights and Measures. It shall have its seat in Paris.

II.—The International Office shall fulfil the function of collecting information as to the progress of infectious diseases. To this end it shall receive information given to it by the chief Health Authorities of the States that are parties to it.

III.—The Office shall periodically set out the results of these labours in official reports which shall be communicated to the contracting Governments. These reports must be made public.

IV.—The Office shall be supported by contributions from the contracting Governments.

V.—The Government, in whose country the International Office is to be established, shall be charged with the submission, within three months of the signing of the proceedings of the Conference, for the approval of the contracting States, of Regulations for the institution and conduct of that Office.

INDEX.

CAMBRIDGE: PRINTED BY JOHN CLAY, M.A. AT THE UNIVERSITY PRESS